FOURTH EDITION

PHTLS

BASIC AND ADVANCED PREHOSPITAL TRAUMA LIFE SUPPORT

Prehospital Trauma Life Support Committee of the National Association of Emergency Medical Technicians in Cooperation with the Committee on Trauma of the American College of Surgeons

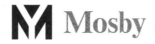 Mosby

An Imprint of Elsevier Science

St. Louis   London   Philadelphia   Sydney   Toronto

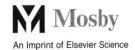

Mosby
An Imprint of Elsevier Science

Mosby, Inc.
11830 Westline Industrial Drive
St. Louis, Missouri 63146

Library of Congress Cataloging-in-Publication Data

PHTLS basic and advanced prehospital trauma life support / Prehospital
    Trauma Life Support Committee of the National Association of
    Emergency Medical Technicians in Cooperation with the Committee on
    Trauma of the American College of Surgeons.—4th ed.
       p.   cm.
    Includes bibliographical references and index.
    ISBN 0–8151–4569–1
    1. Medical emergencies.   2. First aid in illness and injury.
3. Traumatology. I. National Association of Emergency Medical
Technicians (U.S.).   Pre-Hospital Trauma Life Support Committee.
II. American College of Surgeons.   Committee on Trauma.
    [DNLM: 1. Wounds and Injuries—therapy. 2. Emergencies. 3. First
Aid—methods. WO 700P577 1999]
    RC86.7.P48   1999
    616.02′5—dc21
    DNLM/DLC   98-27270

02 / 9 8 7 6 5

Joseph D. "Deke" Farrington, MD, FACS

Father of EMS
January 16, 1909–January 20, 1982

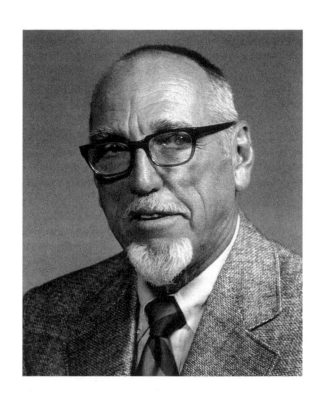

Forty-five years ago, no training program was available to educate prehospital personnel in the management of trauma patients. J.D. "Deke" Farrington, MD, felt that trauma victims deserved better than an unattended ride to the hospital in the back of a hearse. In 1958 he convinced the Chicago Fire Department that firefighters should be trained to manage emergency patients. Along with Dr. Sam Banks, Deke started the Trauma Training program in Chicago. More than four million people have been trained according to the guidelines they developed. Still, no standards for ambulance design and equipment existed, communication systems between physicians and EMTs were missing, and national standards for training and certification had yet to be written. Deke helped write these as well.

Deke was involved in every aspect of the origins of EMS; nothing in the early development of EMS happened without his hand or his influence.

As a member of the National Academy of Sciences/ National Research Council committee, Farrington helped write the famous paper, "Accidental Death and Disability, The Neglected Disease of Modern Society." His ideas and support launched the National Association of EMTs, and

he was one of the major players in the National Registry of EMTs for more than 15 years.

This "Moses" of EMS was the son of a Baptist minister in the deep South. His nickname was short for Deacon. Born in Richmond, Virginia, he lived in every state in the impoverished South. He attended the University of Alabama when it was only a 2-year medical school in Birmingham, before obtaining his MD degree at Rush Medical School in Chicago. He lost his mother at an early age due to a lack of proper medical care. This experience, along with his love for people and his religious training, was most likely the source of his zeal to improve the care of the injured patient.

Thirty-three years prior to the publication of this textbook, "Deke" Farrington published the article that was the focal point for the beginning of EMS. "Death in a Ditch" is the landmark paper most often identified as the point of change in prehospital care. Most people in EMS have heard of it, but many have not read it. In the first few paragraphs it is easy to grasp the state of prehospital care in the 1960s and Deke's vision of what it should be. We have come a long way in doing what he asked. Don't stop now. Continue to improve yourself and the care that you provide.

Contributors

EDITORS

Norman E. McSwain, Jr., MD, FACS, NREMT-P
PHTLS Editor-in-Chief
Professor of Surgery
Department of Surgery
Tulane University School of Medicine
New Orleans, Louisiana

Scott Frame, MD, FACS, FCCM
Associate Professor of Surgery
Director, Division of Trauma/Critical Care
University of Cincinnati Medical Center
Cincinnati, Ohio

James L. Paturas, EMT-P
Director, Department of EMS
Bridgeport Hospital
Bridgeport, Connecticut

EXECUTIVE COUNCIL

Will Chapleau, EMT-P, RN, TNS, CEN
Chairman, PHTLS
Emergency Medical Services Coordinator
Emergency Medical Education
St. James Hospital
Chicago, Illinois

Scott Frame, MD, FACS, FCCM
Associate National Medical Director, PHTLS
Associate Professor of Surgery
Director, Division of Trauma/Critical Care
University of Cincinnati Medical Center
Cincinnati, Ohio

Norman E. McSwain, Jr., MD, FACS, NREMT-P
National Medical Director, PHTLS
Professor of Surgery
Department of Surgery
Tulane University School of Medicine
New Orleans, Louisiana

Steve Mercer, NREMT-P
Education Coordinator, PHTLS
Iowa Department of Public Health
Bureau of Emergency Medical Services
Des Moines, Iowa

James L. Paturas, EMT-P
International Coordinator, PHTLS
Director, Department of EMS
Bridgeport Hospital
Bridgeport, Connecticut

Dennis Rowe, EMT-P
Vice-Chairman, PHTLS
Q/A Education Manager
Rural/Metro Corporation
Knoxville, Tennessee

Jeffrey Salomone, MD
Associate National Medical Director, PHTLS
Emory University School of Medicine
Department of Surgery
Atlanta, Georgia

Elizabeth M. Wertz, RN, BSN, MPM, EMT-P
Immediate Past Chairperson, PHTLS
International PHTLS Committee
Pittsburgh, Pennsylvania

CONTRIBUTING EDITORS

Chip Boehm, RN, EMT-P
EMS Education Officer
Portland Fire Department
Portland, Maine

Will Chapleau, EMT-P, RN, TNS, CEN
Emergency Medical Services Coordinator
Emergency Medical Education
St. James Hospital
Chicago, Illinois

Gregory Chapman, RRT, REMT-P
Instructor Coordinator
Institute of Prehospital Emergency Medicine
Hudson Valley Community College
Troy, New York

Alice "Twink" Dalton, RN, MS,
   NRPM
Trauma Care Coordinator
St. Joseph Hospital
Omaha, Nebraska

Michael D'Auito, MD, FACS
Medical Director
"The Burn Center"
Bridgeport Hospital
Bridgeport, Connecticut

Walter Idol, MS, EMT-P
Chief Flight Paramedic
University of Tennessee Medical
   Center
Knoxville, Tennessee

Richard Judd, PhD, EMT
President
Central Connecticut State
   University
New Britain, Connecticut

Merry McSwain, EMT-P, RN, BSN
Intensive Care Unit
Tulane University Medical Center
New Orleans, Louisiana

Bill Metcalf, EMT
Publisher/General Manager, JEMS
JEMS Communications
Carlsbad, California

Lawrence D. Newell, NREMT-P, EdD
Adjunct Professor
Department of Emergency Medical
   Technology
Northern Virginia Community
   College
Annandale, Virginia

Peter Pons, MD, FACEP
Research Coordinator
Denver Health Medical Center
Denver, Colorado

Jeffrey P. Salomone, MD
Assistant Professor of Surgery
Trauma and General Surgery/
   Critical Care
Department of Surgery
Emory University School of
   Medicine
Atlanta, Georgia

J.J. Tepas III, MD, FACS, FAAP
Chairman, Department of Surgery
University of Florida, College of
   Medicine
Jacksonville, Florida

Michael Werdmann, MD, FACEP
Chairman, Department of
   Emergency Medicine
Diplomat, American Board of
   Pediatrics
Bridgeport Hospital
Bridgeport, Connecticut

MILITARY CONTRIBUTIONS

Gregory H. Adkisson, Capt., MC,
   USN
Commanding Officer
Defense Medical Readiness Training
   Command (DMRTC)
San Antonio, Texas

Morris L. Beard, SFC, USA, NREMT-P
Special Operations Forces Liaison
Joint Medical Readiness Training
   Center (JMRTC)
San Antonio, Texas

Frank K. Butler, Jr., Capt., MC, USN
Biomedical Research Director
Defense Medical Readiness Training
   Command (DMRTC)
San Antonio, Texas

Milton R. Fields III, Tsgt., USAF
   NREMT-P
Military PHTLS Coordinator
Joint Medical Readiness Training
   Center (JMRTC)
San Antonio, Texas

John Mechtel, Capt., USAF, NC
Assistant Chief, Professional
   Programs
Joint Medical Readiness Training
   Center (JMRTC)
San Antonio, Texas

Dale C. Smith, PhD
Chairperson, Department of Military
   History
Uniformed Services University
   Health Sciences
Bethesda, Maryland

Kenneth G. Swan, MD
Professor of Surgery
Chief, Section of General Surgery
UMDNJ/New Jersey Medical School;
Chief, Division of Thoracic Surgery
University Hospital
Newark, New Jersey

K.G. Swan, Jr., BS
1st Year Medical Student
Cornell University Medical College
New York, New York

Steven J. Yevich, LTC, USA, MC
Chief of Staff
Joint Medical Readiness Training
   Center (JMRTC)
San Antonio, Texas

INTERNATIONAL ACKNOWLEDGMENTS

Dr. Jameel Ali
Toronto, Canada

Dr. Nikki Blackwell
Mt. Isa Base Hospital
Mt. Isa, Australia

Dr. Chris Carney
Royal College of Surgeons
London, England

Dr. Ricardo Ferrada
Emergency Department and Trauma
   Unit
Bogota, Columbia

Dr. Fernando Magallenes-Negrete
Hospital Centrar Militar
Lomas de Sotelo, Mexico

Dr. Anna Notander
Stockholm, Sweden

Professor Sergio Olivero
Cattedra di Cirurgia D'urgenza
Turin, Italy

Dr. Renato Poggetti
Brazilian American College of
   Surgeons
Sao Paulo, Brazil

Dr. Oswaldo Rois
Fundacion EMME
Buenos Aires, Argentina

Dr. Mario Uribe
American College of Surgeons-Chile
Santiago, Chile

NATIONAL ASSOCIATION OF EMTs

James B. Allen, NREMT-P
President
National Association of EMTs
Clinton, Mississippi

Deborah Knight-Smith, EMT
Vice President
National Association of EMTs
Clinton, Mississippi

Bruce Shade, EMT-P
Treasurer
National Association of EMTs
Clinton, Mississippi

John Fitzsimmons, NREMT
Secretary
National Association of EMTs
Clinton, Mississippi

Corine Curd
Program Coordinator
International PHTLS Office
Clinton, Mississippi

REVIEWERS

Linda Abrahamson, EMT-P
EMS Education Coordinator
Silver Cross Hospital
Joliet, Illinois

Michael Armacost, MA, NREMT-P
Director of Prehospital Care
Colorado Department of Public
   Health and Environment
Emergency Medical Services
Denver, Colorado

Mark Lockhart, NREMT-P
Deputy Chief
Maryland Heights Fire Protection
   District
Maryland Heights, Missouri

PHTLS Honor Roll

PHTLS continues to prosper and promote high standards of trauma care all over the world. It would not be able to do this without the contributions of many dedicated and inspired individuals over the past two and a half decades. Some of the names below were instrumental in the development of our very first textbook. Others were constantly "on the road" spreading the word. Still others "put out fires" and otherwise problem solved to keep us growing. The PHTLS Executive Council, along with the editors and contributors of this, our fourth edition, would like to express our thanks to all of those listed below. PHTLS lives, breathes, and grows, because of the efforts of those that volunteer their time to what they believe in.

Jameel Ali, MD
J.M. Barnes
Anne Bellows
Don E. Boyle, MD
Susan Brown
Alexander Butman
H. Jeannie Butman
Steve Carden
Edward A. Casker
Bud Caukin
Will Chapleau
Philip Coco
Alice "Twink" Dalton
Judith Demarest
Joseph P. Dineen, MD
Leon Dontigney, MD
Betsy Ewing
Scott Frame, MD
Sheryl G.A. Gabram, MD
Capt. Bret Gilliam
Vincent A. Greco
Len Jacobs
Lou Jordan
Richard Judd
Dawn Loehn
Mark Lockhart
Robert Loftus
William McConnell, DO
Norman E. McSwain, Jr., MD

Fernando Magallenes-Negrete, MD
Scott W. Martin
Don Mauger
Steve Mercer
George Moerkirk, MD
Stephen Murphy
Jeanne O'Brien
Joan Drake-Olsen
Dawn Orgeron
James Paturas
Thomas Petrich
James Pierce
Brian Plaisier, MD
Peter Pons, MD
Mark Reading
John Sigafoos
Paul Silverston, MD
David Skinner, FRCS
Richard Sobieray
Sheila Spaid
Michael Spain
Don Stamper
J.J. Tepas III, MD
Richard Vomacka
Elizabeth Wertz
Roger White, MD
David Wuertz
Kenneth J. Wright, MD
Al Yellin, MD

Again, thanks to all of you. And, thanks to everyone all over the world for making PHTLS work.

PHTLS Executive Council
Editors and Contributors of PHTLS

Acknowledgments

In publishing, there are two groups of workers. One is the group that appears in the listing of the authors. The other is the group that did not necessarily utter the words that showed up on the printed page but who actually made it happen. These unsung worker bees include the editorial staff, the copy editors, the artists, the photographers, and the support staff in our own offices. They are mentioned here. We, the editors, hope that everyone has been included.

Heading the Mosby editorial staff, Jennifer Roche provided her expertise as Executive Editor for the fourth edition. We also thank Jennifer's predecessor, Claire Merrick, for her support on the third edition and as we began this edition.

We would also like to thank members of the Mosby production team: Mark Spann, Project Manager, and Jodi Everding, Production Editor. In addition, we appreciate the efforts of Lisa Nomura, Production Editor with Graphic World.

Photographer Kristin Burke provided excellent work for the third edition, and many of her photographs were carried over into the fourth edition. Many new photographs, including most of the work in the two skills chapters, were taken by Stewart Halperin for this edition. Also, beautiful new illustrations were provided by Nadine Sokol and Jeanne Robertson.

We thank Alex Butman and Rick Vomacka for their work on the first two editions because it was this foundation that made the third and fourth editions possible. We also appreciate the efforts and support of the following: James E. Wilberger, Chairman of the Emergency Services–Prehospital ACS/COT subcommittee; the Advanced Trauma Life Support committee, specifically Chairman Richard Bell, MD, FACS, and Manager Irvene Hughes, RN; the Committee on Trauma Executive Secretary, Carol Williams; and the present and the past Chairman of the Committee on Trauma of the American College of Surgeons, David Hoyt, MD, FACS, and John A. Weigelt, MD, FACS, respectively.

We owe a sincere debt of gratitude to our wives, children, and significant others who have put up with our long hours away from them during the preparation of this material.

One of the most important persons involved throughout the entire project—Kellie White at Mosby—has quietly pushed us, beat on us, rewritten what we did wrong, arranged the illustrations, and spent hours with us on e-mail making sure that everything was on time and achieving a host of other accomplishments to complete this edition. We would never have made it without Kellie. In almost 30 years of academic writing, the editor-in-chief has had the opportunity to work with many other individuals in similar positions, and there has never been anyone better. She will be the marker that I hold up to judge perfection in all future interactions with publishers.

Finally, in my own life, Vanessa Angelety-Lee, my assistant, my confidant, and my support . . . Thanks for everything.

Norman E. McSwain, Jr., MD, FACS, NREMT-P

Preface

When assuming the obligation to be an EMT, one accepts the responsibility to provide patient care as close to absolutely perfect as possible. This cannot be achieved without having a knowledge of the subject that is as complete as possible. We must remember that the patient did not choose to be involved in a traumatic situation. The EMT, on the other hand, *has* chosen to be there to take care of the patient. It is the obligation of the EMT to give 100% all of the time. The patient has had a bad day. The EMT cannot have a bad day. The EMT must be sharp and responsible in the competition between the patient and death and disease.

The patient is the most important person at the scene of an emergency. The EMT does not have time to think about where to transport the injured patient. The EMT does not have time to think about where medications or supplies are housed within the jump kit. The EMT does not have time to think about what order to perform the physical examination in or what treatment should take priority over another. The EMT does not have time to practice a skill that is needed to provide care for the patient. The EMT must have all of this information and more stored in his or her mind and all supplies and equipment present in the jump kit when arriving on the scene. The EMT without the proper equipment or without the proper knowledge may neglect to do things that could potentially increase the patient's chances for survival. The responsibilities of an EMT are too great for this to happen.

The EMT is an integral member of the patient care team, just as the nurse or physician in the emergency department, operating room, intensive care unit, or any other part of the hospital. EMTs must be practiced in their skills so that they can move the patient quickly and efficiently out of the environment of the emergency and transport the patient quickly to the appropriate hospital.

Development of the PHTLS program was started in 1981, immediately on the heels of the ATLS program. It is the responsibility of the working EMT to assimilate this knowledge and these skills in order to use them for the benefit of the patients for whom they are responsible.

This fourth edition of the PHTLS program has been thoroughly revised, based on the 1997 ATLS guidelines for care of the trauma patient. While following the ATLS guidelines, PHTLS is specifically designed for the unique situation in which the trauma patient presents to the EMT. The editors and authors of this material and the PHTLS division of the National Association of Emergency Medical Technicians hope that you will use this information and daily rededicate yourself to the care of those persons who cannot care for themselves . . . *the trauma patient.*

Norman E. McSwain, Jr., MD, FACS, NREMT-P
Editor in Chief, PHTLS

Contents

Note on Terminology

PROVIDER LEVEL

The PHTLS course originally developed by the National Association of EMTs in co-operation with the Committee on Trauma of the American College of Surgeons was written primarily for EMT-Paramedics and EMT-Intermediates. More recently, the PHTLS Basic version for EMT-Bs has been implemented. It is recognized, however, that prehospital care providers, and the readers of this text, vary widely in educational background and certification—from EMT-Bs to physicians. Accordingly, in the interest of simplicity and consistency, a policy decision has been made to use the generic term "EMT" throughout these pages to refer to the person providing the prehospital care described in the text.

Prehospital Trauma Life Support and the National Association of Emergency Medical Technicians

PAST, PRESENT, AND FUTURE

During the late 1970s, management of the trauma patient by hospital and prehospital clinical providers was disjointed and without established clinical standards of care. Most of the EMS providers used the same standards for care of the cardiac patient and the trauma patient. It was not recognized that there was a major difference between the definitive care of the cardiac patient (reestablish the cardiac rhythm, which could be done in the field) and definitive care of the trauma patient (stop hemorrhage, which could be done only in the operating room). As a whole, clinical care providers functioned without understanding of this basic principle. In addition, there was no system of priorities when treating the trauma patient.

In 1978 the Lincoln Medical Education Foundation (LMEF) Physicians Committee on Trauma developed and piloted the first Advanced Trauma Life Support (ATLS) course in cooperation with the Southeast Nebraska Emergency Medical Services. On a national level, the American College of Surgeons Committee on Trauma (ACS/COT) also recognized the fact that better educational opportunities were needed in improving trauma management for physicians. Both organizations agreed to work together and to develop a national trauma educational program for physicians. Out of this relationship developed the national ATLS program in 1979. The ATLS course has become the "gold" standard for trauma care, first in the United States and now throughout most of the world.

Based on the success of the ATLS course in providing physician trauma education, the National Association of Emergency Medical Technicians (NAEMT) decided to provide similar education for its members and other prehospital emergency health care personnel. Gary Labeau, then President of NAEMT, requested that Dr. Norman E. McSwain, Jr., FACS, a member of the NAEMT Board of Directors, the first chairman of the ATLS ad hoc committee for the ACS, and the chairman of the Prehospital Care Subcommittee of the American College of Surgeons Committee on Trauma, work with Robert Nelson, REMT-P, of Michigan, on the feasibility of developing an educational program for EMS, similar to ATLS.

Throughout 1982, with the support of Tulane University School of Medicine where Dr. McSwain was Professor of Surgery, an initial draft curriculum providing the basis for the further development of the course was completed. During the 1983 calendar year, a Prehospital Trauma Life Support (PHTLS) Committee was established, and further refinements of the PHTLS curriculum were implemented. During this same year, pilot courses were conducted at Tulane University School of Medicine in New Orleans, Louisiana; Marian Health Center in Sioux City, Iowa; Yale University School of Medicine in New Haven, Connecticut; and Norwalk Hospital in Norwalk, Connecticut.

In the early part of 1984, the first national faculty PHTLS course was conducted at Tulane University School of Medicine in New Orleans. The graduates of this program formed the backbone for the cadre of PHTLS Affiliate Faculty who would make PHTLS courses accessible throughout the United States. Another milestone was realized when in 1986 development of the PHTLS Basic course was initiated. Since those early beginnings over 200,000 individuals (1999) have successfully completed a PHTLS provider course at either the basic or advanced level. In addition, thousands of EMT-Bs, EMT-Is, EMT-Ps, nurses, and physicians have attended PHTLS Instructor workshops so they too could offer the program locally. Regional, state, and assistant state coordinators were appointed to offer administrative oversight. One feature of the PHTLS program that has been and remains paramount is the quality improvement component. The state and regional leadership along with the state ACS/COT chairman ensure that each course conducted follows the standards of care approved by the American College of Surgeons Committee on Trauma and PHTLS National Committee.

PHTLS IN THE MILITARY

The evolution of the PHTLS program led the PHTLS Committee to begin work in 1988 on the establishment of programs for U.S. military medical personnel. This program has been extremely successful because of the hard work and dedication of both the military and civilian personnel. The authority for the program has been placed with the Military Medical Education Institute (MMEI) of the Uniformed Services University of the Health Sciences (USUHS). MMEI courses for National Guard and Reserve personnel are conducted by the Defense Medical Readiness Training Institute (DMRTI) based at Fort Sam Houston, Texas. PHTLS has become a regular course offering along with Combat Casualty Care Course (C4), ATLS, Advanced Cardiac Life Support (ACLS), Trauma Nurse Core Curriculum (TNCC), Advanced Burn Life Support (ABLS), Combat Anesthesia, and others.

This fourth edition of PHTLS includes the military PHTLS curriculum. This training program is an addition to the regular PHTLS program for those who need this special education.

INTERNATIONAL PHTLS

The sound principles of prehospital trauma management emphasized in the PHTLS course have led prehospital care providers and doctors outside the United States to request the importation of the PHTLS program to their respective homelands. As the PHTLS International faculty has traveled from country to country, two recurring themes have been noted: the diversity of prehospital trauma care and the dedication of prehospital care providers. Although many similarities can be noted between the prehospital trauma care practiced in many countries and the delivery of EMS in the United States, a few significant differences in training levels, equipment, and medical therapy have been identified. But more importantly, without exception we have been truly impressed with the dedication to excellence in care of the trauma victim that has been demonstrated worldwide.

Importing PHTLS

Prior to the introduction of PHTLS to a nation, several requirements must be met. Medical oversight must be established, and a small core of PHTLS instructors from the host country must be trained in the United States.

Medical Oversight

In order for PHTLS to be imported to a foreign country, there must be an established Advanced Trauma Life Support program. Through its Committee on Trauma, the American College of Surgeons provides medical control of the PHTLS program both in the United States and internationally. As the ATLS program has been introduced around the globe (29 countries in 1998), the Committee on Trauma has established a network of doctors who possess a commitment to trauma. These Committees, often an International Chapter of the American College of Surgeons, then promulgate ATLS programs and provide the

medical oversight for PHTLS courses. A memorandum of understanding (MOU) is then signed between NAEMT and this oversight group. The agreement is made to abide by the policies of the PHTLS Division and ensure quality control of all courses taught.

Faculty Training

PHTLS requires that several individuals from the foreign country travel to the United States and attend a PHTLS Provider/Instructor workshop. The PHTLS Provider/Instructor workshop must be at a PHTLS Executive Council approved site. This requirement achieves several goals. First, the sponsors gain insight on how the PHTLS course is organized and learns firsthand of the need for sufficient quantities of EMS equipment. Second, PHTLS instructors are available to aid in delivering lectures and teaching skill stations during the inaugural course.

Inaugural PHTLS Courses

Once a host country has signed the MOU with NAEMT and several PHTLS instructors have been trained, dates are set for that country's inaugural PHTLS course. A 3-day Provider/Instructor workshop and a subsequent 2-day Provider program is scheduled. Students for the Provider/Instructor workshop are selected by the host country.

The host country is required to cover the travel expenses for three members of the PHTLS International Faculty, including one doctor, either the PHTLS Medical Director or one of the Associate Medical Directors. At the inaugural PHTLS Provider program, these three individuals deliver key lectures and oversee the teaching and organization of the course. Upon completion of the Provider course, the superior students complete an Instructor course, taught by the PHTLS International Faculty. Following a 1-day break, the new instructors teach a Provider course, audited by the International Faculty.

The Current Status of International PHTLS

The following countries are currently holding approved PHTLS courses. The organization that signed the MOU for each country is listed as well.

Australia	Queensland Health
Argentina	Fundacion EMME
Barbados	Barbados Defense Force, St. Anne's Fort
Brazil	Brazilian American College of Surgeons
Canada	NAEMT
Chile	American College of Surgeons—Chile
Columbia	Emergency Department and Trauma Unit—Bogota
England	Royal College of Surgeons

Greece	American College of Surgeons—Greece
Ireland	National Ambulance Training School—St. Mary's Hospital
Israel	Director Instruction Department—Magen David Adom
Italy	Cattedra di Cirurgia D'urgenza
Mexico	Hospital Centrar Militar
Sweden	Swedish Anesthesia Society—Sodersjukhuset
Trinidad	Undine West

The Horizon . . .

As this PHTLS text goes to press, Holland, Greece, Hong Kong, and Peru are presently scheduling their inaugural courses. As the program continues to grow, PHTLS should serve as a forum for sharing ideas about trauma care and EMS across international boundaries.

VISION FOR THE FUTURE

Webster's Dictionary defines *success* as ". . . the attainment of wealth, favor or eminence." Clearly, the success that the PHTLS program has witnessed over the past 15 years meets each of these descriptions. Attainment of a *wealth* of knowledge is realized by each prehospital clinician who attends a course. In addition, trauma patients treated following the standards and skills promulgated by the PHTLS program attain *wealth* by improved outcomes. The PHTLS program has also reached a stage of pre-*eminence* throughout the world as the "gold" standard for prehospital trauma management.

All that PHTLS has accomplished would not have been possible without the vision, dedication, and tireless effort of its founder, Norman E. McSwain, Jr., MD, FACS, NREMT-P. Dr. McSwain has spent numerous hours fighting for the improvement of prehospital trauma care. He has done this through continuous development and revisions of the PHTLS program. However, a leader is only as good as the *team* that realizes the vision and makes things happen. With the support of thousands of volunteers across the globe who serve as instructors, instructor trainers, affiliate faculty, national faculty, course coordinators, and course medical directors, PHTLS has reached a stage of maturity that has ensured its survival and that of its patients well into the next century.

In addition, there have been a group of believers who have made the sacrifice of time, and sometimes family, in their support and hard work for the PHTLS program. Since 1981, these individuals, who are too numerous to mention individually, have served in a variety of positions and have formed the backbone of the PHTLS program through the national committees, subcommittees, task forces, and staff.

Having a *vision* is no good if you cannot have that *vision* carried forward by future leaders. Since the beginning of the program, Dr. McSwain's vision has received that support by the elected leaders. The following individuals have served as the elected leadership and deserve special recognition for going above and beyond in their support of the PHTLS program.

National PHTLS Medical Director

| Norman E. McSwain, Jr., MD, FACS, NREMT-P | 1981–Present |

National PHTLS Vice Medical Director

| Scott B. Frame, MD, FACS, FCCM | 1995–Present |

National PHTLS Chairpersons

Richard Vomacka, REMT-P	1983–1985
James L. Paturas, EMT-P	1985–1988
David Wuertz, REMT-P	1988–1990
John Sinclair, EMT-P	1990–1991
James L. Paturas, EMT-P	1991–1992
Elizabeth M. Wertz, RN, BSN, MPM, EMT-P	1992–1996
Will Chapleau, RN, EMT-P, TNS, CEN	1996–Present

International PHTLS

| James L. Paturas, EMT-P, Chairman | 1996–Present |
| Jeffery Salomone, MD, FACS, NREMT-P Medical Associate Director | 1997–Present |

As the world awaits the start of a new century, the challenge for the PHTLS program will be to continue to enhance those values that have been promulgated since the early 1980s. In addition, new programs are under development that specifically target the pediatric and geriatric populations. Pilot programs are being developed for first responder personnel so that the continuity of care is ensured for each and every citizen involved in a traumatic emergency. In addition, new educational methodologies are being considered that will enhance the educational experience for the individual participating in a course and reach the largest possible audience.

PURPOSE AND MISSION

STATEMENT OF PURPOSE

The *Statement of Purpose* for the PHTLS program, as well as this text, is to provide the student or practicing prehospital clinician with the underlying beliefs that constitute the foundation of the program. The fundamental belief, which has not wavered since 1981, is that *definitive care* cannot be provided for the critically injured trauma patient in the field. But, the continuum of care begins at the scene with prehospital trauma management. Transfer of that care then continues in the emergency department with further evaluation and stabilization and surgical intervention in the operating suite. The final step in this continuum is the rehabilitation of the patient back into society.

Deke Farrington, MD, FACS, taught us that patient care is the most important thing that we can provide. It is the premise of the PHTLS course that good patient care is provided by EMTs exercising correct judgment in the field. Correct judgment must be based on a well-found fund of knowledge of anatomy, physiology, pathophysiology, assessment, and management. Patient care should be judgment driven and not protocol driven. Protocols are helpful to direct one's thinking but should not direct patient care. Patient care should be driven by the variables of the patient's condition, the scene, the number of patients, and other factors combined with the EMT's fund of knowledge to make the necessary decisions for patient care.

Since the late 1960s, studies have shown that trauma patient outcomes can have positive effects if the first three steps in this continuum of trauma care are delivered in an expeditious manner. This means that the trauma patient must reach the operating suite intervention within the first critical postinsult "golden hour." Therefore, the role of the prehospital clinician is to practice the three key principles of caring for the critically injured trauma patient: rapid assessment, effective stabilization, and safe transportation.

The PHTLS program attempts to increase each participant's understanding and skills in prehospital trauma management. This increased understanding of the kinematics, pathophysiology, systemic impact, and intervention techniques will result in improving the assessment and treatment of the multisystem trauma patient and offer a perspective into the patient's individual needs. The PHTLS program enhances the philosophy that care of the multisystem trauma patient is unique and requires specific needs that may exceed traditional treatment modalities. Therefore, the PHTLS program stresses the need for:

- Rapid and accurate assessment
- Identification of shock and hypoxemia
- Initiation of intervention techniques
- Rapid and safe transportation

MISSION STATEMENT

The PHTLS mission continues to provide the highest quality prehospital trauma education to all who wish to avail themselves of this opportunity. The PHTLS mission also enhances the achievement of the NAEMT mission (see page xxi). The PHTLS program is committed to quality and performance improvement. As such, PHTLS is always attentive to changes in technology and methods of delivering prehospital trauma care that may be used to enhance the clinical and service quality of this program.

The PHTLS fourth edition text and supporting materials demonstrate the continuous evolution and improvement of this program. The primary objective of NAEMT and the PHTLS program is to continue to embrace change and develop enhancements to the program that are in the best interest of prehospital clinicians and, most importantly, of their patients.

SPECIAL NOTE

This text, although a valuable tool in itself, is the text for the PHTLS program. Each PHTLS course reinforces the material presented herein through interactive assessment labs, lecture presentations, intervention technique skill stations, open discussion, and evaluation stations. For positive outcomes to be realized for the critical trauma patient, intelligent prehospital trauma management is required. Unless that care focuses on the critical components of trauma management and transportation, potentially salvageable patients may die. The purpose of this program is to prevent such needless deaths.

NATIONAL ASSOCIATION OF EMERGENCY MEDICAL TECHNICIANS

NAEMT HISTORY

The National Association of Emergency Medical Technicians was founded in 1975, with support of the National Registry of EMTs and numerous leaders in emergency medicine. It serves as the national voice for prehospital emergency health care professionals. Throughout NAEMT's history, association leadership and membership have comprised primarily EMT-Bs, EMT-Is, EMT-Ps, EMS educators, and EMS administrators. In addition, nurses and physicians have served in both leadership and general membership positions.

NAEMT's prime objective is to promote the professional status of the EMT at all levels (B, I, and P), EMS educator, and EMS administrator. NAEMT actively participates in the development of EMS education standards and accreditation, develops and promulgates continuing education programs for members and nonmembers, participates in legislative initiatives, and produces career information for the public and the EMS industry.

NAEMT has developed ongoing liaison relationships with over 28 federal agencies and professional organizations servicing the emergency/trauma medicine and public safety community. The American College of Surgeons, American College of Emergency Physicians, National Registry of Emergency Medical Technicians, Commission on Accreditation of Ambulance Services, Emergency Nurses Association, and the Federal Emergency Management Agency are a few of these liaison organizations. The PHTLS program was developed by the NAEMT in cooperation with the American College of Surgeons, Committee on Trauma as a natural extension of the Association's "mission" and one example of the benefit of these liaison relationships.

NAEMT MISSION ──────────────

The mission of the National Association of Emergency Medical Technicians, Inc., is to be a professional representative organization that will receive and represent the views and opinions of prehospital care personnel and to thus influence the future advancement of EMS as an allied health profession. NAEMT will serve its professional membership through educational programs, liaison activities, development of national standards and reciprocity, and the development of programs to benefit prehospital care personnel.

Introduction

Our patients did not choose us. We have chosen to treat them. We could have chosen another profession, but we did not. We have accepted the responsibility for patient care in some of the worst situations: when we are tired or cold, when it is rainy and dark, and often when conditions are unpredictable. We must either accept this responsibility or surrender it. We must give to our patients the very best care that we can—not while we are daydreaming, not with unchecked equipment, not with incomplete supplies, not with yesterday's knowledge, and not with indifference. We cannot know what medical information is current, and we cannot purport to be ready to care for our patients if we do not read and learn each day. The Prehospital Trauma Life Support (PHTLS) course provides a part of that knowledge to the working EMT but, more important, it ultimately benefits the person who needs our all—the patient. At the end of each run, we should feel that the patient received nothing short of our very best.

TRAUMA CARE IN THE 1990s

The opportunity for the EMT (EMT-B, I, P) to provide a service for a fellow human being is greater in the management of trauma patients than in any other kind of patient encounter. Not only is the number of trauma patients larger than most other patient populations, but the chance of survival of the trauma patient who has been provided good hospital care is greater than that of any other patient. The EMT can lengthen the life span of the trauma patient and benefit society because of the number of productive years saved. Therefore, the EMT's influence on the trauma patient is greater than on any other patient.

Understanding, learning, and practicing the principles taught in the PHTLS course will be more beneficial to your patients than any other educational program you have completed since you finished your initial training. This sounds like an ambitious statement, but the facts are there.

Trauma is the leading cause of death in persons age 1 through 44. Eighty percent of teenage deaths are secondary to trauma. Sixty percent of childhood deaths are secondary to trauma. Three times more Americans die of trauma each year than died in the Vietnam war. Every 10 years more Americans die of trauma than have died in all U.S. military conflicts combined. Furthermore, 11 million people are temporarily disabled and 450,000 are permanently disabled each year. Only in the over-50 age group do cancer and heart disease begin to compete with trauma as a leading cause of death.

The EMT can do very little to increase the cancer patient's survival. Yet for the trauma patient the EMT's action can often make the difference between life and death or between temporary, minimal disability and serious, permanent disability. Sixty million injuries occur each year in the United States alone. Thirty million will require medical care, and 9 million of these injuries are disabling. Three hundred thousand will be permanently disabled, and 8.7 million will be temporarily disabled.

The cost is staggering: 40% of the U.S. health care spending, or over $100 billion, is for management of these trauma patients. In addition, another $300 billion is lost in wages, insurance administration costs, property damage, and employer costs.

Lost productivity from trauma patients' disabilities is the equivalent of 5.1 million years at a cost of over $65 billion. For patients who are killed, 5.3 million years of life are lost (34 years per person) at a cost of over $50 billion. Comparatively, the costs (measured in dollars and in years lost) for cancer and heart disease are much less, as illustrated in Figure I-1.

Trauma care is divided into three phases: preincident, incident, and postincident. The EMT has responsibilities in each phase, although it is during the postincident phase that the EMT is trained to work.

PREINCIDENT PHASE

Trauma is no accident. This familiar idea can be captured in one word: prevention. Webster's Dictionary defines an *accident* as "an event occurring by chance or arising from unknown causes." Yet most trauma deaths and injuries do not fit this definition; rather, they are preventable. Traumatic incidents fall into two categories: intentional and unintentional. In working toward prevention in both of these areas, EMTs must educate the public to increase the use of automobile occupant restraint systems, promote legislation to reduce the use of weapons in criminal activities, and promote nonviolent conflict resolution. In addition to caring for the trauma patient, all members of the health care delivery team have a responsibility to reduce the number of victims. Currently, violence and unintentional trauma cause more deaths annually in the United States than all diseases combined. Violence accounts for over one-third of these deaths (Figure I-2). Motor vehicle and firearms are involved in more than one-half of

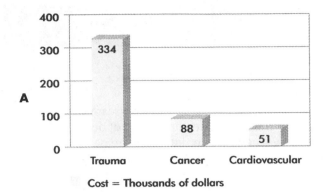
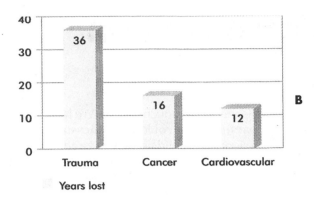

Figure I-1 A, Comparative costs in thousands of dollars to United States citizens for victims of trauma, cancer, and cardiovascular disease each year. B, Comparative number of years lost due to trauma, cancer, and cardiovascular disease.

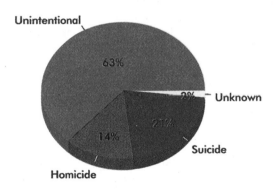

Figure I-2 Unintentional trauma and violence account for more deaths than all others combined.

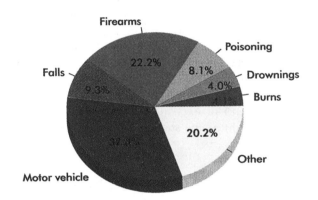

Figure I-3 Motor vehicle trauma and firearms account for more than half of the deaths that occur as a result of unintentional trauma and violence.

all trauma deaths. Most of these are preventable (Figure I-3).

Motorcycle helmet usage laws are one example of legislation that has had an effect on injury prevention. In 1966 Congress gave the Department of Transportation the authority to mandate that states pass legislation requiring the use of motorcycle helmets. The use of helmets subsequently increased to almost 100%, and the fatality rate decreased dramatically. In 1975 Congress rescinded this authority. More than half of the states repealed or modified the existing legislation, and there was an increase in related fatalities. As some states reinstate these laws, the rate is dropping again. This change is demonstrated in Figure I-4.

INCIDENT PHASE

In our own lives, we should make sure that we "practice what we preach." Whether driving our own automobile or an emergency vehicle, we should both protect ourselves and teach by the example of always using the protective devices we have available, such as lap and diagonal life belts, both in the driving compartment and in the patient care compartment. We should drive safely at all times.

POSTINCIDENT PHASE

Donald Trunkey, MD, has proposed a trimodal categorization of trauma deaths. Deaths that occur during the first few minutes after an incident are mostly unpreventable, except for improved airway management. Deaths that occur during the second phase may be prevented by good prehospital care and by good hospital care (Figure I-5).

R. Adams Cowley, MD, founder of the Maryland Institute of Emergency Medical Services, described and defined what he called "the golden hour." Based on computer studies of patients brought into one of the first trauma centers in the United States (MIEMS), Dr. Cowley discovered that patients who received definitive care (usually hemorrhage control in the operating room) within 1 hour after the injury had a much higher survival rate than those who received their care later. An average urban EMS system has a response time from the time the incident occurs until arrival on the scene of 6 to 8 minutes. The usual transport time back to the hospital is another 8 to 10 minutes. Thus 15 to 20 minutes of that magic golden hour are used just to get to the scene and to transport the patient to the hospital. If the EMTs at the scene are not efficient, well organized and well trained, they can spend 30 to 40 minutes on the scene. Add this to the transport time, and it is apparent that the golden hour has already passed before any physician has an opportunity to treat the patient.

One of the most important responsibilities of the EMT is to spend as little time on the scene as possible to evaluate the patient, perform lifesaving maneuvers, and prepare the patient for transportation to the hospital.

A second responsibility is to transport the patient to the appropriate hospital. The factor most critical to any patient's survival is the length of time that elapses between the incident and definitive care. For a cardiac arrest patient, definitive care is the restoration of normal heart rhythm. CPR, of course, is merely a holding pattern. For a patient whose airway is compromised, definitive care is the management of the airway and restoration of adequate ventilation. The reestablishment of either ventilation or normal cardiac rhythm by defibrillation is usually easily achieved in the field; therefore, transportation time is not as critical in the cardiac patient.

The management of trauma patients is different. Definitive care is hemorrhage control. Hemostasis cannot always be achieved in the field or in the emergency department, but it must be achieved in the operating room. Therefore, to determine which hospital is the most appropriate, the EMT must consider both the transport time to a given hospital and the capabilities of the facility.

A trauma center that has an in-house surgical team, OR team, and trauma team can often place a trauma patient with hemorrhage in the operating room within 10 to 15 minutes after the patient's arrival. On the other hand, a hospital without in-house surgical capabilities must await the arrival of the surgeon, the operating room staff, and the anesthesiologist before the patient can be transported from emergency department to operating room. Additional time may then elapse before the hemorrhage can be controlled (Figure I-6).

HISTORY OF EMS

This book, the PHTLS course, and our care of the trauma patient are based on the objectives developed and taught to us by the early pioneers of prehospital care. The list of these innovators is long. A few, however, especially deserve our recognition:

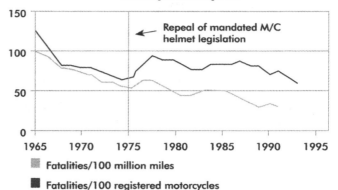

Motorcycle fatality rate

■ Fatalities/100 million miles
■ Fatalities/100 registered motorcycles

Figure I-4 Motor helmet legislation and therefore the mandated use of helmets has significantly reduced the motorcycle fatality rate. Repeal of this law in 1975 produced a marked increase in these numbers of fatalities. The number of fatalities for registered motorcyclists has just now dropped as low as prior to the repeal of this law as many states reinstate their own laws.

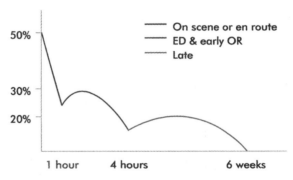

Figure I-5 Trimodal groups of trauma deaths. Those in the first hour phase can be significantly reduced only by adequate prevention with seat belts, motorcycle helmets, respecting the speed limit, and decreased alcohol use by drivers. Those in the second phase can be significantly reduced by good prehospital care and development of good trauma systems to adequately care for these patients, both in the hospital and out. Those in the third phase will be reduced as the trauma system provides prompt in-hospital definitive care.

J.D. "Deke" Farrington, MD, the father of modern emergency medical services, stimulated the development of improved prehospital care with his landmark article "Death in a Ditch" and with his work as chairman of all three of the initial documents establishing the basis of EMS: the essential equipment list for ambulances of the American College of Surgeons, the KKK standards of the Department of Transportation, and the first EMT basic training program. Robert Kennedy, MD, was the author of "Early Care of the Sick and Injured Patient." Sam Banks, MD, who along with Dr. Farrington taught the first prehospital training course to the Chicago Fire Department

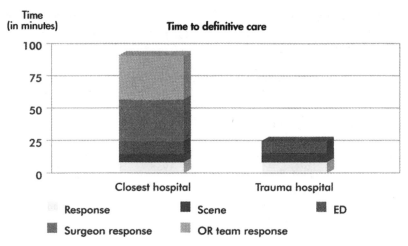

Figure I-6 In locations where trauma centers are available, bypassing hospitals not committed to the care of the trauma patient can significantly improve patient care. In severely injured trauma patients, definitive patient care must occur in the operating room. An extra 5 to 10 minutes spent en route to a hospital with an in-house surgeon and in-house operating room staff will significantly reduce the time to definitive care. The green indicates surgical response from home. The yellow indicates operating team response from home. In hospitals with in-house surgical and operating room staff, these delays do not exist.

in 1957, started us off in the proper care of the trauma patient. But as early as the late 1700s, Baron Dominick Jean Larrey, Napoleon's physician-in-chief, recognized the need for prompt prehospital care. He developed the "flying ambulance" for timely retrieval of men injured on the battlefield and introduced the premise that individuals in these flying ambulances should be trained in medical care to provide on-scene and en route care for the patients. There was minimal change between this period and the time that Dr. Farrington and the early leaders, such as Oscar Hampton, MD, and Curtis Arts, MD, brought us out of the "dark ages" and into the modern era of emergency medical services and prehospital care.

In a 1965 text edited and compiled by George J. Curry, MD, a leader of the American College of Surgeons and its Committee on Trauma, he stated the following: "Injuries sustained in accidents affect every part of the human body. They range from simple abrasions and contusions to multiple complex injuries involving many body tissues. This demands efficient and intelligent primary appraisal and care, on an individual basis, before transport. It is obvious that the services of trained ambulance attendants are essential. . . . If we are to expect maximum efficiency from ambulance attendants, a special training program must be arranged." Although prehospital care was rudimentary when Dr. Curry wrote this passage, the words still hold true today as we address the specific area of prehospital trauma care rather than the broad field of general emergency medical services.

Dr. Curry's call for specialized training of "ambulance attendants" has been answered during the past 25 years, by this text and by the landmark white paper "Accidental Death and Disability—the Neglected Disease of Modern Society," which the National Academy of Science's National Research Council issued just 1 year later. We are reminded how primitive our efforts were and how far we have come in a brief time. Yet despite the continual rush of new developments, procedures, equipment, provider levels, and standards, there seems to be a need to go back and rethink issues to fill in the spaces left by the march of progress through the field of EMS.

All of these individuals teach several basic principles that have been expanded upon and refined over time. Simply stated, these are (1) rapidly respond to the patient; (2) stabilize the patient on the scene by providing efficient but prompt care to reestablish ventilation and provide adequate oxygenation; and (3) rapidly transport the patient to the most appropriate facility.

Rapid access to the victim is dependent on an EMS system that offers easy access to the system, especially with a single emergency phone number (usually 9-1-1), a good communication system to dispatch the unit, and well prepared and trained EMTs.

Efficient on-scene medical care requires EMTs who are well trained in rapid identification of the victim's problem and skilled in airway management, proper immobilization procedures, and shock management. Finally, the EMT must exercise good judgment to decide what action should be taken on the scene, how it can be performed efficiently, and which steps should be carried out en route to the hospital.

Lastly, the EMT must ensure that the patient is transported to the appropriate facility. This facility is the one that can most promptly and appropriately provide definitive care for the patient. In a rural area, there is often no choice because there is usually only one hospital available in the community. The next hospital may be miles away, and the trauma center could be even farther.

In this instance, the prehospital provider must decide whether helicopter transport from the scene is warranted. This is a fairly simple calculation. The approximate time of ground transportation is on one side of the equation. On the other side is the time necessary for helicopter alert and lift off, travel to the scene, management on the scene, and travel back to the hospital. The means of transportation chosen is determined by which of the two times is shorter.

CHAPTER OBJECTIVES

CHAPTER 1

Kinematics of Trauma

At the completion of this course the student will be able to:

- Define energy and force as they relate to trauma.

- Define laws of motion energy and understand the geometric role increased speed plays in causing injuries.

- Describe each type of auto collision and its effect on unrestrained victims (e.g., "down-and-under," "up-and-over," compression, deceleration).

- Describe the pathophysiology of the head, spine, thorax, and abdomen that result from the above named forces.

- List specific injuries and their causes as related to interior and exterior vehicle damage.

- Describe the function of supplemental restraint systems (air bags).

- Describe the kinematics of penetrating injuries.

- List the motion and energy considerations of mechanisms other than motor vehicle collisions (e.g., blasts, falls).

- Define the role of kinematics as an additional tool for patient assessment.

Scenario

It is a warm, clear Saturday afternoon in June, and a small private aircraft has just taken off from Coronado Airfield. On board is the pilot, his wife, and two friends. They plan to fly over the Rocky Mountains for a sight-seeing trip.

As the plane achieves its rotation speed, the pilot maneuvers the aircraft into a gentle climb with full power. At 600 feet the engine suddenly quits, and the plane loses lift. In an attempt to control the crash, the pilot rapidly lowers the nose into a step glide so that the wings regain some lift.

Thanks to the pilot's skill, the plane hits the ground on its belly. "Pancaking" into the hard desert ground, it bounces twice before a tree rips off its right wing. Three hundred gallons of fuel begin to pour out behind the plane. The plane continues forward, where it is finally stopped by a large radio transmission tower. Witnesses on the ground estimate the forward speed of the aircraft at the time of impact to be approximately 30 miles per hour.

Your unit is the first to arrive on the scene. You smell aviation fuel and observe that the ground behind the plane is soaked with gasoline. The left wing is still intact and does not appear to be leaking gasoline at this time. The fuselage of the plane is badly damaged from repeatedly hitting and bouncing on the ground. The front of the aircraft is displaced approximately 3 feet rearward. All four occupants are still in the cabin in their seats, with lap and diagonal straps in place.

What injuries do you wish to consider region by region, for example, head, neck, chest, abdomen, pelvis, or extremities?

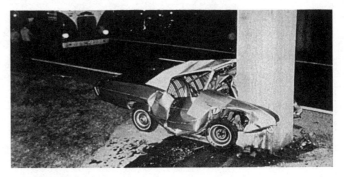

Figure 1-1 Evaluating the scene of the incident is critical. Such information as direction of impact, passenger compartment intrusion, and amount of energy exchange will provide valuable insight in the possible injuries of the occupants.

Box 1-1   Injury Prevention: Our Responsibility

Part of our job as members of the medical care team is to become active in injury prevention. Our words can have important implications. For example, Webster's *Dictionary* defines an "accident" as "an event occurring by chance or arising from unknown causes," although the second definition is "an unfortunate event resulting from carelessness, unawareness, or ignorance." The EMT should strive to be careful, aware, and informed. Part of the EMT's responsibility is to educate patients and potential victims regarding prevention. The EMT should use the terms "motor vehicle collision" or "crash," not "motor vehicle accident" to describe the event. An accident is an Act of God, not caused by man. Therefore, we should have no responsibility for it. On the other hand, a collision is man-made, therefore we do have responsibility and can prevent them. We must work to reduce drinking and driving and conflict resolution with guns.

Unexpected traumatic injuries are responsible for more than 125,000 deaths in the United States each year. Automobile collisions alone accounted for 41,907 deaths in 1996. Successful management of trauma patients depends on identifying injuries or potential injuries; good assessment skills are a necessity. But even with good assessment skills, many injuries can be missed if they are not suspected. An emergency medical technician (EMT) may overlook an injury simply because he or she does not know where to look. Even if obvious injuries are treated, injuries that are not obvious can be fatal because they are not managed at the scene. Knowing where to look and how to assess for injuries is as important as knowing what to do after injuries are found.

A complete, accurate history of a traumatic incident and proper interpretation of this information can allow the EMT to predict more than 90% of the patient's injuries before he or she ever lays a hand on the patient. The medical care of a trauma patient can be divided into three phases: precrash, crash, and postcrash. The term "crash" does not necessarily mean an automotive crash. The crash of an auto into a pedestrian, of a missile (bullet) into the abdomen, or of a construction worker into the asphalt after a fall from a four-story building are all crashes. In

each case, there is an energy exchange between a moving object and the tissue of the trauma victim or between the moving trauma victim and a stationary object.

The precrash phase includes all of the events that precede the incident, such as the ingestion of alcohol or drugs. Conditions that predate the incident are also part of the precrash phase, such as a patient's acute or pre-existing medical conditions or state of mind. Typically, young trauma patients do not have chronic illnesses. However, with older patients, medical conditions that are present before the trauma can cause serious complications in the prehospital management of the patient and can significantly influence the outcome. For example, the elderly driver of a car that has struck a utility pole may have chest pain indicative of a myocardial infarction

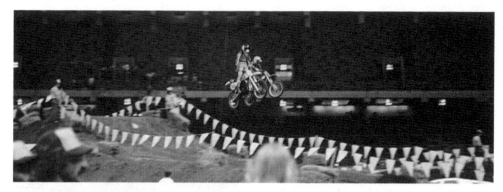

Figure 1-2 A motorcycle going over a jump does not suddenly stop when contact is lost with the ground. The momentum of the motorcycle and the previously existing energy carry both the motorcycle and the rider forward unless obstructions stop the motion.

(heart attack). Did the driver hit the utility pole and have a heart attack, or did he have a heart attack and then strike the utility pole? As medical personnel, we have the responsibility to reduce the amount of trauma just as we have the responsibility to treat the patients once they are injured (Box 1-1).

The second phase in the history of a trauma incident is the crash phase, which begins at the time of impact between one moving object and a second object. The crash phase ends when all motion has stopped. The second object in the crash can be either stationary or in motion, and one or both objects can be a human being. The directions in which the energy exchange occurred, the amount of energy that was exchanged, and the effect these forces had on the patient are all important considerations for medical providers.

The information gathered about the crash and precrash phases is used by the prehospital provider to manage the patient in the postcrash phase. This phase begins as soon as the energy from the crash is absorbed and the patient is traumatized. The onset of life-threatening trauma can be slow or fast, depending in part on the action taken by the EMTs. In the postcrash phase the EMT's understanding of the kinematics of trauma, his or her index of suspicion regarding injuries, and the EMT's strong assessment skills all become crucial to the outcome of the patient.

To understand the effects of the forces that produce bodily injury, two components must be understood: energy and anatomy. Anatomic implications are discussed system-by-system later in the chapter.

OVERVIEW OF KINEMATICS: UNDERSTANDING ENERGY

The EMT's first step in obtaining a history is to evaluate the events that occurred at the collision scene (Figure 1-1). In a motor vehicle crash, for instance, what does the scene look like? Who hit what and at what speed? How long was the stopping time? Were the victims restrained by seat belts, or were they unrestrained and thus able to be thrown about the vehicle? Were occupants thrown from the vehicle? Did they strike objects? If so, how many objects? These and many other questions must be answered if the EMT is to understand the exchange of forces that took place and then translate this information into a prediction of injuries and appropriate patient care.

The process of surveying the scene to determine what injuries might conceivably have resulted from the forces and motion involved is called kinematics. Because kinematics is based on fundamental principles of physics, an understanding of the pertinent laws of physics is necessary.

LAWS OF ENERGY AND MOTION

Newton's first law of motion states that a body at rest will remain at rest and a body in motion will remain in motion unless acted upon by some outside force. The motorcycle in Figure 1-2 was stationary until the energy from the engine started it moving along the dirt track. Once in motion, although it leaves the ground, it remains in motion until it hits something or returns to the ground and the brakes are applied. The same is true of the person sitting in the front seat of an automobile. Even if the car hits a tree and stops, the unrestrained person continues in motion until he or she hits the steering column, dashboard, and/or the windshield. The impact with these objects stops the forward motion of the torso or head, but not the organs.

Why does the sudden starting or stopping of motion result in trauma and injury to an individual? This question is answered by a second principle of physics, the law of conservation of energy, which states that energy cannot be created or destroyed but can be changed in form. The motion of the vehicle is a form of energy, and when the motion starts or stops the energy must be changed to another form. It may take on the form of mechanical, thermal, electrical, or chemical energy.

An example of energy changing form when motion is stopped occurs when a driver brakes and the car decelerates. The energy of motion is converted into the heat of friction (thermal energy) on the brake drum and on the roadway as rubber is "burned" onto the asphalt. Similarly, the mechanical energy of a car crashing into a wall is dissipated by the bending of the frame or other parts of the car and by the transfer of energy to the occupants.

Kinetic energy is a function of an object's weight and speed. In humans, the victim's weight and mass are the same thing. Likewise, speed and velocity are the same. The relationship between weight and speed as it affects kinetic energy is:

$$\text{Kinetic energy} = 1/2 \text{ of the mass} \times \text{the velocity squared, or}$$
$$KE = M/2 \times V^2.$$

Thus, the kinetic energy involved when a 150-pound (lb) person travels at 30 miles per hour (mph) is:

$$150 \text{ lb at } 30 \text{ mph} = 67,500 \text{ KE units.}$$

For the purpose of this discussion, no specific physical unit of measure (such as foot-pounds) is given. The formula is used merely to illustrate the change in force. As just shown, a 150-lb person traveling at 30 mph would have 67,500 units of kinetic energy to convert to another form of energy when he or she stops. This change takes the form of damage to the vehicle and injury to the person in it, unless the energy can take some less harmful form.

A significant question that arises in a discussion of kinetic energy is, which factor has a greater effect on the amount of kinetic energy produced: mass or velocity? To answer this question, consider a 160-lb person traveling at 30 mph:

$$160 \text{ lb at } 30 \text{ mph} = 72,000 \text{ KE units.}$$

And if we go back to our previous example of a 150-lb person but increase the velocity by 10 mph:

$$150 \text{ lb at } 40 \text{ mph} = 120,000 \text{ KE units.}$$

As these calculations show, velocity (speed) increases the rate of production of kinetic energy more so than mass. Much greater damage will occur in a high-speed or high-velocity collision than in a collision at a slower speed. Differences in mass (weight) among occupants of the same vehicle have relatively little effect on their vulnerability to injury. For example, a small child and a 200-lb adult are quite different in size and weight, but if they are both in a vehicle that is traveling at 55 mph, the most significant determinant of the amount of force that will be applied to them is their common speed (velocity)—not their weight difference.

The following example illustrates this principle. Imagine that a car traveling at 35 mph hits a brick wall. The

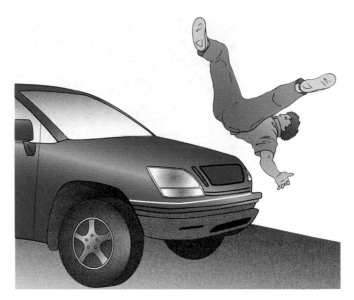

Figure 1-3 The energy exchange from a moving vehicle to a pedestrian crushes tissue and imparts speed and energy to the pedestrian to knock the victim a distance from the point of impact. Injury to the patient can occur at the point of impact as the pedestrian is hit by the car and as the pedestrian is thrown onto asphalt or into another vehicle. (From American College of Emergency Physicians. *Paramedic Field Care: A Complaint Based Approach.* St. Louis: Mosby, 1997.)

wall stops the car, but the 150-lb driver continues to travel at 35 mph until stopped by impact with the steering wheel. When impact occurs, the G forces (G = force of gravity) will approximate 30G. The driver will be moving forward with approximately 4,500 foot-pounds (ft-lb) of force, because:

$$\text{Force (ft-lb)} = \text{mass (weight)} \times$$
$$\text{G (deceleration or acceleration).}$$

In reality, actual deceleration (G force) would depend on the rate of deceleration as well as other factors that are not presented or discussed here. However, this example shows the importance of the force generated by an impact.

Stated differently, the impact of the steering column against the chest of the driver would be equivalent to a standing person having a telephone pole driven into her chest at 35 mph.

The other factor that must be considered in a collision is the stopping distance. Before a crash, the driver is moving at the same speed as the car. At the split second of the crash, car and driver both decelerate to a speed of zero. This great deceleration force is transmitted to the driver's body. If the stopping distance is increased, the force of deceleration is decreased and the resulting damage is proportionately decreased.

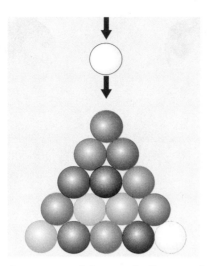

Figure 1-4 The energy of the cue ball is transferred to each of the other balls.

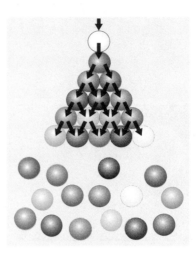

Figure 1-5 The energy exchange described above pushes the balls apart or creates a cavity.

This inverse relation between stopping distance and injury also applies to falls. A person may survive a fall if he or she lands on a compressible surface, such as deep powder snow. The same fall terminating on a hard surface, such as concrete, can be devastating. The compressible material increases stopping distance and absorbs at least some of the energy, rather than allowing it all to be absorbed by the body. The result is decreased injury and damage to the body. This principle also applies to other kinds of collisions. For instance, a car that hits an unyielding bridge abutment will be damaged more seriously than a car that hits another car from behind. In the latter example both vehicles absorb a significant amount of the energy, thus reducing the amount of energy that must be absorbed by the occupant(s). In addition, an unrestrained driver will be more severely injured than a restrained driver, because the restraint system, rather than the body, absorbs a significant portion of the "damage energy."

Therefore, once an object is in motion and has a specific energy of motion, in order to come to a complete rest the object must lose all of its energy by converting the energy to another form or transferring it to another object. If, for example, an automobile strikes a pedestrian, the pedestrian is crushed by the vehicle and knocked away from it (Figure 1-3). The vehicle is slowed by the impact, but this reduced velocity is transferred to the pedestrian, resulting in injury and creating velocity. Loss of motion of a moving object translates into tissue damage to the victim.

Although blunt and penetrating trauma are considered separate, the only real difference is "penetration" of the skin. If an object's entire energy is concentrated on one small area of skin, it is likely that the skin will tear and the object will enter the body and create a more concentrated energy exchange. This can result in greater destructive power to one area. On the other hand, a larger object whose energy is dispersed over a much larger area of skin may not penetrate the skin. In this instance, the damage will be distributed over a larger area of the body, with the injury pattern less localized.

CAVITATION

The basic mechanics of energy exchange are relatively simple. Driving a cue ball down the length of a pool table into the racked balls at the other end transfers the kinetic energy of the cue ball to each of the racked balls (Figures 1-4 and 1-5). The cue ball gives up its energy and slows or even stops, while the other balls move away from the impact point. The same kind of energy exchange occurs when a bowling ball rolls down the alley, hitting the set of pins at the other end. The pool balls and bowling pins are knocked out of their positions. The same thing happens when a moving object strikes the human body or when the human body is in motion and strikes a stationary object. The tissue of the human body is knocked out of its normal position, creating a cavity. This process is called cavitation.

Two types of cavities may be created. A temporary cavity forms at the time of impact, but the tissue returns to its previous position, and the cavity cannot be seen when the EMT or physician examines the patient later. A temporary cavity is caused by stretch. A permanent cavity also forms at the time of impact and is caused by compression or tearing of tissue. It is also caused partly by stretch, but since it does not rebound to its original shape, it can be seen later (Figure 1-6).

The difference between the two cavities is related to the elasticity of the tissue involved. For example, forcefully swinging a baseball bat into a steel drum leaves a dent, or "cavity," in its side. Swinging the same baseball bat with the same force into a similarly sized and

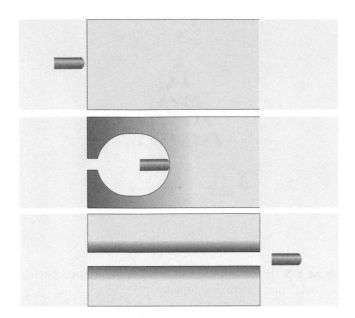

Figure 1-6 A permanent cavity is seen as the patient is examined in the emergency department or operating room.

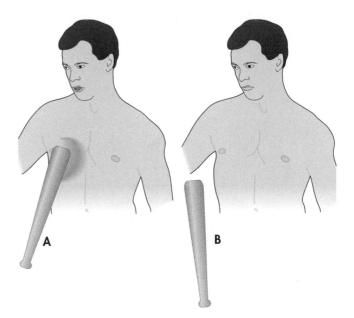

Figure 1-7 A, As a baseball bat crashes into the chest, a definitive temporary cavity is seen by the user of the bat and felt by the receiver of the blow. B, As soon as the bat rebounds from the thoracic wall, no evidence of the injury is visible. The astute EMT must recognize that this cavity existed at the time of impact and that the expansion of the cavity into the chest may have caused internal damage.

shaped mass of foam rubber will leave no dent once the bat is removed. The difference is elasticity: the foam rubber is more elastic than the steel drum. The human body is more like the foam rubber than the steel drum. If you drove your fist into another person's abdomen, you would feel it go in. Yet when you pull your fist away, you would not see a dent. Similarly, a baseball bat swung into the chest will leave no obvious cavity in the thoracic wall, but it certainly would cause some damage (Figure 1-7). The EMT is obligated to obtain a complete history to determine the approximate size of the cavity at the time of impact so that injuries can be accurately predicted.

ENERGY EXCHANGE

Density

The amount of energy exchange that occurs during an impact depends on how many tissue particles are hit. The denser a tissue (measured in particles per volume), the greater the number of particles that will be hit by a moving object. Similarly, enlarging the front surface area of the object will increase the number of tissue particles hit. Driving your fist into a feather pillow and driving your fist at the same speed into a brick wall will produce very different effects on the hand. The fist absorbs more energy with the dense brick wall than with the less dense feather pillow.

Surface Area

Wind exerts pressure on a hand when it is extended out of the window of a moving car. When the palm of the

hand is parallel to the street and parallel to the direction of the flow through the wind, some backward pressure is exerted on the front of the hand (fingers) as the particles of air strike the hand. Rotating the hand 90°, to a vertical position, places a larger surface area into the wind; thus more air particles make contact with the hand, increasing the amount of force on it.

As the body collides with an object, the number of tissue particles affected by the impact determines the amount of energy exchange and, therefore, the amount of damage that results. The number of tissue particles affected is determined by the density of the tissue and by the size of its front surface area.

The front surface area of a small object, such as a knife or bullet, may penetrate both the skin and organs as well as other tissues inside the body. This penetration creates a cavity (temporary or permanent) along the pathway of the object. Conversely, an object with a larger front surface area that cannot penetrate the skin, such as an automobile, will produce a cavity in the direction of the impact. The cavity is analogous to the visible damage on a car involved in a collision: the occupants of the vehicle will have damage on the same side as the vehicle damage and will experience a similar amount of energy exchange. Whether that energy exchange is completely transmitted to the body depends on whether the occupant is using a restraining device (safety belt or belt and air bag).

BLUNT AND PENETRATING TRAUMA

In general, trauma can be classified as blunt or penetrating. These two types of trauma are distinguished by the types of injuries produced and the types of cavities created. Recall that energy exchange is directly related to the density and to the size of the frontal area at the point of contact between the object and the victim's body. In blunt trauma, injuries are produced as the tissues are compressed, decelerated, or accelerated, whereas in penetrating trauma, injuries are produced as the tissues are crushed and separated along the path of the penetrating object. Both types create a cavity, forcing the tissues out of their normal position.

In blunt trauma, only a temporary cavity is created. In penetrating trauma (such as a gunshot wound), both a permanent and a temporary cavity exist. The energy of a rapidly moving object with a small frontal projection will be concentrated in one area and may exceed the tensile strength of the tissue and penetrate it. The temporary cavity that is created will spread away from the pathway of this missile in both frontal and lateral directions.

USING KINEMATICS IN ASSESSMENT

The assessment of a trauma patient must involve knowledge of kinematics. For instance, a driver who hits the steering column (blunt trauma) will have a large cavity in his or her anterior chest at the time of impact; however, the chest rapidly returns to, or near, its original shape as he or she rebounds from the steering wheel. Suppose two EMTs examine the patient separately. One understands kinematics and the other does not. The one without such understanding will be concerned only with the bruise visible on the patient's chest. The EMT who understands kinematics will recognize that there was a large cavity at the time of impact; that the ribs had to bend in for the cavity to form; and that the heart, lungs, and great vessels were compressed by the formation of the cavity. Therefore, the knowledgeable EMT will suspect injuries to the heart, lungs, great vessels, and chest wall, whereas the other EMT will not be aware of these possibilities.

The knowledgeable EMT will assess the injuries, manage the patient, and initiate transport more aggressively because he or she suspects serious intrathoracic injuries, rather than react to what otherwise appears to be only a minor closed, soft tissue injury. The early identification, adequate understanding, and appropriate treatment of the underlying injury will significantly influence whether the patient lives or dies.

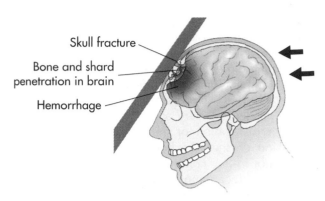

Figure 1-8 As the skull impacts some movable object, pieces of bone are fractured and are pushed into the brain substance.

BLUNT TRAUMA

In blunt trauma, two forces are involved in the impact: shear and compression. Both are a result of one organ or object (or part of an organ or object) changing speed faster that another object, organ, or part of an organ. Injury can result from any type of impact, such as a collision on the athletic field, a fall, a motorcycle or automobile crash, or a pedestrian accident.

BLUNT TRAUMA INJURIES

In the following section, the injuries sustained by various parts of the body during blunt trauma are discussed.

Head

When the body is traveling forward, such as in a frontal vehicular collision or a head-first fall, the head becomes the lead point of the "human missile." The initial energy exchange will occur on the scalp and the skull. The skull can be compressed and fractured, pushing the broken bony segments of the skull into the brain (Figure 1-8). The brain will continue to move forward, becoming compressed against the intact or fractured skull and producing a concussion, contusions, or lacerations. The brain is soft and compressible; therefore, its length will be shortened. The posterior part of the brain may separate from the skull, stretching or breaking (shearing) any vessels in the area (Figure 1-9). Hemorrhage into the epidural, subdural, or subarachnoid space can result. If the brain separates from the spinal cord, it will most likely occur at the brain stem. The only indication the EMT may have that any of these injuries have occurred is a soft tissue injury to the scalp, a bull's-eye fracture of the windshield (Figure 1-10), or a contusion of the patient's scalp.

Neck

The dome of the skull is fairly strong and can absorb the impact of a collision quite well; however, the cervical spine is much more flexible and cannot tolerate the pressure of the impact without significant angulation or compression (Figure 1-11). Hyperextension or hyperflexion of the neck produces severe angulation, often resulting in fracture or dislocation of the vertebrae. Direct in-line compression crushes the bony vertebral bodies. Either angulation or in-line compression can result in an unstable spine, which can impinge upon the spinal cord in the spinal canal (Figure 1-12).

The skull's center of gravity is anterior to and cephalad to the point at which the skull attaches to the bony spine. Therefore, a lateral impact on the torso when the neck is unrestrained will produce lateral flexion and rotation of the neck (Figure 1-13). Cervical flexion or hyperextension may also occur and cause significant damage to the soft tissues of the neck.

Thorax

If the impact of a collision is centered on the anterior part of the chest, the sternum will receive the initial energy ex-

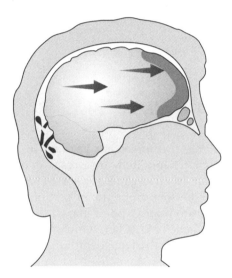

Figure 1-9 As the skull stops its forward motion, the brain does not. This is similar to the motorcyclist going over the jump in Figure 1-2. The brain continues to move forward. The part of the brain nearest the impact is compressed, bruised, and perhaps even lacerated, while the portion furthest away from the impact is separated from the skull with tearing and lacerations of the vessels involved.

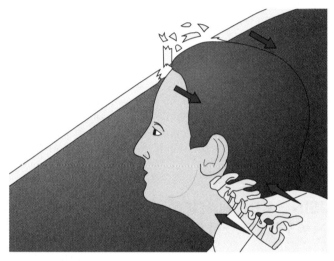

Figure 1-11 The skull frequently stops its forward motion, but the torso does not. Just as the brain compresses within the skull as in Figure 1-19, the torso continues in its forward motion until its energy is absorbed. The weakest point of this forward motion is the cervical spine.

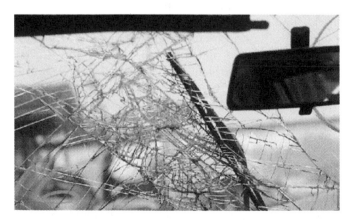

Figure 1-10 A bull's-eye fracture of the windshield is the EMT's major indication that there has been skull impact and energy exchange both to the skull and the cervical spine.

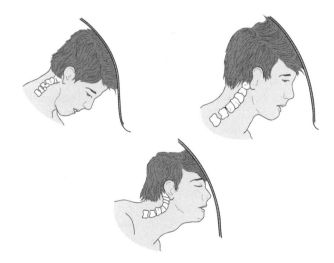

Figure 1-12 The spine can be compressed directly along its own axis or angled either into hyperextension or hyperflexion.

change. When the sternum stops moving, the posterior thoracic wall (muscles and thoracic spine) and all the organs in the thoracic cavity will continue to move toward the anterior chest wall.

The heart, ascending aorta, and aortic arch are relatively unrestrained within the thorax. The descending aorta tightly adheres to the posterior thoracic wall and the vertebral column. The resultant motion is analogous to holding the flexible tubes of a stethoscope just below where the rigid tubes from the earpiece end and swinging the acoustic head of the stethoscope from side to side (Figure 1-14). As the skeletal frame stops abruptly in

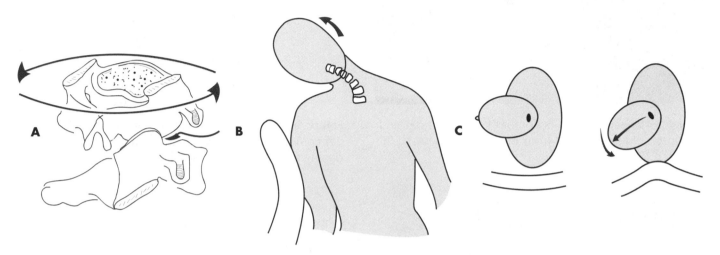

Figure 1-13 A through C, The center of gravity of the skull is anterior and superior to its pivot point between the skull and cervical spine. During a lateral impact when the torso is rapidly accelerated out from under the head, the head turns toward the point of impact, both in the lateral and anterior-posterior angles. Such motion separates the vertebral bodies from the side of opposite impact and rotates them apart. Jumped facets, ligaments, tears, and lateral compression fractures result.

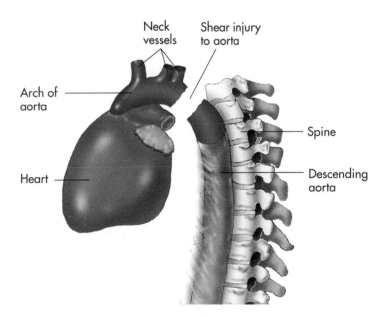

Figure 1-14 The descending aorta is a fixed structure that moves with the thoracic spine. The arch, aorta, and heart are freely movable. Acceleration of the torso in a lateral impact collision or rapid deceleration of the torso in a frontal collision produces a different rate of motion between the arch-heart complex and the descending aorta.

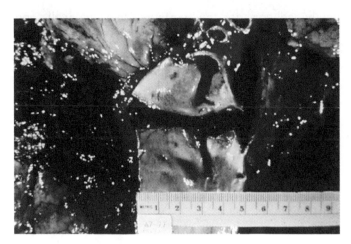

Figure 1-15 Tears at the junction of the arch and descending aorta frequently result from the actions discussed in Figure 1-14.

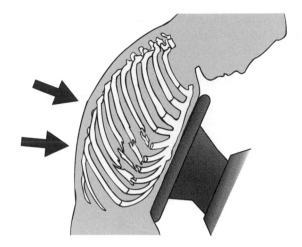

Figure 1-17 Ribs forced into the thoracic cavity by external compression usually fracture in multiple places, producing the clinical condition known as flail chest.

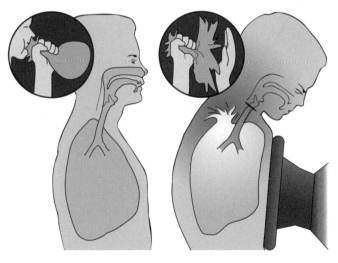

Figure 1-16 Compression of the lung against a closed glottis, by impact either on the anterior or lateral chest wall, produces an effect like that of compressing a paper bag when the opening is closed tightly by the hands. The paper bag ruptures, and so does the lung.

a collision, the heart and the initial segment of the aorta continue their forward motion. The shear forces produced can tear off the aorta at the junction of the portion of free motion and the tightly bound portion (Figure 1-15).

An aortic tear may result in an immediate, complete transection of the aorta. More commonly, aortic tears are only partial, and one or more layers of tissue remain intact. The remaining layers are under great pressure, however, and a traumatic aneurysm often develops, much like the bubble that can form on a weak part of a tire. The aneurysm eventually ruptures within minutes, hours, or days after the original injury. Approximately 80% of these patients will die on the scene at the time of initial

impact. Of the remaining 20%, one third will die within 6 hours, one third within 24 hours, and one third will live 3 days or longer. The EMT must recognize the potential for such injuries and relay this information to the hospital personnel.

Compression of the chest wall is common with frontal and lateral impacts and produces an interesting phenomenon called the "paper bag" effect, which may result in a pneumothorax. As the victim sees the accident coming, he or she instinctively takes a deep breath and holds it. In doing so, the glottis closes, sealing off the lungs. With a significant energy exchange on impact, the lungs may burst like a paper bag full of air that is popped (Figure 1-16).

Compression injuries of the external thorax may produce fractured ribs, leading to either a pneumothorax, flail chest, or both (Figure 1-17). Compare this mechanism to what happens when a car stops suddenly against a dirt embankment. The frame of the auto bends, which absorbs some of the energy. However, the rear of the car continues to move forward until all the energy is absorbed by the embankment. The posterior thoracic wall also continues to move until all the energy is absorbed by the ribs, resulting in multiple fractures, pneumothorax, flail chest, or all three.

Compression injuries to the internal structures of the thorax may include a cardiac contusion, which occurs as the heart is compressed between the sternum and the spine. Significant dysrhythmias can result. The lungs can also become compressed and contused, which will compromise respirations.

Abdomen

Injury to the abdominal organs occurs at their points of attachment to the mesentery. During a collision, the

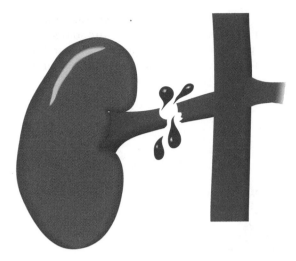

Figure 1-18 Just as the heart and arch of the aorta tear away from the fixed descending aorta during thoracic acceleration-deceleration injury, producing shear fractures of the aorta (see Figure 1-15), so do other organs tear away from their point of attachment to the abdominal wall. The spleen, kidney, and small intestine are particularly susceptible to these types of shear forces.

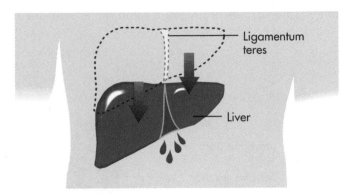

Figure 1-19 The liver is not supported by any fixed structure. Its major support comes from the diaphragm. The diaphragm is freely movable. As the body travels in a down-and-under pathway (see Figure 1-23), so does the liver. When the torso stops but the liver does not, the liver continues downward onto the ligamentum teres (a remnant of the uterine vessels), tearing the liver. This is much like pushing a tight cheese-cutting wire into a block of cheese.

forward motion of the body stops, but the organs continue to move forward, causing tears at the points of attachment of organs to the abdominal wall. If the organ is attached by a pedicle (a stalk of tissue), the tear can occur where the pedicle attaches to the organ, where it attaches to the abdominal wall, or anywhere along the length of the pedicle (Figure 1-18). Organs that can shear this way are the kidneys, the small intestine, the large intestine, and the spleen.

Another kind of injury that often occurs during deceleration is laceration of the liver caused by its impact with the ligamentum teres. The liver is suspended from the diaphragm but only minimally attached to the posterior abdomen near the lumbar vertebrae. The ligamentum teres attaches to the anterior abdominal wall at the umbilicus and to the left lobe of the liver in the midline of the body. (The liver is not a midline structure. It lies more on the right than on the left.) A "down-and-under" pathway in a frontal-impact collision, or feet-first fall, causes the liver to bring the diaphragm with it as it descends into the ligamentum teres (Figure 1-19). The ligamentum teres will fracture or bisect the liver, like a cheese slicer slices cheese.

Pelvic fractures are the result of damage to the external abdomen and may cause injury to the bladder or lacerations of the blood vessels in the pelvic cavity. Approximately 10% of patients with pelvic fractures also have a genitourinary injury.

Organs pressed by the vertebral column into the steering column or dashboard during a frontal-impact collision may rupture. The effect of this pressure is similar to the effect of placing the organ on an anvil and striking it with a hammer. Solid organs frequently injured in this manner include the pancreas, spleen, liver, and kidneys.

Injury may also result from a build-up of pressure in the abdomen. The diaphragm is a 5-millimeter (5 mm = approximately 1/4 inch) muscle located across the top of the abdomen, and it separates the abdominal cavity from the thoracic cavity. Its contraction causes the pleural cavity to expand for ventilation. The anterior abdominal wall comprises two layers of fascia and one very strong muscle. There are three lateral muscle layers with associated fascia, and the lumbar spine and its associated muscles provide strength to the posterior abdominal wall. The multi-layered perineum lies inferior to the diaphragm (Figure 1-20). The diaphragm is the weakest of all the walls and structures surrounding the abdominal cavity. It may be torn or ruptured as the intra-abdominal pressure increases (Figure 1-21). This injury has four common consequences: (1) the "bellows" effect normally created by the diaphragm as an integral part of breathing is lost; (2) the abdominal organs can enter the thoracic cavity and reduce the space available for lung expansion; (3) the displaced organs can become ischemic from compression of their blood supply; and (4) if intra-abdominal hemorrhage is present, blood can also cause a hemothorax. The diaphragm can be compressed from any direction, but compression most commonly occurs from the direction of the anterior abdominal wall.

Another injury caused by increased abdominal pressure is a rupture of the aortic valve as a result of retrograde blood flow (Figure 1-22). Although this injury is rare, the EMT should be aware of the possibility. It occurs when a collision with the steering column or involvement in another kind of accident (e.g., ditch or tunnel cave-in) has produced a rapid increase in intra-abdominal pressure. This rapid pressure increase results in a sudden increase of aortic blood pressure. Blood is pushed back (retrograde) against the aortic valve with enough pressure to cause rupture of the valve cusps.

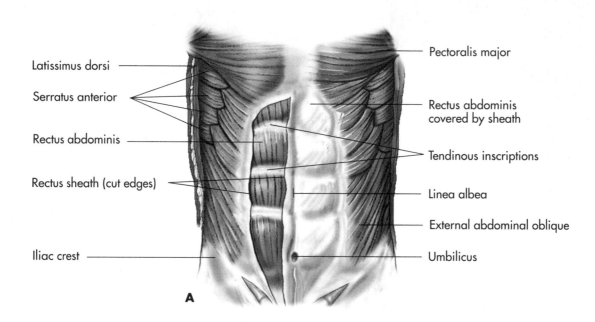

Latissimus dorsi

Serratus anterior

Rectus abdominis

Rectus sheath (cut edges)

Iliac crest

Pectoralis major

Rectus abdominis covered by sheath

Tendinous inscriptions

Linea albea

External abdominal oblique

Umbilicus

A

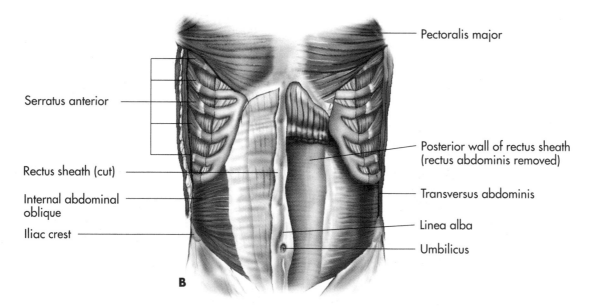

Serratus anterior

Rectus sheath (cut)

Internal abdominal oblique

Iliac crest

Pectoralis major

Posterior wall of rectus sheath (rectus abdominis removed)

Transversus abdominis

Linea alba

Umbilicus

B

Figure 1-20 The anterior, lateral, posterior, and inferior walls of the abdomen are extremely strong with multiple layers of fascia and muscle. The superior component of the abdominal cavity (the diaphragm) is only a 5-mm muscle and the weakest part of the abdominal cavity. (From Seeley, R.R.; Stephens, T.D.; and Tate, P. *Essentials of Anatomy and Physiology,* St Louis: Mosby–Year Book, Inc. 1991.)

MOTOR VEHICLE COLLISIONS

There are many kinds of blunt trauma, but motor vehicle collisions (MVCs)—including motorcycle collisions—are the most common, with pedestrian/motor vehicle collisions a close second. Compression and shear injuries often result from MVCs but are not limited to this type of crash.

Automobile collisions can be divided into five types:

- head-on or frontal impact
- rear impact
- lateral or side impact
- rotational impact
- rollover

Although there are variations on each pattern, being able to identify the five patterns will nevertheless provide insight into other similar types of crashes.

In motor vehicle collisions and other rapid deceleration mechanisms, such as snowmobile, motorcycle, and boating collisions as well as falls from heights, three collisions occur: (1) the vehicle collides with an object or with another vehicle; (2) the unrestrained occupant collides with the inside of the vehicle; and (3) the occupant's internal organs collide with one another or with the wall of the cavity that contains them. An automobile hitting a tree serves as an example.

The first collision occurs when the automobile strikes the tree. Although the vehicle stops, the unrestrained driver keeps moving forward (consistent with Newton's first law of motion). The second collision occurs when the driver hits the steering wheel and windshield. Although the driver stops moving forward, many internal organs keep moving (Newton's first law again) until they strike another organ or cavity wall or are suddenly stopped by a ligament, fascia, vessel, or muscle. This is the third collision.

Each of these collisions causes different kinds of damage, and each must be considered separately to analyze the incident. One easy way to estimate the injury pattern to the occupant is to look at the car to determine which of the five types of collisions the car was involved in. The occupant receives the same kinds and amounts of forces as does the vehicle. The energy exchange will be similar and will take place in a similar direction.

Head-on or Frontal Impact

In head-on impacts, forward motion is stopped abruptly. In a frontal impact involving a motor vehicle, such as a car hitting a brick wall, the first collision occurs when the car hits the wall, resulting in damage to the front of the car. The amount of damage to the car indicates the approximate speed of the car at the time of impact. A severely damaged car, for example, was probably moving at a high speed and will probably contain severely injured victims.

Although the vehicle suddenly ceases to move forward, the occupant, if unrestrained and therefore not slowed with the car, continues to move and will follow one of two possible paths: either down-and-under or up-and-over.

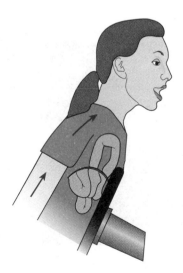

Figure 1-21 With increased pressure inside the abdomen, the diaphragm can rupture.

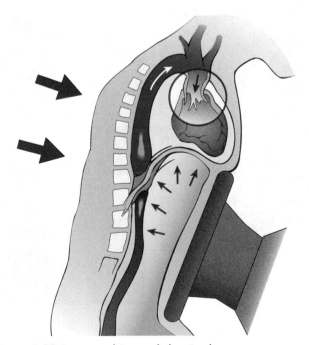

Figure 1-22 Increased intra-abdominal pressure can force blood in a retrograde fashion up the aorta and against the aortic valve. The aortic valve may then tear.

The Down-and-Under Path

In a down-and-under path, the occupant continues to move downward into the seat and forward into the dashboard or steering column (Figure 1-23). The importance of understanding kinematics can be illustrated by what hap-

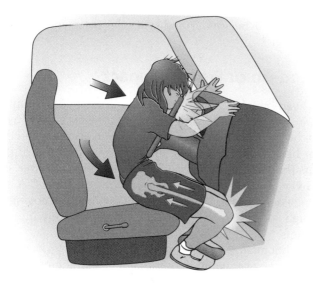

Figure 1-23 The occupant and vehicle travel forward together. The vehicle stops, and the unrestrained occupant continues forward until something retards that motion. (From American College of Emergency Physicians. *Paramedic Field Care: A Complaint Based Approach.* St. Louis: Mosby, 1997.)

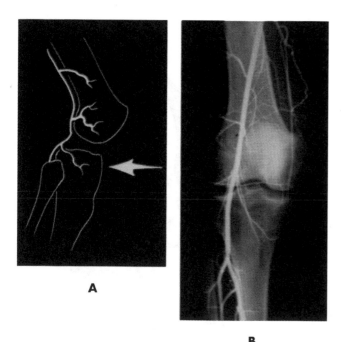

A

B

Figure 1-24 A and B, The popliteal artery lies in close proximity to the joint, tightly tied to the femur above and the tibia below. Separation of these two bones stretches, kinks, and/or tears the artery.

pens to the knee in this pathway. The foot can twist if planted on the floor panel or on the brake pedal with a straight knee, resulting in a fracture at that joint. In most cases, however, the knees are most often the lead point of the human missile, which will strike the dashboard.

The knee has two possible impact points against the dash: the femur and the tibia. If the tibia hits the dash and stops first, the femur remains in motion and overrides it. A dislocated knee, with torn ligaments, tendons, and other supporting structures, can result. Because the popliteal artery is so tightly attached to the femur and the tibia, the opening of the joint stretches the vessel at this point (Figure 1-24), tearing the lining of the artery or causing complete disruption. Such popliteal artery injuries are frequently associated with knee dislocations.

This kind of injury must be recognized early, before edema and hemorrhage make an accurate assessment impossible. If recognition is delayed, surgical repair carries a less favorable prognosis than surgery performed earlier. In addition, a clot may develop in an unrecognized damaged popliteal artery when the patient is in surgery for management of other injuries or in bed with the legs covered up. If the loss of perfusion to the extremity is not detected within several hours, amputation may be necessary. A delay in recognizing this possible injury increases the risk of an adverse outcome for the patient.

A knee imprint on the dashboard is the key indicator of knee impact (Figure 1-25). The EMT must look for this and other impact points on the inside of the vehicle as well as on the outside. These imprints often shrink spontaneously either shortly after impact or during extrication. Unless the dents in the dashboard caused by the knee impact are observed and recognized, this injury may not be suspected and thus not reported to the emergency department physicians.

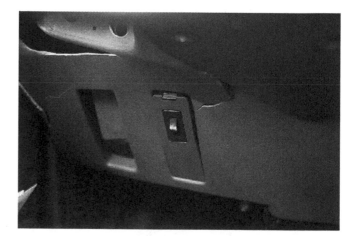

Figure 1-25 The impact point of the knee on the dashboard indicates both a down-and-under pathway and a significant absorption of energy along the lower extremity.

When the femur is the point of impact, the energy must be absorbed on the bone's shaft, which can break (Figure 1-26). In addition, the continued forward motion of the pelvis onto the femur, which remains intact, can override the femur's head, resulting in a posterior dislocation of the acetabular joint.

After the knees' impact, the upper body rotates forward into the steering column or dashboard. The pattern of injury in this latter phase of the "down-and-under" sequence is the same as in the "up-and-over" sequence (Figure 1-27). The chest or abdomen may hit the steering wheel or dash.

The Up-and-Over Path

In this sequence, the body's forward motion carries it up and over the steering wheel (Figure 1-28). The head is usually the lead body portion striking the windshield or windshield frame. The chest or abdomen collides with the steering wheel. If the chest strikes the column, serious injury to the thoracic cage or soft tissues or organs may occur. If the abdomen strikes it, compression injuries can occur, most often to the solid abdominal organs (kidneys,

liver, pancreas, and spleen). Hollow organs are also susceptible to injury.

The kidneys, spleen, and liver are also subject to shear injury as the abdomen strikes the steering wheel and stops abruptly. An organ may be torn from its normal anatomic restraints and supporting tissues. The continued forward motion of the kidneys after the vertebral column has stopped moving may cause tears in the renal vessels near the points at which they join the inferior vena cava and the descending aorta. These great vessels adhere so tightly to the posterior abdominal wall and vertebral column that the continued forward motion of the kidneys can stretch the renal vessels to the point of rupture.

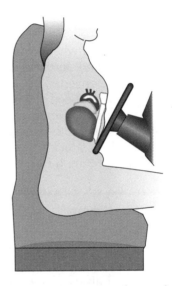

Figure 1-27 The upper torso rotates forward onto the steering column at the lower extremity as it stops its forward motion.

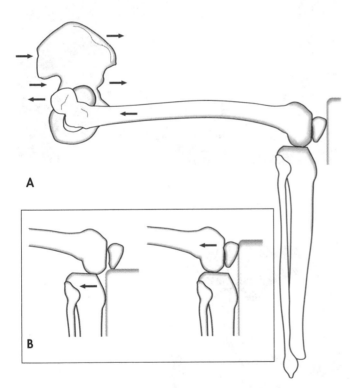

Figure 1-26 A, If the tibia impacts the dashboard, the femur overrides it, tearing the supporting structures of the knee and the popliteal artery. If the femur is the impact point, energy absorption is distributed along the length of the femur. B, If the femur stops its forward motion because of impact on the dash, the continued forward motion of the pelvis stretches the supporting ligaments at the joints and surrounding muscle, resulting in a posterior dislocation of this joint.

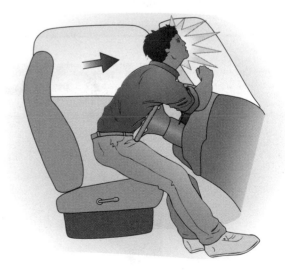

Figure 1-28 The configuration of the seat and the position of the occupant can direct the initial force on the upper torso with the head as the lead point. (From American College of Emergency Physicians. *Paramedic Field Care: A Complaint Based Approach.* St. Louis: Mosby, 1997.)

As the body continues to rotate forward and upward, the chest strikes the steering wheel or dashboard. The victim will have compression injuries to the anterior chest, which may include broken ribs, flail chest, pulmonary contusion, myocardial contusion, or damage to the great vessels. If the impact is low on the chest wall, rupture of the higher solid abdominal organs (liver and spleen) can occur.

The head is also a point of impact. When its forward motion stops, the momentum of the still-moving torso following it must be absorbed. One of the most easily bent or fractured parts of the body lies between the head and the torso—the cervical spine (see page 8).

Rear Impact

Rear-impact collisions occur when a moving or stationary object is struck from behind. In these collisions, the energy of the impact is converted to acceleration. The greater the difference in the speed of the two vehicles, the greater the force of the initial impact and therefore the more energy available to create damage. For example, when a stopped vehicle is struck from behind by a second vehicle traveling at 55 mph (55 − 0 = 55), the im-

pact will be far greater than that produced when a vehicle going 30 mph is struck by another vehicle traveling at 55 mph (55 − 30 = 25). In forward collisions, the sum of both vehicles' speeds becomes the velocity at which damage is produced. In rear-end collisions, the velocity is the difference between these speeds.

Upon impact, the vehicle in front shoots ahead, like a bullet discharged from a gun, as does everything in contact with the car. If the headrest is not positioned to prevent hyperextension of the neck over the top of the seat, tearing of the neck's ligaments and supporting anterior structures often occurs (Box 1-2; Figure 1-29).

If the headrest is up, the head moves with the seat (Figure 1-30). If the car is allowed to move forward without interference until it slows to a stop, the occupant probably will not be injured. However, if the car strikes another

---

Box 1-2 Head Restraints

If it can be proved that the victim's headrest was not properly positioned when the neck injury occurred, some courts consider reducing the liability of the party at fault in the collision on the grounds that the victim's negligence contributed to his own injuries (contributory negligence). Similar measures have been considered in cases of failure to use occupant restraints.

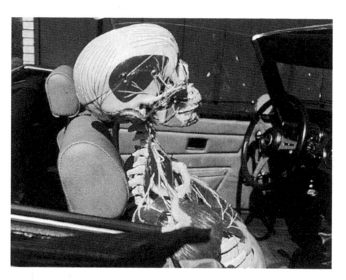

Figure 1-29 A rear-impact collision forces the torso forward. If the head restraint is in a down position, the head is hyperextended over the top of the seat.

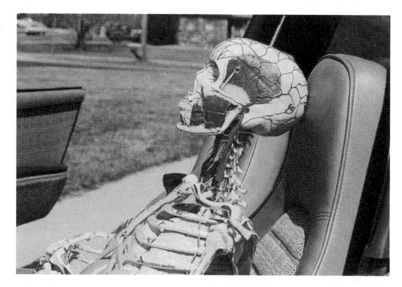

Figure 1-30 If the head restraint is up, the head moves forward with the torso, and neck injury is prevented.

car or object or if the driver slams on the brakes and stops suddenly, the occupants are thrown forward, following the characteristic pattern of a front-impact collision. The accident then involves two impacts—rear and frontal. The double impact increases the likelihood of injury. When dealing with this kind of accident, the EMT should look for two sets of injuries: those caused by the rear impact and those caused by the (secondary) frontal impact.

Lateral or Side Impact

Lateral-impact collisions occur when a vehicle is struck from the side. The vehicle that is hit is propelled away from the impact in the direction of the impact. The entire side of the vehicle is thrust against the side of the occupant. The occupant, then, may be injured in two ways: (1) by the movement of the car (Figure 1-31), and (2) by the door's projection into the passenger compartment as it is bent inward (Figure 1-32). Injury caused by the car's movement is less severe if the occupant is belted and moves with the car.

As the chest receives the impact, lateral compression injuries result, fracturing the ribs on the side of the impact. Other injuries may include a lateral flail chest, pulmonary contusion, or injury to solid organs (Figure 1-33). Occupants on the driver's side are vulnerable to splenic injuries, since the spleen is a left-sided organ, whereas those on the passenger side are more likely to receive an injury to the liver.

If the victim's arm is at her side, it can rotate posteriorly out of the way. If the arm is pinned between her chest and the door, it absorbs the impact and transfers the force both to the clavicle and to the chest wall. As a result, the clavicle is usually fractured outward along the curve of its medial one third (Figure 1-34).

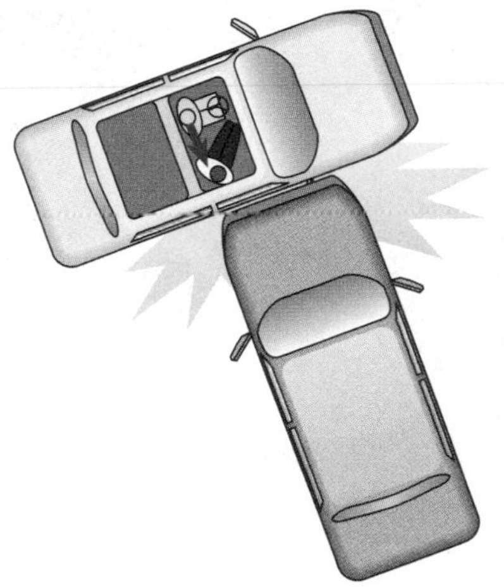

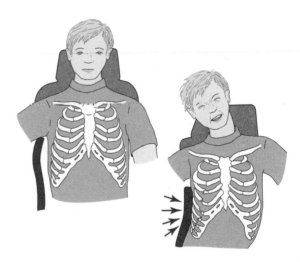

Figure 1-33 Compression against the lateral chest and abdominal wall injures the underlying spleen, liver, and kidney.

Figure 1-31 Lateral impact of the vehicle pushes the entire automobile into the unrestrained passenger. The restrained passenger is moved laterally with the vehicle.

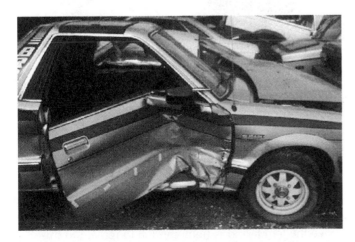

Figure 1-32 Intrusion of the side panels into the passenger compartment provides another source of basic injury.

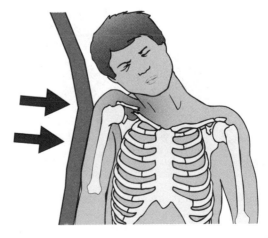

Figure 1-34 Compression of the shoulder against the clavicle produces midshaft fractures of this bone.

The pelvis and femur are also frequently struck by the door. The impact forces the head of the femur to move medially through the pelvis at the acetabulum (Figure 1-35). The wing of the ilium (pelvis) can be pushed in, fracturing the pelvis both anteriorly and posteriorly.

Head or scalp injuries can occur as the door, side window, or door post strikes the side of the head. These injuries range from simple facial lacerations to cerebral contusions and hemorrhage.

When the vehicle is moved by the force of the impact, it is as if the car is suddenly moved out from under its occupants. In this case, the use of seat belts will reduce the severity of injury. Because of the lap belt, the occupant begins lateral motion with the car and is "pulled" away from the impact point. The head is supported by the spine but in an off-center position. The center of gravity is forward and superior to the point of support. As the trunk is pushed laterally by the side impact, the tendency of the head to remain in its original position until pulled by the neck (according to Newton's first law of motion) will

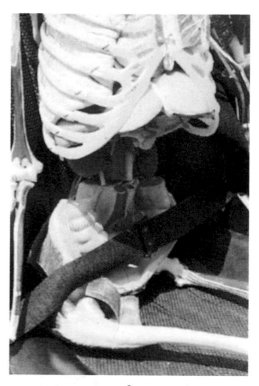

A

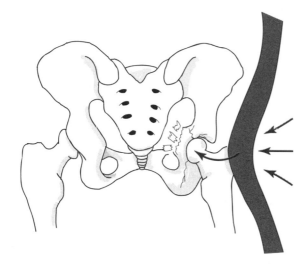

Figure 1-35 Lateral impact on the femur pushes the head through the acetabulum or fractures the pelvis.

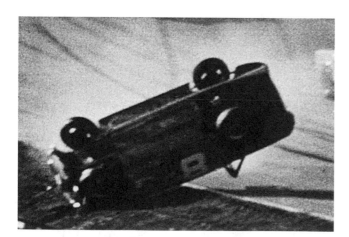

Figure 1-36 During a rollover, the unrestrained occupant can be wholly or partially ejected out of the car or can bounce around inside the car. This action produces multiple and somewhat unpredictable injuries, but they are always severe.

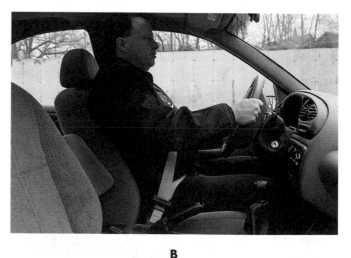

B

Figure 1-37 A properly positioned seat belt is located below the anterior superior iliac spine on each side, above the femur and is tight enough to remain in this position. The bowl-shaped pelvis protects the soft intra-abdominal organs.

produce both lateral flexion and rotation of the cervical spine (see Figure 1-13 on page 9). The combination of these movements leads to more frequent and more severe cervical injuries than is produced by either of the two movements alone. The result will be tears or strains of the ligaments and supporting structures of the neck. Fractures of the spine are more common with lateral collisions than with rear collisions. Injury to the spinal cord caused by this kind of impact may result in a neurologic deficit.

During a side-impact crash, the occupants are also subject to injury from a secondary collision with other passengers, such as when the head of one occupant strikes the head or shoulder of the person sitting next to him or her. The presence of an injury on the side of the patient opposite the side hit by the other vehicle should alert the EMT to check the adjacent occupant for injuries resulting from the collision of the two persons. Another form of secondary collision can occur when the occupant(s) of the vehicle are projected about the vehicle and strike the opposite side of the vehicle from the initial collision point. The EMT who is aware of the kinematics of energy will be alert to the possibility of these types of injuries.

Rotational Impact

Rotational-impact collisions occur when one corner of a car strikes an immovable object, the corner of another vehicle moving 90° to it, or a vehicle moving slower or in the opposite direction of the first car. Following Newton's first law of motion, this corner of the car will stop while the rest of the car continues its forward motion until its energy is completely transformed.

Rotational-impact collisions result in injuries that are a combination of those seen in head-on and lateral-impact collisions: the victim continues to move forward and then is hit by the side of the car (as in a lateral collision) as the car rotates around the point of impact.

Rollover

During a rollover, the car may undergo several impacts at many different angles, as may the occupant's body and internal organs (Figure 1-36). Injury and damage can occur with each one of these impacts. It is almost impossible to predict the injuries these victims may receive.

Restraints

In the injury patterns previously described, the victims were assumed to be unrestrained, as are the majority of automobile occupants in the United States (55% in 1992). The effectiveness of occupant protection laws in the various states is significant: the national seat belt usage rate increased from 11% in 1982 to 45% in 1988. In 1996, seat belt usage by drivers in fatal crashes was 51%;

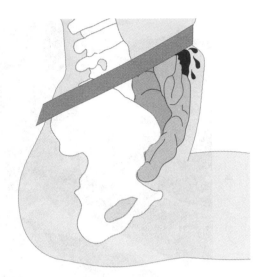

Figure 1-38 A seat belt that is incorrectly positioned above the brim of the pelvis allows the abdominal organs to be trapped between the moving posterior wall and the belt. Injuries to the pancreas and other retroperitoneal organs as well as blowout ruptures of the small intestine and colon result.

in injury crashes, 79.6%; and in property crashes, 79.5%. Ejection from vehicles accounts for 27% of the 125,000 trauma deaths that occur each year. One out of thirteen ejection victims suffers a spine fracture. After ejection from the automobile, the body is subjected to a second impact as the body strikes the ground (or another object) outside the car. This second impact can result in injuries that are even more severe than the initial impact. In fact, the risk of death for ejected victims is six times greater than for those who are not ejected. Clearly, seat belts save lives.

But what occurs when the victims are restrained? If a seat belt is positioned properly, the pressure of the impact is absorbed by the pelvis and the chest, resulting in few or no serious injuries. The proper use of restraints transfers the force of the impact from the patient's body to the restraint belts and restraint system. With restraints, injuries are not life threatening, or at least the chance of receiving life-threatening injuries is greatly reduced (Figure 1-37).

However, in order to be effective, restraints must be worn properly. An improperly worn restraint may not protect against injury in the event of a crash, and it may even cause injury. When lap belts are worn loosely or are strapped above the anterior iliac crests, compression injuries of the soft abdominal organs can occur. Compression injuries of the soft intra-abdominal organs (spleen, liver, and pancreas) result from compression between the seat belt and the posterior abdominal wall (Figure 1-38). Increased intra-abdominal pressure can cause diaphragmatic rupture and herniation of abdominal

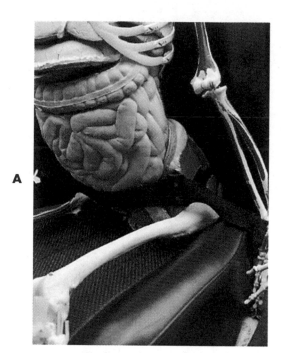 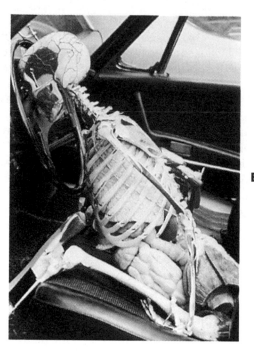

A   B

Figure 1-39 When worn alone, the diagonal strap retards forward motion but produces an excessive force on the neck. Neck injuries as severe as decapitation have been reported. (From McSwain, N.E. *The Basic EMT: Comprehensive Prehospital Patient Care Text.* St. Louis: Mosby, 1996.)

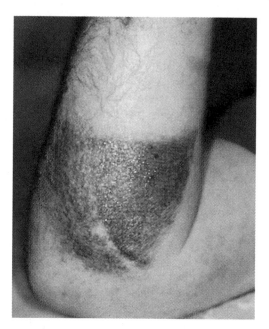 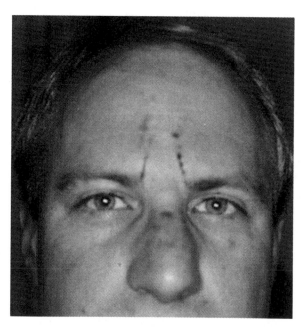

Figure 1-40 Abrasions of the forearm are secondary to rapid expansion of the air bag when the hands are tight against the steering column. (From McSwain, N.E. *The Basic EMT: Comprehensive Prehospital Patient Care Text.* St. Louis: Mosby, 1996.)

Figure 1-41 Expansion of the air bag into eyeglasses produces abrasions. (From McSwain, N.E. *The Basic EMT: Comprehensive Prehospital Patient Care Text.* St. Louis: Mosby, 1996.)

organs. Anterior compression fractures of the lumbar spine can also occur as the upper and lower parts of the torso pivot over the restrained T12, L1, and L2 vertebrae.

Even when worn properly, lap belts ideally should not be worn alone. Without the diagonal shoulder strap to

stop the forward movement of the upper body, severe facial, head, and neck injuries may occur as the head strikes the dashboard or steering wheel (Figure 1-39). As was initially shown in Europe, diagonal straps worn alone can produce severe neck injuries, including decapitation.

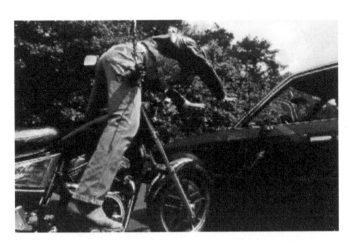

Figure 1-42 The position of a motorcycle driver is above the pivot point of the front wheel as the motorcycle impacts an object head-on.

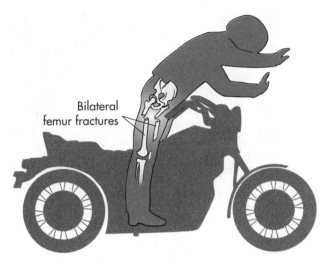

Bilateral femur fractures

Figure 1-43 The body travels forward and over the motorcycle, impacting the thighs and femurs into the handlebars. The driver can also be ejected.

MOTORCYCLE COLLISIONS ————

Motorcycle collisions account for a significant number of the motor vehicle deaths that occur in the United States each year. The laws of physics are the same as in other kinds of collisions, but the mechanism of injury varies slightly from automobile and truck collisions. This variance occurs in each of the following types of impacts: head-on, angular, or ejection.

A head-on collision into a solid object stops the forward motion of the cycle (Figure 1-42) because the motorcycle's center of gravity is above and behind the front axle, which is the pivot point in such a collision. The motorcycle will tip forward and the rider will crash into the handlebars. The rider may receive injuries to the head, chest, abdomen, or pelvis depending on what part of the anatomy strikes the handlebars. If the rider's feet remain on the pegs of the motorcycle and the thighs hit the handlebars, the forward motion will be absorbed by the midshaft femur, commonly resulting in bilateral femur fractures (Figure 1-43).

In an angular-impact collision, the bike hits an object at an angle. The cycle will then collapse on the rider or cause the rider to be crushed between the cycle and the object struck. Injuries to the upper or lower extremities may occur, resulting in fractures and/or extensive soft tissue injury (Figure 1-44). Injuries may also occur to organs of the abdominal cavity due to energy exchange.

In an ejection-impact collision, the rider is thrown from the bike like a missile. The rider will continue in flight through the air until his or her head, arms, chest, abdomen, or leg strikes another object, such as a motor vehicle, a telephone pole, or the road. Injury will occur at the point of impact and will radiate to the rest of the body as the energy is absorbed. As with the occupant ejected from an automobile, the potential for serious injury is very high for this essentially unprotected rider.

In the United States, automatic diagonal straps are still being worn without the manual lap strap, resulting in an increasing frequency of neck injuries. One suit against an auto manufacturer was settled for $1.6 million when the automatic diagonal strap was worn alone.

As mandatory seat belt usage laws are passed in the United States, injuries caused by improperly worn restraints have become more frequent, and the EMT must evaluate for these injuries. However, because a seat belt is being used (even if improperly), the overall severity of the injuries will be lessened, and the number of fatal collisions will be significantly reduced.

Originally, air bags were designed to cushion only the forward motion of the occupant. They absorb energy slowly by increasing the body's stopping distance. They are extremely effective in the first collision of head-on impacts, the 65% to 70% of collisions that occur between the headlights. Because they deflate immediately after the impact, they are not effective in multiple-impact collisions, nor are they effective in lateral or rear-impact collisions. Once the air bag has deployed and deflated (>0.5 seconds), if the car veers into the path of an oncoming car or off the road into a tree, there is no air bag protection left. Because air bags are of little or no use in lateral and rollover collisions, several manufacturers have now developed driver side door air bags. Air bags should always be used in combination with seat belts for maximum protection.

Recently, air bags have been shown to be dangerous to children and small adults especially when children are placed in incorrect positions in the front seat.

When air bags deploy, they can produce minor but noticeable injuries that must be managed by the EMT. These include abrasions of the arms, chest, and face (Figure 1-40), foreign bodies to the face and eyes, and injuries caused by the occupant's eyeglasses (Figure 1-41).

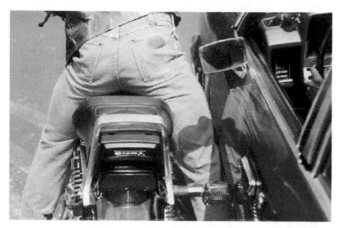

Figure 1-44 If the motorcycle does not hit an object head-on, it collapses like a scissors, trapping the rider's lower extremity between the object impacted and the motorcycle.

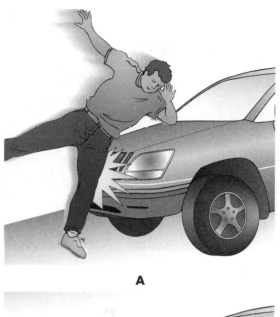

A

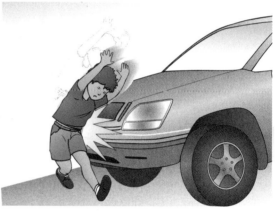

B

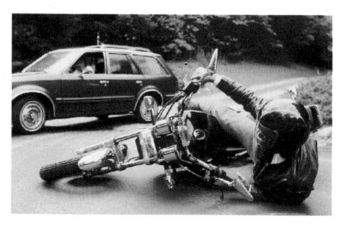

Figure 1-45 To prevent being trapped between two pieces of steel (motorcycle and automobile), the rider will frequently lay the motorcycle down to dissipate the injury. This often causes abrasions (road burns) as the rider's speed is slowed on the asphalt.

Figure 1-46 A and B, The initial impact between a vehicle and a pedestrian is the bumper of the vehicle against the pedestrian's lower extremities. (From American College of Emergency Physicians. *Paramedic Field Care: A Complaint Based Approach.* St. Louis: Mosby, 1997.)

"Laying the bike down" is a protective maneuver used by professional racers and some street bikers to separate themselves from the bike in an impending collision. In this maneuver, the rider turns the bike sideways and drags his or her inside leg on the pavement or grass. This action slows the rider more than the bike so that the bike will move out from under the rider. The rider will then slide along on the pavement but will not be trapped between the bike and the object it hits. These riders usually end up with abrasions (road rash) and minor fractures but avoid the severe injuries associated with the other kinds of impacts (Figure 1-45).

Motorcyclists' protection includes boots, leather clothing, and helmets—when they are worn. Of the three, the helmet affords the best protection. It is built like the skull: strong and supportive externally and energy-absorbent internally. The helmet's skull-like structure absorbs much of the impact, thereby decreasing injury to the face, skull,

and brain. The helmet provides only minimal protection for the neck but does not cause neck injuries. Failure to use helmets has been shown to increase head injuries by more than 300%. Most states that have passed mandatory helmet legislation have found an associated reduction in motorcycle accidents. Louisiana had a 60% reduction in head injuries in the first 6 years after passage. Helmet usage is very important for injury prevention.

PEDESTRIAN INJURY

Two patterns commonly seen in pedestrian versus motor vehicle collisions demonstrate different injury patterns. The difference is associated with the age group of the victim: adult or child. When an adult sees that he is about to be struck by an oncoming vehicle, he tries to protect

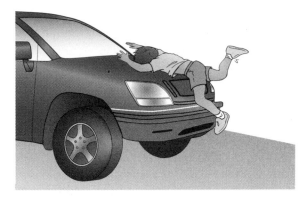

Figure 1-47 The torso then rolls on top of the vehicle impacting the hood, windscreen, or roof of the car.

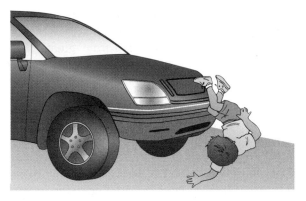

Figure 1-48 Finally, the torso falls off the car onto the asphalt producing compression injuries to the head, cervical spine, and the torso. A child, being closer to the ground, is impacted higher on the body by the bumper or hood of the car.

himself by turning away. The injuries are frequently lateral or even posterior. Children, on the other hand, will face the oncoming vehicle. This most often results in anterior injuries. Due to the varying heights of a child and an adult relative to the bumper and hood of a car, the striking patterns will also be different.

There are three separate phases of a pedestrian versus motor vehicle crash. Each phase has its own injury pattern:
1. The initial impact is to the legs and sometimes to the hips (Figure 1-46).
2. The torso rolls onto the hood of the auto (Figure 1-47).
3. The victim falls off the auto and onto the asphalt, usually head first, with possible cervical spine trauma (Figure 1-48).

Adults are usually struck first by the car's bumper in the lower legs, fracturing the tibia and fibula and driving the legs out from under the pelvis and torso. As the victim folds forward, the pelvis and upper femur are struck by the front of the vehicle's hood. As the abdomen and thorax fall forward, they strike the top of the hood. This substantial second strike can result in fractures of the upper femur, pelvis, ribs, and spine and produce serious intra-abdominal or intrathoracic damage. Injury to the head and face at this point will depend upon the victim's ability to protect them with his or her arms. If the victim's head strikes the hood, or if the victim continues to move up the hood so that his or her head strikes the windshield, injury to the face, head, and spine can occur.

The third impact occurs as the victim falls off the auto and strikes the pavement. The victim can generally receive a significant blow on one side of the body to the hip, shoulder, and head. Head injury commonly occurs when striking either the car or the pavement and must always be considered. Similarly, because all three impacts produce sudden, violent movement of the torso, neck, and head, an unstable spine must always be assumed to be present. An evaluation of the mechanism of injury should also include a determination if the victim, after

hitting the roadway, was struck again by a second vehicle traveling next to or behind the first.

Children, because they are shorter, are initially struck higher on the body than adults. The first impact generally occurs when the bumper strikes the child's legs (above the knees) or pelvis, damaging the femur or pelvic girdle. The second impact occurs almost instantly afterward: the front of the vehicle's hood continues forward and strikes the child's thorax. The head and face strike the front or top of the vehicle's hood. Because of the child's smaller size and weight, the child may not be thrown clear of the vehicle, as usually happens with an adult. Instead, the child can be dragged by the car while partially under the car's front end. If the child falls to the side, the lower limbs may also be run over by a front wheel. If the child falls backward, ending up completely under the car, almost any injury can occur—being dragged, struck by projections, or run over by a wheel.

As would an adult, any child struck by a car usually receives some head injury and, because of the sudden, violent forces acting on the head, neck, and torso, the child must be assumed to have an unstable spine. Additionally, the force of the impact, which is usually midthoracic, should raise suspicion of significant intrathoracic injury even in children who initially appear asymptomatic. Any child who is struck by a car should be considered to have suffered multisystem trauma, requiring rapid transport to the closest appropriate hospital (trauma center).

Knowing the specific sequence of multiple impacts in pedestrian versus vehicle collisions and understanding the multiple underlying injuries they can produce are the keys to making the initial assessment and to determining the appropriate management of the patient.

FALLS

Victims of falls may also suffer injury from multiple impacts. To properly assess a fall victim, the EMT should estimate the height of the fall, evaluate the surface on which the victim landed, and determine which part of the body struck first. Victims who fall from greater heights have a higher incidence of injury because their velocity increases as they fall. In general, falls from greater than three times the height of the victim are severe. The kind of surface on which the victim lands, and particularly its degree of compressibility (ability to be deformed by the transfer of energy), also has an effect on stopping distance.

Determining which part of the body hit first is important because it will help the EMT to predict the injury pattern. The pattern that often occurs when victims fall or jump from a height and land on their feet is called the "Don Juan" syndrome. Only in the movies can the character Don Juan jump from a balcony, land on his feet, and walk painlessly away. In real life, bilateral calcaneus (heel bone) fractures, fractures of the ankles, or distal tabula/fibula fractures are often associated with this syndrome. After the feet land and stop moving, the legs are the next body part to absorb energy. Knee fractures, long bone fractures, and hip fractures can result. The body is forced into flexion by the weight of the still-moving head and torso and can cause compression fractures of the spinal column in the thoracic and lumbar areas. Hyper-

flexion occurs at each bend of the S-shaped spine, producing flexion injuries. These victims are often described as breaking the "S" (Figure 1-49).

If the victim falls forward onto his or her outstretched hands, the result can be bilateral Colles' fractures of the wrists. If the victim did not land on his or her feet, the part of the body that struck first should be assessed, the pathway of energy displacement evaluated, and the injury pattern determined.

If the falling victim lands on his or her head with the body almost in line, such as commonly occurs in shallow water diving injuries, the entire weight and force of the moving torso, pelvis, and legs are brought to bear (compression) on the head and cervical spine. A fracture of the C-spine can result, just as with the up-and-over pathway of the frontal impact collision.

SPORTS INJURIES

Many sports or recreational activities such as skiing, diving, baseball, and football are capable of causing severe injury. These injuries may be caused by sudden deceleration forces or by excessive compression, twisting, hyperextension, or hyperflexion. In recent years, a variety of sports activities have become available to a wide spectrum of occasional, recreational participants who often lack the necessary training and conditioning or the proper protective equipment. Recreational sports and activities today include participants of all ages. Sports, such as downhill skiing, waterskiing, bicycling, and skateboarding, involve potentially high-velocity activities. Others, such as trail biking, all-terrain vehicle (ATV) riding, and snowmobiling, may produce velocity, deceleration, collisions, and impacts similar to motorcycle or motor vehicle accidents.

The potential injuries of a victim who is in a high-speed collision and is then ejected from a skateboard, snowmobile, or bicycle are similar to those sustained when a person is ejected from an automobile at the same speed because the amount of energy is the same. The specific mechanisms of car and motorcycle accidents have been described earlier in this chapter.

The potential mechanisms commonly associated with each sport are too numerous to list in detail. The general principles, however, are the same. In assessing the mechanism of injury, the EMT needs to consider the following:
- What forces acted on the victim, and how?
- What are the apparent injuries?
- To what object or part of the body was the energy transmitted?
- What other injuries are likely to have been produced by this energy transfer?
- What was compressed (by either cavitation or the "second collision" of internal organs)?
- How sudden was the deceleration or acceleration?

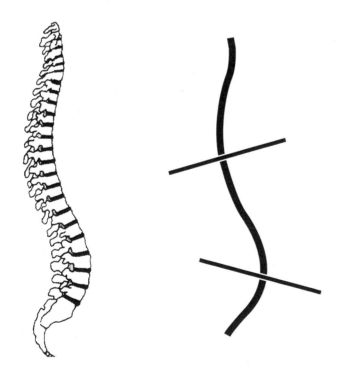

Figure 1-49 As the lower part of the spine stops its forward motion, the continued motion of the upper torso and head compress the spine. This motion tends to produce compression injuries on the side of the concavity and extraction injuries on the side of the convexity.

- What injury-producing movements occurred (such as hyperflexion, hyperextension, compression, or excessive lateral bending)?

When the mechanism of injury involves a high-speed collision between two participants, such as in a collision between two skiers, it is often difficult to reconstruct the exact sequence of events from witnesses. In such crashes, the injuries sustained by one skier are often guidelines for examining the other. In general, the EMT needs to know what part struck what, and what injury resulted from the energy transfer. For example, if one victim sustains an impact fracture of the hip, a part of the other skier's body must have struck with substantial force and therefore must have suffered a similar high impact. If the second skier's head struck the first skier's hip, the EMT should suspect potentially serious head injury and an unstable spine for the second skier.

Broken or damaged equipment may also be an important indicator of injury and must be included in the evaluation of the mechanism of injury. A broken sports helmet is evidence of the force with which it struck. Because today's skis are made of highly durable compositions and metals, a broken ski indicates that extreme localized force came to bear even when the mechanism of injury may appear unimpressive. The severely dented front of a snowmobile indicates the force with which a tree was struck. The presence of a broken stick after an ice hockey skirmish raises the question of whose body broke it, how, and specifically what part of the victim's body was struck by it or fell on it.

The injuries caused by these forces must be taken seriously, and the victim must be evaluated thoroughly before he or she is moved from the scene. The patient should be evaluated:

- for life-threatening injury
- for mechanism of injury (what happened and exactly how?)
- to determine whether protective gear was worn (it may have been removed prior to the EMT's arrival)
- to determine how the forces that produced injury in one victim affected any other person

- by assessing damage to equipment (what are the implications of this damage relative to the body?)
- for possible associated injuries

High-speed falls, collisions, and falls from heights without serious injury are common in many sports of violent contact. The ability of athletes to sustain incredible collisions and falls with only minor injury—which is due largely to impact-absorbing equipment—may cloud the EMT's assessment. The EMT may overlook the potential for injury in sports injury victims. By applying the principles of kinematics and carefully considering the exact sequence and mechanism of injury, the EMT can better recognize those sports collisions in which greater forces than usual came to bear. Kinematics is an essential tool for identifying possible underlying injuries and for determining which patients require further evaluation and treatment at the hospital.

BLAST INJURIES

The incidence of blast injuries increases during warfare, but these injuries are also becoming more common in the civilian world as terrorist activities and hazardous material incidents increase. Blasts may injure 70% of the people in the vicinity, whereas an automatic weapon used against the same size group may injure only 30%. Mines, shipyards, chemical plants, refineries, fireworks firms, factories, and grain elevators are some of the areas in which explosions are a particular hazard. However, because many volatile materials are transported by truck or rail, and domestic and bottled gas are common household items, an explosion can occur almost anywhere.

An explosion can be divided into three phases: primary, secondary, and tertiary (Figure 1-50). Different types of injuries occur during these three phases.

Primary injuries are caused by the pressure wave of the blast. They usually occur in the gas-containing organs, such as the lungs and the gastrointestinal tract. Primary injuries include pulmonary bleeding, pneumothorax, air emboli, or perforation of the gastrointestinal organs.

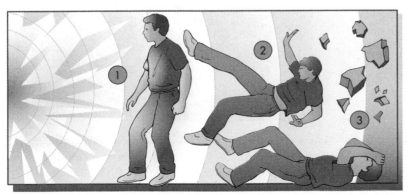

Figure 1-50 In a blast there are three phases of injury. Heat and light first reach the victim. This is followed by a pressure wave that compresses body parts and knocks the victim to the ground. Lastly, falling debris can become missiles that produce injury. (From American College of Emergency Physicians. *Paramedic Field Care: A Complaint Based Approach.* St. Louis: Mosby, 1997.)

Pressure waves rupture and tear the small vessels and membranes of the gas-containing organs (cavitation) and may also injure the central nervous system. These waves may cause severe damage or death without any external signs of injury. Burns from the heat wave are also a common primary injury. Burns occur on unprotected body areas that are facing the source of the explosion.

Secondary injuries occur when the victim is struck by flying glass, falling mortar, or other debris from the blast. Secondary injuries include lacerations, fractures, and burns.

Tertiary injuries occur when the victim becomes a missile and is thrown against an object. Injury will occur at the point of impact, and the force of the blast will be transferred to other organs of the body as the energy from the impact is absorbed. Tertiary injuries are usually apparent, but the EMT must look for associated injuries according to the type of impact that the victim suffered. The injuries that occur in the tertiary phase are similar to those sustained in ejections from automobiles and falls from significant heights.

Secondary and tertiary injuries are the most obvious and are usually the most aggressively treated. Primary injuries are the most severe, but they are often overlooked and sometimes never suspected. Adequate assessment of the various kinds of injuries is vital if the EMT is to manage the patient properly. Blast injuries often cause severe complications that may result in death if they are overlooked or ignored.

PENETRATING TRAUMA

THE PHYSICS OF PENETRATING TRAUMA

The principles of physics discussed at the beginning of this chapter are equally important when dealing with penetrating injuries.

The kinetic energy that a striking object transfers to body tissue is represented by:

$$\text{Kinetic energy} = \frac{\text{mass}}{2} \times \text{velocity}^2.$$

Recall that energy cannot be created or destroyed, but it can be changed in form. This principle is important in understanding penetrating trauma. For example, while a lead bullet is in the brass cartridge casing, which is filled with explosive powder, the bullet has no force. But when the primer explodes, the powder burns, producing rapidly expanding gases that are transformed into force. The bullet then moves out of the gun and toward its target.

According to Newton's first law of motion, after this force has acted upon the missile, the bullet will remain at that speed and force until it is acted upon by some outside force. When the bullet hits something, such as a human body, it strikes the individual tissue cells. The energy

(speed and mass) of the bullet's motion is exchanged for the energy that crushes these cells and moves them away (cavitation) from the path of the bullet.

The larger the frontal area of the moving missile, the greater the number of particles that will be hit; therefore, the greater the energy exchange that occurs and the larger the cavity that is created.

The size of the front surface area of a projectile is influenced by several factors: its initial size, whether the size changes at the time of impact, whether the object tumbles and assumes a different angle inside the body than the angle assumed as it entered the body, and whether the object fragments. Therefore, energy exchange or potential energy exchange can be analyzed based on the following considerations.

Factors that Affect the Size of the Frontal Area

As just mentioned, the factors affecting the size of the frontal area include profile, tumble, and fragmentation.

Profile

The profile or frontal area of an ice pick is much smaller than that of a baseball bat, which in turn is much smaller than that of a truck. A pointed missile (such as a dum-dum type bullet), if crushed and deformed as a result of striking a body, will have a much larger frontal area

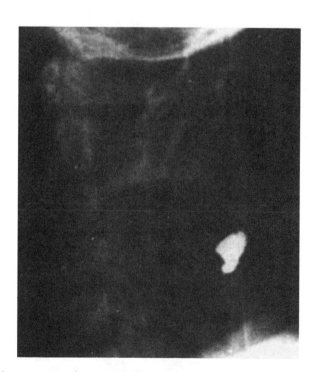

Figure 1-51 Changes in the profile or trauma projection increase the particles hit and therefore the amount of energy dispersal. (From McSwain, N.E., Jr. "Pulmonary Chest Trauma." In *Principles of Trauma Surgery*, edited by J.A. Moylan. New York: Gower, 1992.)

than before its shape was changed. A hollow-point bullet flattens and spreads on impact. This change enlarges the frontal area so that it hits more tissue particles and produces greater energy exchange. A larger cavity forms, and more injury results (Figure 1-51).

In general, as a bullet travels through the air after being discharged from a weapon, it will strike fewer air particles and maintain most of its speed if its frontal area is kept small and streamlined by its conical shape. If that missile strikes the skin and becomes deformed, covering a larger area, there will be a much greater energy exchange than if its front surface area does not expand (Box 1-3).

Tumble

A wedge-shaped bullet's center of gravity is located nearer to the base than to the nose of the bullet. When the nose of the bullet strikes something, it slows rapidly. Momentum continues to carry the base of the bullet forward; in other words, the center of gravity seeks to become the leading point of the bullet. This movement causes an end-over-end motion, or tumble. As the bullet tumbles, the normally horizontal sides of the bullet will become its leading edges, thus striking far more particles than when the nose was the leading edge (Figure 1-52). More energy exchange is produced and, therefore, greater tissue damage.

Box 1-3   Expanding Bullets

A munitions factory in Dum Dum, India, manufactured a bullet that expanded when it hit the skin. Ballistic experts recognized this design as one that would cause more damage than is necessary in war; therefore, these bullets were prohibited in military conflicts. The Geneva Convention (1880) and the Petersburg Treaty (1899) both affirmed this principle, denouncing these "dum-dum" projectiles and other expanding missiles, such as silver tips, hollow points, scored lead cartridges or jackets, and partially jacketed bullets.

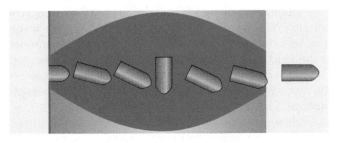

Figure 1-52 The tumble motion of a missile maximizes its damage at 90°.

Fragmentation

Bullets such as those with soft noses, vertical cuts in the nose, and safety slugs that contain many small fragments increase body damage by breaking apart on impact. The mass of fragments produced comprises a larger frontal area than the single solid bullet, and energy is dispersed rapidly into the tissue. If the missile shatters, it will spread out over a wider area, with two results: (1) more tissue particles will be struck by the larger frontal projection, and (2) the injuries will be distributed over a larger portion of the body because more organs will be struck (Figures 1-53, 1-54, and 1-55). The multiple pieces of shot from a shotgun blast produce similar results. Shotgun wounds are an excellent example of the fragmentation injury pattern.

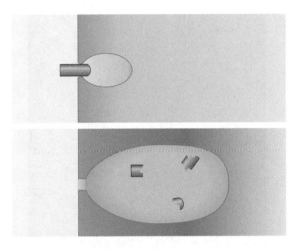

Figure 1-53 A missile that is made of soft lead or another component that breaks up will cause damage over a wider area as well as creating maximum absorption of the energy as many more tissue particles are impacted.

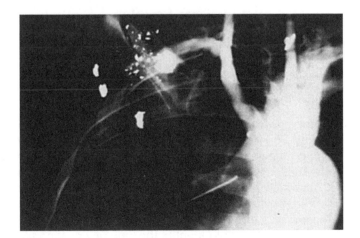

Figure 1-54 When the missile breaks up into smaller particles, this fragmentation increases its frontal area and increases the energy distribution. (From McSwain, N.E., Jr. "Pulmonary Chest Trauma." In *Principles of Trauma Surgery,* edited by J.A. Moylan. New York: Gower, 1992.)

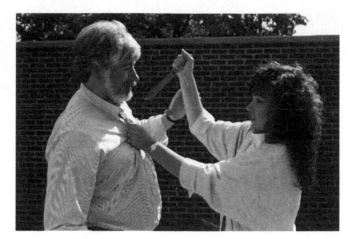

Figure 1-56 Women tend to stab down, with the knife held on the little-finger side of the hand.

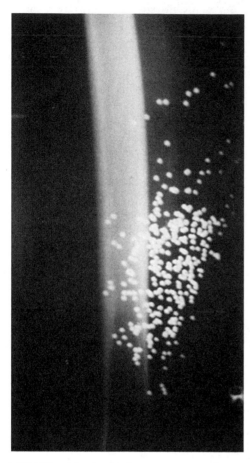

Figure 1-55 The ultimate in fragmentation damage is caused by a shotgun.

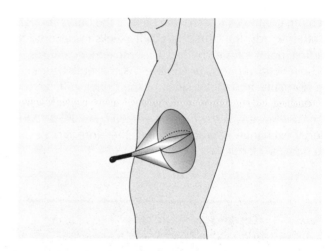

Figure 1-57 The damage produced by a knife depends on the movement of the blade inside the victim.

Damage and Energy Levels

Damage caused in a penetrating injury can be estimated by classifying penetrating objects into three categories according to their energy capacity.

Low-energy Weapons

Low-energy weapons include hand-driven weapons such as a knife or ice pick. These missiles produce damage only with their sharp points or cutting edges. Since these are low-velocity injuries, they are usually associated with less secondary trauma (i.e., less cavitation will occur). Injury in these victims can be predicted by tracing the path of the weapon into the body. If the weapon has been removed, the EMT should identify the type of weapon used and the gender of the attacker whenever possible. Men tend to stab with the blade on the thumb side of the hand and with an upward thrust, whereas women tend to stab downward and hold the blade on the little-finger side (Figure 1-56).

When evaluating a patient with a stab wound, it is important to look for more than one wound. Multiple stab wounds are possible and should not be ruled out until the patient is completely exposed and closely examined. This close inspection may take place at the scene or en route to or at the hospital, depending on the circumstances surrounding the incident and the condition of the patient.

The attacker may stab his victim and then move the knife around inside the body. A simple entrance wound may therefore give the EMT a false sense of security. The entrance wound may be small, but the damage inside may be extensive. Internal injuries cannot be determined in the field, but the possibility must always be suspected, even in seemingly minor injuries. The potential scope of the movement of the inserted blade is an area of possible damage (Figure 1-57).

Evaluation of the patient for associated injury is important. For example, the diaphragm can reach as high as the nipple line on deep expiration. A stab wound to the lower

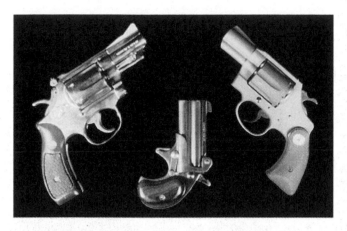

Figure 1-58 Medium-energy weapons are usually guns that have short barrels and contain cartridges with lesser power. High-energy weapons are assault rifles and hunting rifles.

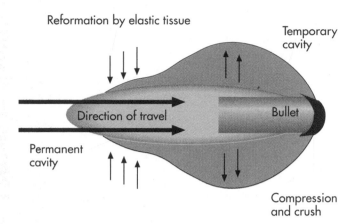

Figure 1-59 A bullet crushes tissues directly in its path. A cavity is created in the wake of the bullet. The crushed part is permanent. The temporary expansion can also produce injury.

chest can injure intrathoracic and intra-abdominal structures as well.

Medium- and High-energy Weapons

Firearms fall into two groups: medium energy and high energy. Medium-energy weapons include handguns and some rifles. As the amount of gunpowder in the cartridge increases, the speed of the bullet, and therefore its kinetic energy, increases (Figure 1-58).

Medium- and high-energy weapons, in general, damage not only the tissue directly in the path of the missile but also the tissue on each side of the missile's path. The variables of tumble, fragmentation, and profile will influence the extent and direction of the injury. The pressure on tissue particles, which are moved out of the direct path of the missile, compresses and stretches the surrounding tissue. A temporary cavity is always associated with weapons in the medium-energy classification. This cavity is usually three to six times the size of the missile's front surface area (Figure 1-59).

High-energy weapons include assault weapons, hunting rifles, and other weapons that discharge high-velocity missiles. These missiles not only create a permanent track but produce a much larger temporary cavity than lower-velocity missiles. This temporary cavity expands well beyond the limits of the actual bullet track and damages and injures a wider area than is apparent during the initial assessment. Tissue damage is far more extensive with a high-energy penetrating object than with one of medium energy. The vacuum created by this cavity pulls clothing, bacteria, and other debris from the surrounding area into the wound.

Another consideration in predicting the damage from a gunshot wound is the range or distance from which the gun (either medium- or high-energy) is fired. Air resistance slows the bullet; therefore, increasing the distance will decrease the velocity at the time of impact and

will result in less injury. Most shootings are carried out at close range with handguns, so the probability of serious injury is high.

ENTRANCE AND EXIT WOUNDS

When evaluating the victim of a penetrating trauma, the EMT should evaluate entrance and exit wounds. The EMT should be aware that tissue damage will occur at the site of entry into the body, in the path of the weapon's entrance, and upon exit from the body. Knowledge of the victim's position, the attacker's position, and the weapon used is essential in determining the path of injury.

Evaluating wound sites can provide the EMT with valuable information to direct the management of the patient and to relay to the receiving hospital. Do two holes in the victim's abdomen indicate that a single missile entered and exited or that two missiles are both still inside the patient? Did the missile cross the midline (usually causing more severe injury) or remain on the same side? In what direction did the missile travel? What organs are likely to have been in its path?

Entrance and exit wounds usually produce identifiable injury patterns to soft tissue. An entrance wound from a gunshot lies against the underlying tissue, but an exit wound has no support (Figure 1-60). The former is a round or oval wound and the latter is a stellate (starburst) wound (Figure 1-61). Because the missile is spinning as it enters the skin, it leaves a small area of abrasion (1 to 2 mm in size) that is black or pink. No abrasion is present on the exit side (Figures 1-60 and 1-62). If the muzzle was placed directly against the skin at the time of discharge, the expanding gases will enter the tissue and produce crepitus on examination. Within 5 to 7 centimeters (cm) the burning gases will burn the skin (Figure 1-63); at 5 to 15 cm, the smoke will adhere to the skin; and inside

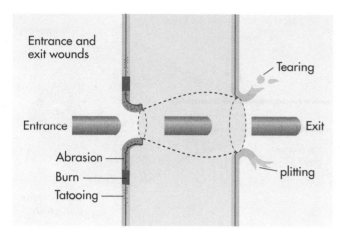

Figure 1-60 A spinning missile produces a 1- to 2-mm abraded edge along the wound if it enters straight. If it enters at an angle, the abraded side is on the bottom of the missile, where there is more contact with the skin, and covers a much wider area.

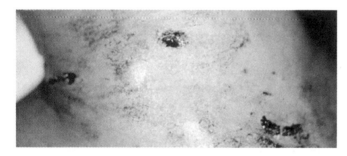

Figure 1-61 The entrance wound is round or oval in shape, and the exit wound is stellate or linear.

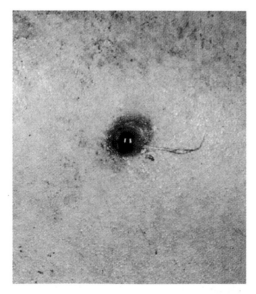

Figure 1-62 The abraded edge indicates that the bullet traveled from top right to bottom left.

25 cm the burning cordite particles will tattoo the skin with small (1 to 2 mm) burned areas.

PENETRATING TRAUMA INJURIES

In the following section, the injuries sustained by various parts of the body during penetrating trauma are discussed.

Head

After the missile penetrates the skull, its energy must be distributed within a closed space. Particles accelerating away from the missile are forced against the unyielding skull, which cannot expand as skin can. Thus the brain tissue is compressed against the inside of the skull, producing more injury than if it could expand freely. If the forces are strong enough, the skull may explode from the inside out.

A bullet may follow the curvature of the interior of the skull if it enters at an angle and has insufficient force to exit the skull. This path can produce significant damage. It is characteristic of medium-velocity missiles, such as the .22 caliber or .25 caliber pistol, which has for this reason been called the "assassin's weapon."

Thorax

Three major groups of structures inside the thoracic cavity must be considered in evaluating a penetrating injury to the chest: the pulmonary, vascular, and gastrointestinal tracts.

Pulmonary

Because lung tissue is less dense than blood, solid organs, or bone, a penetrating object does less damage to it than

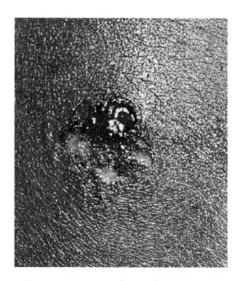

Figure 1-63 Gases coming from the end of a muzzle held in close proximity to the skin produce partial- and full-thickness burns on the skin.

to other thoracic tissue. Because much of the area traversed by the missile is air, there are fewer particles to be hit and less energy to be transferred, so less damage is produced. However, the damage to the lung can be clinically significant (Figure 1-64).

Vascular

Smaller vessels that are not attached to the chest wall may be pushed aside without significant damage. However, if larger vessels, such as the aorta and vena cava, are hit, they cannot move aside easily and are more susceptible to damage.

The myocardium stretches as the bullet passes through and then contracts, leaving a smaller defect. The thickness of the muscle may control a low-energy penetration such as a knife or .22 caliber bullet, preventing immediate exsanguination and allowing time to get the victim to a hospital.

Gastrointestinal Tract

The esophagus, the part of the gastrointestinal tract that traverses the thoracic cavity, can be penetrated and can leak its contents into the thoracic cavity. The signs and symptoms of such an injury may be delayed for several hours or several days.

Abdomen

The abdomen contains structures of three types: air-filled, solid, and bony. Penetration by a low-energy missile may not cause significant damage; only 30% of knife wounds penetrating the abdominal cavity require surgical exploration to repair damage. A medium-energy injury (handgun wound) is more damaging—85% to 95% require surgical repair. However, even with injuries caused by medium-energy missiles, the damage to solid and vascular structures may not produce immediate exsanguination. Often the hemorrhage can be temporarily controlled and the patient resuscitated by EMTs using the pneumatic

antishock garment and intravenous fluids, and the patient can be transported to the hospital in time for effective surgical intervention.

Extremities

Penetrating injuries to the extremities can include damage to bones, muscles, or vessels. When bones are hit, bony fragments become secondary missiles, lacerating surrounding tissue (Figure 1-65). Muscles often expand away from the path of the missile. This stretching causes hemorrhage (Figure 1-66). Vessels can be penetrated by the missile, or a near-miss can damage the lining of a blood vessel, causing clotting and obstruction of the vessel within minutes or hours.

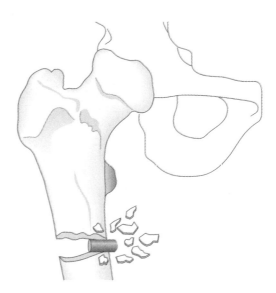

Figure 1-65 Bone fragments become secondary missiles themselves, producing damage by the same mechanism as the original penetrating object. (From McSwain, N.E., Jr. "Pulmonary Chest Trauma." In *Principles of Trauma Surgery*, edited by J.A. Moylan. New York: Gower, 1992.)

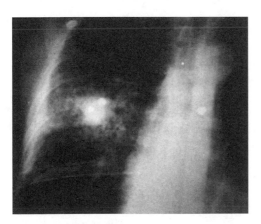

Figure 1-64 Lung damage produced by the cavity at a distance from the point of impact is easily appreciated from this radiograph.

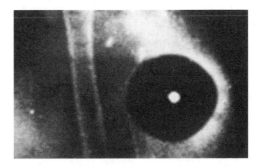

Figure 1-66 The more energy that the penetrating object has, the greater the energy exchange and therefore the greater the size of the temporary cavity. (From McSwain, N.E., Jr. "Pulmonary Chest Trauma." In *Principles of Trauma Surgery*, edited by J.A. Moylan. New York: Gower, 1992.)

• Summary •

Kinematics must be considered at every accident scene. Proper evaluation of the kinematics and mechanism of injury will help the EMT predict the injuries a patient has sustained. This evaluation will lead to proper assessment and management of the patient. Important questions for the EMT to ask in assessing the trauma scene are listed in Box 1-4.

Box 1-4:   Important Questions to Ask Yourself at the Trauma Scene

Asking the following questions will guide your assessment of the victim and ultimately improve the quality of patient care.

Impacts

What type of impact occurred—frontal, lateral, rear, rotational, rollover, angular, or ejection?
At what speed or velocity did the crash occur?
What was the stopping distance?
Were the victims using protective devices?
Where are the most severely injured victims likely to be?
What forces were involved (blunt vs. penetrating; compression vs. shear)?
What path did the energy follow; what organs may have been injured on that path?
Is the victim a child or an adult?

Falls

How long was the fall?
Onto what type of surface did the patient fall? Was it hard or soft? Was the surface able to absorb any residual energy?
What part of the body struck first?

Blasts

How close to the explosion was the patient?
What primary blast injuries are likely?
What secondary blast injuries are likely?
What tertiary blast injuries are likely?

Penetrating Trauma

Where is the assailant?
Who was the assailant? (Male or female? How tall?)
What weapon was used?
If a gun was used, what type?
What type of bullet struck the victim?
What was the range?
What was the angle?

Scenario Solution

Your first actions, upon arrival at the scene, are to ensure that the hazardous materials team has been dispatched with fire/rescue and to request that two additional units be dispatched plus a field supervisor. You also notify dispatch that you have a low-level mass casualty incident (MCI) and request they contact the trauma center and have the helicopter launched. Finally, you request that the power company be dispatched to the scene.

As you approach the plane from the front, to avoid the contaminated ground behind the aircraft, you observe that no wires have fallen to the ground; it appears that all wires have remained intact on the tower. As you perform your global assessment of the scene, the fixed base operations manager from the airport approaches and offers her assistance in disconnecting the plane's power supplies. This reduces the immediate threat of fire from a spark or active circuit on the plane and allows you to continue with your initial assessments.

All four passengers are in their seats with both lap and diagonal belts on and intact. The engine, while being displaced rearward approximately 3 feet, does not appear to have intruded into the passenger compartment. The windscreen is intact with the exception of the pilot's side, left front. It appears that something has penetrated through the left side of the windscreen. Your only access is through the single door which is located on the right front side of the fuselage.

Passenger #1, the pilot's wife in the right front seat, has no pulse or respirations and appears to have a broken neck. You notice that the headrest on her seat is broken to the rear. Your understanding of kinematics supports your linking the sudden deceleration of the aircraft and broken headrest with significant transfer of energy to the patient. You and your partner rapidly remove her from the passenger compartment to the front of the plane and away from your access area.

While you are extricating passenger #1, the fire department and hazardous materials teams arrive and take control of the fuel spill and are available to assist with extrication. Additionally, the field supervisor has arrived and taken control of the scene, establishing a vehicle staging area and triage area. He has also notified the medical investigator's office due to the fatality.

You are able to remove the passenger's seat and get better access to the pilot. He is responsive to voice, nonpurposeful, and has the following injuries as identified during your primary survey; an open pneumothorax on his left lateral chest wall, point tenderness and guarding of the upper left quadrant, and bilateral tibia/fibula fractures with moderate hemorrhage. Your review of the interior damage, exterior forces applied to the aircraft body, and an understanding of energy transfer lead you to rapidly extricate this patient on a long backboard. You anticipate significant injuries to the thorax and abdomen based on deceleration and shear forces. He is moved to the staging area as the helicopter is landing.

Passenger #3 is in the right rear seat and appears to be alert and oriented, complaining only of a headache. He is aware of all events and his primary survey is unremarkable. He wants to exit the plane on his own, but due to the mechanism of the crash you correctly elect to remove him on a long backboard using standard precautions for spine injury. Even though he is presenting as uninjured, you are concerned that he could have a head injury of significance. His safety belts have prevented him from being thrown about the cabin, but he was subjected to significant energy forces to his neck from the plane bouncing on the ground and from deceleration forces when it struck the tower. Masked or hidden injuries are a major concern to this patient.

Passenger #4 is found in her seat awake but clearly confused. While she responds to voice, it is nonpurposeful. Her primary is unremarkable except for a laceration and hematoma to the right parietal area of her head. You observe that the left rear window casing is deformed and appears to be the probable contact point for her head. Her left pupil is dilated, and she is apparently becoming more confused and combative. Here again, your concern is that she struck her head on the window casing, and the crash exposed her cervical spine to major deceleration and lateral forces. Her head injury could be caused by the same mechanism or could have been sustained during one of the other energy transfers (deceleration). You rapidly extricate her on a long backboard and move her to the triage area. She is quickly reassessed and immediately loaded into a ground vehicle for transport to the trauma center.

Due to your understanding of the kinematics of trauma, you made rapid assessments and correct decisions as to how to handle the patients in this MCI. You were aware of energy transfer occurring at the time of the plane's impact on the ground (down-and-under) as well as at the time of impact with the radio tower (deceleration, shear). Because of your understanding of the kinematics of trauma, your proper scene management, and your patient care decisions, all three of the plane's occupants who survived the initial crash survived their hospitalizations and necessary surgery for their life threatening injuries.

Review Questions

Answers provided on page 333.

1 One of the first concepts of energy and trauma injuries that an EMT must understand comes from Newton's first law of motion. This law states:
  A A body in motion will become a body at rest without any influence of outside forces.
  B A body in motion or at rest will remain that way until acted upon by some outside force.
  C Energy can be created as easily as it can be destroyed.
  D For every force of acceleration a patient experiences, they will experience an equal and opposite deceleration force.

2 Kinetic energy is defined as being a function of an object's weight and speed. The kinetic energy production rate is influenced to a greater degree by which factor?
  A the patient's body weight
  B the stopping distance after impact
  C the speed at the time of collision
  D the angle at which the impact occurs and energy is transferred

3 The mechanics of energy exchange between two objects is relatively simple. When one object strikes another, energy is transferred. In evaluating energy exchange in a patient, the EMT must remember the concept of cavitation. When an object strikes the patient it displaces particles (tissue). If this displacement of tissue is more forceful than the elasticity of the tissue, _____ will result.
  A a temporary cavity
  B a permanent cavity
  C deformation of the object

4 Motor vehicle collisions take on five (5) different impact types. The type known as "head-on" or "frontal impact" can result in two possible paths for the occupants of the vehicle. The down-and-under path will generally result in the unrestrained occupants of the front seat experiencing their first impact with the vehicle on which part of the body?
  A abdomen
  B chest
  C head
  D knees

5 Lateral or side impact type collisions can often produce more severe energy transfer patterns to an occupant of the vehicle. This is due in large part to the fact that the head is supported in an off-center position by the spine. This off-center positioning places the center of gravity forward and superior to the point of support. This places the neck at greatest risk for injuries from:
  A lateral extension and rotation
  B lateral flexion and rotation
  C hyperextension and rotation
  D hyperflexion and rotation

6 Life belts (lap and diagonal) and supplemental restraint systems (air bags) have clearly demonstrated that they reduce serious injury and death in automobile collisions. Tests have shown, however, that the use of one of these devices by itself can result in serious injury or even death. This single restraint device is the:
  A supplemental restraint system
  B lap belt
  C diagonal belt
  D lap belt without a diagonal belt

7 Injuries to patients from energy transfer can occur in many different ways. One of these is a fall. The EMT would consider as potentially serious to the patient, any fall from a height that is _____ the height of the patient.
A twice
B three times
C four times
D five times

8 Blast injuries (explosions) have three phases associated with them. In general, any one of the phases can produce serious or even fatal injuries to victims. The EMT who is knowledgeable in kinematics would be most concerned with injuries occurring in which of the phases?
A the first phase only
B the first and second phase
C the first and third phase
D the second and third phase

9 In assessing patients secondary to penetrating injuries, the EMT with a knowledge of kinematics will remember that the profile and energy of the penetrating object directly influence the degree of cavitation, either temporary or permanent, that will be formed. High-energy missiles will create both a temporary and permanent cavity. This degree of cavitation will result in:
A less damage to tissues due to absorption of the energy by the temporary cavity
B more damage in the permanent cavity, but less damage in the temporary cavity
C greater damage not only in the permanent cavity but also in the temporary cavity due to greater energy exchange
D lesser damage to tissues in the permanent cavity and more damage to tissues in the temporary cavity due to greater energy transfer

10 Evaluation of patients who have been shot is a critical step in determining both the potential severity of injury and treatment options. Evaluation of the wound site(s) includes determining several vital pieces of information. Of the questions listed in the chapter, the one that would be most indicative of a more serious injury to the thorax or abdomen would be:
A Do two holes in the victim's body indicate one entrance and one exit wound or two entrance wounds?
B What direction did the missile take in the body?
C What organs are likely to have been hit?
D Did the missile cross the midline?

CHAPTER OBJECTIVES

CHAPTER 2

Patient Assessment and Management

At the completion of this course the student will be able to:

- Explain the importance of the patient assessment process in the overall management of the trauma patient.

- Identify the discrete steps involved in the process of assessing and managing the trauma patient.

- Explain why evaluation of safety, scene, situation, and kinematics are vitally important when performing an assessment.

- Describe the 15-second global evaluation followed by the rest of the primary survey/initial assessment using the A B C D E method.

- Describe the rapid examination skills necessary to evaluate respiration, circulation, and level of consciousness/responsiveness.

- Identify life-threatening conditions that require immediate attention.

- Identify the steps in the secondary survey/focused history and physical examination.

- Understand the importance of the question "Why?"

Scenario

It is hot—one of those summer days, without a cloud in the sky, when the sun beats down like a high-powered heat lamp, warming everything to flashpoint. You and your partner are dispatched to a motorcycle/automobile crash at a major intersection, located about 10 minutes away. Fire units are also responding, and dispatch informs you that the helicopter is available if needed for rapid transport. No other units are on the scene, and no additional information is available at this time.

As you respond, you and your partner don gloves and agree that it will be your job to grab the trauma bag and go immediately to the patient upon arrival, while your partner will follow with a spine board, suction, and oxygen.

Your unit is the first to arrive on the scene and as you pull up, you see a motorcycle under a car in the middle of the intersection. A crowd is standing around a helmeted figure, who is lying on the ground, wearing what looks like a tank top, shorts, and sandals. You quickly grab the trauma bag and start toward the patient.

- What actions should you accomplish as you move toward the patient?
- Based on the information that you already know, what are some initial issues that will need to be addressed as soon as possible?
- Once you reach the patient, what will your actions be?

Assessment is the cornerstone of excellent patient care. For the trauma patient, as for other emergent patients, assessment is the foundation upon which all management and transportation decisions are based.

The first goal in assessment is to determine the patient's current condition—where the patient is along the continuum between life and death. An overall impression of the patient's status is developed, and baseline values for the patient's respiratory, circulatory, and neurologic status are established. Next, life-threatening conditions are rapidly found, and urgent intervention and resuscitation is initiated. Any conditions requiring attention before the patient can be moved are identified and addressed. Finally, a detailed assessment of non–life- or limb-threatening injuries is conducted, only if time allows, most often while transportation is underway. All of these steps are performed quickly and efficiently, with a goal of minimizing time spent on the scene. Critical patients cannot be allowed to remain in the field for care other than that needed to stabilize them for transport, unless they are trapped or other complications exist that prevent early transportation. By applying the principles learned in this course, the EMT will be able to minimize on-scene delay and rapidly move patients to the appropriate medical facility. Successful assessment and inter-

vention requires a strong knowledge base of trauma physiology and a well thought-out plan for management that is carried out quickly and effectively.

Throughout the trauma management literature, constant mention is made of the need to get the trauma patient to definitive surgical care within an absolute minimum amount of time following the onset of the injury. This obsession with scene time is based on the fact that the critical trauma patient is most likely bleeding. This blood loss will continue until the hemorrhage can be controlled. Except in the instance of the most basic external bleeding, this hemorrhage control can only be accomplished in the operating room (OR).

The primary concerns for assessment and management of the trauma patient are:

Oxygenation
  Airway
  Ventilation
Perfusion
  RBC deliver to the tissue cells
Hemorrhage control
  Temporary in the field
  Permanent in the operating room
    Rapid transportation
    Trauma team immediately available

Landmark research, performed by R. A. Cowley, M.D., in Maryland, established that the time between injury occurrence and definitive care is critical. During this period, when bleeding is uncontrolled and inadequate tissue oxygenation is occurring due to reduced circulation, damage is being done throughout the body. If bleeding is not controlled and tissue oxygenation restored within one hour of the injury onset, the patient's chances of survival plummet. This 60-minute period has come to be called the **golden hour.** In order to get the trauma patient to definitive care in the hospital emergency department, critical care unit, or operating room, the EMT must quickly identify the patient's serious condition, provide only essential, lifesaving care at the scene, and provide for rapid transportation to an appropriate medical facility. In many urban EMS systems, the average time from occurrence of an incident to the arrival of EMTs on the scene is 8 to 9 minutes. Another 8 to 9 minutes will be spent transporting the patient to the hospital. If time on the scene is kept to only 10 minutes, one-half of that golden hour will have passed by the time the patient arrives in the emergency department. Every additional minute spent on the scene is additional time that the patient is bleeding, and valuable time is taken away from the golden hour. To address this critical trauma management issue, it is absolutely essential that quick, efficient evaluation and management of the patient is the ultimate objective. Field time should not exceed 10 minutes. In fact, the shorter the better. The longer the patient is kept in the field, the more blood will be lost, and the likelihood of survival will decrease.

This chapter will cover the essentials of patient assessment and initial management. The basic principles that are described here are identical to those learned in the initial EMT-Basic or Paramedic training program, although different terminology may occasionally be used. For example, the phrase "primary survey" is used in the Advanced Trauma Life Support (ATLS) and PHTLS programs to describe the patient assessment activity known as "initial assessment" in the EMT-Basic course. What is called the "secondary survey" in this course is essentially the same activity that the EMT learned as the "focused history and physical exam of the trauma patient." For the most part, the activities performed in each phase are exactly the same, the various courses simply use different terminology. See Box 2-1 for a comparison of the assessment terminology used in the PHTLS program and the EMT national standard curricula.

SCENE ASSESSMENT

As all prehospital personnel learn in their initial training courses, patient assessment starts long before the patient is actually reached. Dispatch begins the process by providing the EMT with initial information about the incident and the patient, based on bystander reports or information provided by other units first on the scene. The EMT then begins the on-scene information-gathering process by evaluating the scene, immediately upon arrival, before actually reaching the patient's side.

The scene's appearance creates an impression that influences the EMT's entire assessment. Evaluating the scene correctly is important. There is a wealth of information to be gathered by simply watching, listening, and cataloging as much information from the environment as possible. The scene can often provide information about mechanisms of injury, the preincident situation, and the overall degree of safety.

Three components are included in an evaluation of the scene:

1. *Safety*—evaluating all possible dangers to ensure that none still exists for rescuers or the patient.
2. *Scene*—evaluating the number of vehicles involved, determining the forces involved, and ascertaining the degree and type of damage to each vehicle.
3. *Situation*—What really happened here? Why? Are there unanswered questions suggesting other medical possibilities (e.g., a car crash caused by a heart attack)? How many people are involved, and what are their ages?

Although it is important to reach the patient quickly, the first priority for everyone involved at a trauma incident must be safety—of both rescuers and patients. Injured rescuers will only compound the problem. The second

---

Box 2-1 Assessment Terminology

PHTLS	EMT National Standard Curricula
Scene assessment	Scene assessment
Primary survey	Initial assessment
Secondary survey	Focused history and physical exam
Regional surveys	Rapid trauma assessment
Monitoring and reassessment	Ongoing assessment

---

priority is to identify the patient who is in greatest need of emergency medical care or to recognize the existence of a multiple casualty incident. In this case the priority shifts to saving the maximum number of patients rather than focusing all resources on a single patient (see "Triage," p. 52). The third priority is to begin assessment and management of the patient(s) who have been identified as being most needy. This could be the most critically injured of the individual patients or the patient with the greatest chance for survival given the supplies and equipment at hand.

The first two priorities are accomplished with a survey of the scene and an understanding of the history of the incident, including the mechanism of injury (kinematics). The scene survey is discussed only briefly in this chapter, but this does not indicate that it is of minimal importance. Rather, it is a recognition that every prehospital provider should already clearly understand the importance of an effective scene survey immediately upon arrival. Therefore, this chapter can focus on the third priority, assessment and management of the individual patient. Excellent review information concerning the scene survey can be found in any EMT-B, I, or P text.

To re-emphasize, the primary consideration when approaching any scene is the safety of the rescuers. The EMT should not become a victim. If the scene is unsafe, the EMT should stand clear until the scene has been secured by appropriate personnel. The EMT should not attempt a rescue unless trained to do so. An injured EMT reduces the number of providers available to care for the patients present and increases the number of patients for which care must be provided.

Scene safety is not just about rescuer safety; patient safety is also a consideration. Any patient in a hazardous situation must be moved to a safe area before assessment and treatment can begin. Evaluate the hazards that may endanger the patient: extreme temperatures, rain or snow, water, fire, location of the accident, and proximity to highways and cars. Severe weather can be as much of a hazard as the danger of fire, explosion, or electrical shock.

Once scene safety has been clearly established, evaluation of the patient can proceed in an orderly manner. Emphasis is placed first on conditions that may result in loss of life, second on those that may cause loss of limb, and third on all other conditions. Depending upon the severity of the injury and the number of injured patients, "all other conditions" may never be considered until after the patient has arrived at the hospital. This process is known as establishing priorities.

PRIMARY SURVEY (INITIAL ASSESSMENT)

In the critical multisystem trauma patient, the rapid identification and management of life-threatening conditions is the paramount priority. More than 90% of trauma patients have only **simple injuries** (those without systemic impact). For these patients, there is time to be thorough in both the primary (initial assessment) and the secondary survey (focus assessment). For the critically injured patient, the EMT may never conduct more than a primary survey. Instead, the emphasis is on rapid evaluation, starting resuscitation, and transportation to the hospital. This does not obviate the need for any prehospital management. It means, simply: do it faster, do it more efficiently, and do it en route to the hospital.

Quickly establishing priorities and conducting the initial evaluation of life-threatening injuries must be automatic. Therefore the components of the primary and secondary surveys must be memorized. The EMT must think about the pathophysiology of the patient's injuries and conditions—time cannot be wasted trying to remember what comes next.

The basis of life-threatening injuries is most often lack of adequate tissue oxygenation leading to anaerobic (without oxygen) metabolism. This condition is known as shock. Normal body metabolism (aerobic) requires several essential components. The Fick principle identifies the three components necessary for normal metabolism: (1) oxygenation of the red blood cells (RBCs) in the lung; (2) delivery of RBCs to the tissue cells throughout the body; and (3) offloading of oxygen to the tissue. The activities involved in the primary assessment are aimed at identifying and correcting problems with the first two components described in the Fick principle (see Chapter 6).

IMMEDIATE (SIMULTANEOUS) EVALUATION

In discussing the process of patient assessment, management, and decision making, it is necessary to present information in a linear format. That is, step A is followed by

step B, is followed by step C, etc. While presentation of information in this matter makes explanation easier and, perhaps, makes the concepts easier for the student to understand, that is not how the real world functions. The rescuer's brain is like a computer that can receive input from several sources at once—cerebral multi-tasking, if you will. These input data can be assessed simultaneously. The brain is also capable of prioritizing the information from all the input sources, sorting them in such a way that orderly decision making follows.

The A B C D E steps, described later in this chapter, or the sequence of assessment events learned in initial EMT training, are the priorities but not necessarily the order in which the information is collected or received. Most of the data can be gathered in about 15 seconds, and simultaneous processing of these data and appropriate prioritization of the information by the EMT's brain reveals the component that must be managed first.

The primary survey (initial assessment) addresses life-threatening conditions; the secondary survey (focused history and physical exam) of the patient identifies possible limb-threatening injuries first, as well as other, less significant problems.

GENERAL IMPRESSION

The primary survey begins with a simultaneous, or global, overview of the patient's respiratory, circulatory, and neurologic status to identify any obvious significant external problems with oxygenation, circulation, hemorrhage, or gross deformities. As the EMT approaches the patient, he or she can see whether the patient appears to be moving air effectively, whether the patient is awake or unresponsive, whether the patient is holding himself up, and whether he moves spontaneously. Once at the patient's side, a quick check at the radial pulse in the wrist will allow the EMT to evaluate the presence, quality, and rate (very fast, very slow, or generally normal) of circulatory activity. The EMT can simultaneously feel the temperature and moisture of the skin and ask the patient what happened. The patient's verbal response indicates to the EMT the overall status of the airway, whether ventilation is normal or labored, approximately how much air is being moved with each breath, the level of consciousness and mentation (if the patient responds verbally), the urgency of the situation, and perhaps even how many people were involved. "Where do you hurt?" is a follow-up question the EMT can ask while checking the skin color and the rate of capillary refill. The patient's answer will indicate whether the EMT can localize the pain and may help to identify the most likely points of injury. The EMT then scans the patient from head to foot, looking for signs of hemorrhage while gathering all the preliminary data for the primary survey. During this time, the EMT has taken a quick overall look at the patient, making the first few seconds with the patient a global survey of his condition and an evaluation of life-threatening possibilities. The brain has classified all the information according to priorities, classified the severity of the patient's injuries and condition, and identified which injury or condition needs to be managed first. Within 15 to 30 seconds, the EMT has gained a general impression of the patient's overall condition. This part of the primary survey has established whether the patient is presently or imminently in critical condition, and the patient's overall systemic condition has been rapidly evaluated. The general impression will often provide all of the necessary information the EMT needs to determine whether additional sophisticated resources may be necessary to manage the patient. If advanced life support resources are not present but are available in the area, this is the time to consider whether or not they should be called. If helicopter transportation to a trauma facility is going to be appropriate, this is often the time when the decision to request the helicopter can be made. Delay in deciding that additional resources are necessary will only extend on-scene time. Early decision making will ultimately meet the objective of shortening scene time. Once this general impression of the patient's condition has been ascertained, the primary survey can be immediately completed unless there has been a complication that requires more care or evaluation.

The rest of the primary survey must proceed very rapidly. Our remaining discussion of the primary survey will address the specific components that have been identified (or should have been identified) and how they should be prioritized for optimal patient management.

The five steps involved in the primary survey and their order of priority follow:

    A—Airway management and cervical spine control
    B—Breathing (ventilation)
    C—Circulation and bleeding
    D—Disability
    E—Expose and protect from the environment

STEP A—AIRWAY AND CERVICAL SPINE CONTROL
Airway

The airway should be quickly checked to ensure that it is open and clear (patency) and that no danger of obstruction exists. If the airway is compromised, it will have to be initially opened using manual methods (trauma chin lift or trauma jaw thrust) (Figure 2-1). Eventually, as equipment and time is available, airway management can advance to mechanical means (oral, nasal airways, or endotracheal intubation) or to transtracheal methods (percutaneous jet insufflation) (see Chapter 3: Airway Management and Ventilation).

Cervical Spine

As the EMT learned in his or her initial training program, for every trauma patient with a significant mechanism of injury, the EMT must suspect spinal cord injury until it has been conclusively ruled out. Therefore, when establishing an open airway, the EMT must remember that there is a possibility of a cervical spine injury. Excessive movement could cause neurologic damage (or additional neurologic damage) because bony compression may occur in the presence of a fractured spine. The solution is to make sure that the neck is manually maintained in the neutral position (for that patient) during the opening of the airway and the administration of necessary ventilation. This does not mean that the necessary airway maintenance procedures just described cannot or should not be carried out. Instead, it means that they must be performed while protecting the spine from unnecessary movement.

STEP B—BREATHING (VENTILATION)

As described in the earlier discussion of the Fick principle, oxygen must be effectively delivered to the lungs as the first step in the metabolic process. Hypoxia results from inadequate ventilation of the lungs and lack of oxygenation of the patient's tissues. Once the airway is open, the quality and quantity of the patient's ventilation must be evaluated.

Check to see if the patient is breathing. If breathing is not present, the assessment is stopped and EMT-provided ventilation is administered immediately.

If the patient is breathing, estimate the adequacy of the respiratory rate and depth to determine whether the patient is moving enough air. Quickly observe chest rise and listen to the patient talk if he or she is conscious. The respiratory rate can be divided into four levels: a rate of

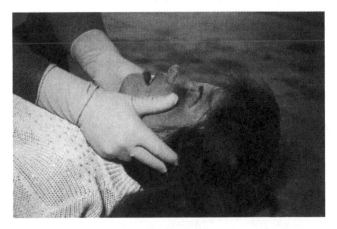

Figure 2-1 If the airway appears compromised, it must be opened while continuing to protect the spine.

<12 breaths per minute is very slow. A rate of 12 to 20 is normal for the adult patient. A rate of 20 to 30 is intermediate-fast; a rate of >30 is abnormally fast and may indicate hypoxia, acidosis, or hypoperfusion (or all three).

Although this function is called the respiratory rate, it is actually an incorrect name. It should be called the ventilation rate. Respiration is the term to describe the entire physiologic process of the uptake of oxygen. Both terms are used interchangeably.

The drive for the respiratory rate is the increased accumulation of CO_2 in the blood and a low level of O_2. When the patient displays an abnormal respiratory rate the EMT should ask "why?" A rapid rate will indicate that there is not enough oxygen reaching the tissue, producing anaerobic metabolism (see Chapter 6: Shock and Fluid Resuscitation) and a build up of acid that the buffer system in the body changes to CO_2 and H_2O. The body's detection system recognizes the increased CO_2 and tells the ventilatory system to speed up to blow off this excess. The faster the ventilatory rate, the higher the level indicating the severity of the metabolic acidosis. This indicates that the patient needs more oxygen or better perfusion or both. A very low rate may indicate ischemia of the brain. If the respiratory rate has dropped to <12, the EMT must either assist the patient or completely take over breathing for him or her. Assisted or total ventilatory support should include supplemental oxygen that achieves an oxygen concentration of 85% or greater (FiO2 of 0.85 or greater).

If the ventilatory rate is normal (12 to 20), watch the patient closely. Although the patient appears stable for the present, consider supplemental oxygen.

If the respiratory rate is intermediate (20 to 30), this patient must be watched closely. Determine whether the patient is improving or deteriorating. Administration of supplemental oxygen (FiO2 > 0.85) is indicated for this patient, at least until it can be determined what his or her overall status is. In such patients, the EMT should be suspicious of the patient's ability to maintain adequate respiration and should remain alert for any deterioration in overall condition (Table 2-1).

Tachypnea, a respiratory rate in excess of 30 breaths per minute, indicates hypoxia, anaerobic metabolism, or both with resultant acidosis. Assisted ventilation with

supplemental oxygen (FiO2 of 0.85 or greater) should be started immediately. The EMT should also begin the search for the cause of the rapid ventilatory rate at once. Oxygenation problem or RBC delivery problem? If the cause is identified, the EMT must intervene immediately. If a respiratory problem is suspected, the chest should be rapidly exposed, observed, and palpated. Auscultate for breath sounds at this point. Required respiratory support should be initiated at once rather than waiting until the end of the primary assessment.

STEP C—CIRCULATION AND BLEEDING

Circulatory system failure is just as life threatening as failure of the respiratory system. Oxygenation of the RBCs without delivery to the tissue cells is of no benefit to the patient. In the initial evaluation of a trauma patient, an adequate overall estimate of the cardiac output and cardiovascular status can be obtained simply by checking the pulse, capillary refilling time, skin color, and skin temperature.

Pulse

Evaluate the pulse for presence, quality, and regularity. Remember that the presence of a palpable peripheral pulse also provides an estimate of blood pressure. This quick check will reveal whether the patient has tachycardia, bradycardia, or an irregular rhythm. It can also reveal information about the systolic blood pressure. If the radial pulse is not palpable, the patient has likely entered the decompensated phase of shock, a late sign of the patient's critical condition. In the primary survey, determination of an exact pulse rate is not necessary. Instead, a gross estimate is obtained rapidly and the assessment quickly moves on to other gross evaluations. The actual pulse rate will be calculated later in the process.

Skin

Capillary-refilling Time

A quick check of the capillary-refilling time is accomplished by pressing over the nail beds or hypothenar eminence (the fleshy part of the palm along the ulnar margin on the little-finger side of the hand). This removes the blood from the visible capillary bed. The rate of return of blood to the beds (refilling time) is a useful tool in estimating blood flow through this most distal part of circulation (Figure 2-2). The cutaneous capillary beds are among the first areas to shut down when the body's compensatory mechanisms begin to work to offset shock. A capillary-refilling time of greater than 2 seconds indicates that the capillary beds are not receiving adequate perfusion. However, capillary refill is a poor indicator of

Table 2-1 Airway management based on spontaneous ventilation rate

Respiratory Rate	Management
<12	Assisted or total ventilation with oxygen (FiO2 > 0.85)
12–20	Observation
20–30	Administer oxygen (FiO2 > 0.85)
>30	Assist ventilation (FiO2 > 0.85)

circulatory status all by itself, because it is influenced by so many other factors. For example, advanced age, cold temperatures, the use of pharmacologic vasodilators or constrictors, or the presence of spinal shock can skew the result. It becomes a less useful check of cardiovascular function in these instances. Capillary refilling time certainly has a place as a method for evaluating circulatory adequacy, but it should be used in conjunction with other techniques.

Color

Adequate perfusion produces a pinkish hue in the skin. Dark skin colors can make this determination difficult. Examination of the color of nail beds and mucous membranes can serve to overcome this challenge. Bluish coloration indicates incomplete oxygenation, while pale coloration is associated with poor perfusion.

Temperature

As with other parts of skin evaluation, temperature is influence by environmental conditions. However, cool skin indicates decreased perfusion, regardless of the cause.

Moisture

Dry skin indicates good perfusion. Moist skin is associated with shock and decreased perfusion.

Bleeding

In cases of external hemorrhage, application of direct pressure will control most or all major hemorrhage until the patient can be moved to a location where an operating room and adequate equipment are available. Pressure bandages, which may include pneumatic compression from either an air splint or the pneumatic antishock garment (PASG), are also an excellent means of hemorrhage control. If internal hemorrhage is suspected, the EMT should quickly expose the abdomen and look and palpate for signs of injury. The pelvis should also be palpated because a pelvic fracture is a major source of intra-abdominal bleeding. This injury should be managed with rapid transport, use of the PASG, and rapid, warm intravenous fluid replacement. Rapid control of blood loss is one of the most important goals in the care of the trauma patient.

Many causes of hemorrhage are not easy to control outside the hospital. The prehospital treatment is rapid delivery of the patient to a hospital equipped and staffed for rapid control of hemorrhage in the operating room.

STEP D—DISABILITY

Having evaluated and corrected, to the extent possible, the factors involved in delivering oxygen to the lungs and circulating it throughout the body, the next step is a direct measurement of cerebral function, which is an indirect

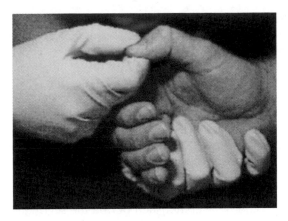

Figure 2-2 Capillary refill time is evaluated by pressing on the nail bed to remove blood and then timing how long it takes for normal color to return.

measurement of cerebral oxygenation. The goal is to determine the patient's level of consciousness (LOC).

The patient's level of consciousness can be accurately evaluated by applying a stimulus to the patient (pinch, squeeze, or sound) and describing the patient's response by using the acronym AVPU, which stands for:

A—Alert
V—Responds to verbal stimulus
P—Responds to painful stimulus
U—Unresponsive

A decreased LOC should alert the EMT to four possibilities:

- decreased cerebral oxygenation (due to hypoxia and/or hypoperfusion)
- central nervous system (CNS) injury
- drug or alcohol overdose
- metabolic derangement (diabetes, seizure, cardiac arrest)

A belligerent, combative, or uncooperative patient should be considered to be hypoxic until proven otherwise. Most patients want help when their lives are threatened. If the patient is refusing help, one must question the reason. Why does the patient feel threatened by the presence of an EMT on the scene? If the patient seems to feel threatened by the situation itself, the EMT should do something to establish enough rapport so that the patient will trust her. If there is nothing in the situation that seems to be threatening, one must consider that the source is medical. Hypoxia is the only condition of those just listed that can quickly and easily be addressed. The rest will require medication not usually available in the field, time to metabolize the toxic agent, or a surgical procedure to relieve intracranial pressure. During the examination, the EMT should determine from the history whether the patient lost consciousness at any time since the injury occurred, what toxic substances might be involved, and whether the patient has any preexisting conditions that might have produced the decreased LOC or aberrant behavior.

The pupils play a major role in the evaluation of the cerebral function at this stage. Are the pupils PEARRL (Pupils Equal And Round, Reactive to Light)? Are the pupils equal to each other? Is each pupil round and of normal appearance, and does it appropriately react to light by constricting, or is it unresponsive and dilated?

The Glasgow Coma Scale (GCS) is a very important evaluative tool both in the short-term and long-term management of the patient. However, assignment of a GCS score should be accomplished during the secondary survey. Its short-term benefit is as an additional factor in determining the severity of the injury. The long-term benefit is in providing a prognosis for patient recovery.

STEP E—EXPOSE AND PROTECT FROM THE ENVIRONMENT

It is impossible to see through clothes while evaluating a trauma patient. Therefore, an early step in the assessment process is to get the clothes out of the way. Exposure of the trauma patient is critical to finding all the injuries. The saying that "the one part of the body that is not exposed will be the most severely injured part" may not always be true, but it is true often enough to warrant total body examination. Also, blood can collect in and be absorbed by clothing and thereby go unnoticed. At some time during

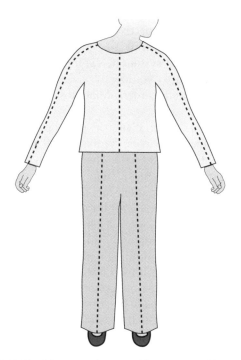

Figure 2-3 Clothing can be quickly removed by cutting as indicated by the dotted lines.

the evaluation of the patient, all of the patient's clothes must be removed (Figure 2-3) and the patient rolled to examine the entire body. When everything has been seen, the patient should be recovered to conserve body heat. Only the necessary parts of the patient should be exposed when the patient is outside of the transport unit, both to preserve the body temperature and to respect the patient's modesty.

How much of the patient's clothing should be removed during an assessment will vary, depending on what conditions or injuries are found. The general rule is to remove as much clothing as necessary to determine the presence or absence of a condition or injury. The EMT should not be afraid to remove clothing if it is the only way the assessment and treatment can be properly completed.

Although it is important to expose a trauma patient's body in order to complete an effective assessment, hypothermia is a serious problem in the management of a trauma patient. Expose only what is necessary in the outside environment. Once inside the warm EMS unit, complete the examination and then re-cover the patient as quickly as possible.

VITAL SIGNS

The quality of the pulse and respiration and the rest of the components of the primary survey must be continually reevaluated because significant changes may occur rapidly. Quantitative vital signs should be measured and motor and sensory status evaluated in all four extremities as soon as possible, but this is not normally accomplished until after the conclusion of the primary survey. Depending on the situation, vital signs may be obtained simultaneously by a second EMT to avoid further delay. Exact "numbers" for pulse, respiration, and blood pressure, however, are not critical in the initial management of the patient with severe multisystem trauma. Therefore, measurement of the exact numbers can be delayed until the essential steps of resuscitation and stabilization have been completed.

RESUSCITATION

Resuscitation describes treatment steps taken to correct life-threatening problems identified in the primary survey. The most important step in resuscitation is rapidly correcting hypoxia and shock (anaerobic metabolism). Airway maintenance and ventilatory support should be initiated as soon as a problem is identified. Ventilatory support should include administration of high concentrations of oxygen ($FiO_2 > 0.85$) as early as possible. If the patient is exhibiting signs of distress and lowered levels of air exchange, ventilatory assistance is needed by way of bag-valve-mask. Similarly, procedures for cardiac arrest management and hemorrhage control should also be implemented as soon as a problem with the circulatory system is identified.

Another important step in resuscitation is the restoration of the cardiovascular system to an adequate perfusing status as quickly as possible. This is accomplished by establishing two large-bore intravenous lines en route to the hospital and the initiation of volume replacement with lactated Ringer's infusion. Whole blood should be added as soon as possible but is usually available only at the emergency department. Therefore, rapid transportation of the severely injured patient to a hospital that is appropriately equipped and staffed is an absolute necessity. However, if time and other factors permit, 1 to 2 liters of warm lactated Ringer's solution should be administered en route to the hospital. (See Chapter 6 for details of the fluid/no fluid controversy.)

At the EMT-Basic level, immediate control of major external hemorrhage, rapid packaging of the patient for transportation, and quickly initiated, rapid but safe transport of the patient to the closest appropriate facility at which fluid replacement and surgical intervention can be accomplished are the key steps in resuscitating the critical trauma patient. These measures must accompany conventional shock treatment measures, such as maintaining adequate body temperature and positioning the patient appropriately (e.g., a modified Trendelenburg position). If transportation time is prolonged, it may be appropriate to call for mutual aid from a nearby advanced life support service that can intercept the basic unit en route to the hospital or helicopter evacuation to a trauma center and thus begin advanced airway and ventilatory management and fluid replacement therapy earlier.

The use of the PASG should be considered for the patient with circulatory insufficiency due to trauma, because it is an effective device for restoring the perfusion of the heart, brain, and lungs when a low cardiovascular volume exists. Most current studies conclude that the PASG is particularly useful for managing decreased RBC delivery from abdominal injuries when the patient's blood pressure is below 50 to 60 mm Hg. An additional application of the PASG is for hemorrhage control for intra-abdominal or pelvic bleeding.

Except in very specialized EMS services, initial central intravenous lines are not appropriate in the field management of patients. Although the benefit of central lines for monitoring fluid replacement has certainly been well proven, it has also been shown that there is a slower rate of fluid administration when a catheter of the length necessary for central line placement is chosen. The time necessary for placement of a central intra-

venous line is greater than that needed for insertion of a peripheral intravenous line and has an in-hospital complication rate of 15%. The extra time spent inserting the central intravenous line often causes the neglect of other important aspects of patient care. Even in the emergency department only a few exceptional situations warrant the use of a central line for the management of a trauma patient.

Any intravenous line for a critical trauma patient is better started en route to the hospital, not at the scene as this will increase scene time. The rare exceptions are those cases, such as entrapment, when the patients simply cannot be moved immediately. Prehospital fluid replacement is a challenge due to the limitations of the tools that EMTs have to use. Specifically, with very few exceptions, EMS providers depend on the use of crystalloid solutions for fluid replacement (see Chapter 6: Shock and Fluid Resuscitation). One to 2 liters of fluid replacement en route to the hospital are generally beneficial to overall patient care.

Consider, for example, a patient with an injury to the spleen who is losing 50 cc/min of blood. Each additional minute that delays the patient's arrival in the OR will add an additional 50 cc of blood loss.

Besides the fact that it takes a lot of volume of crystalloid solution to replace blood, the other problem with the use of crystalloids for volume replacement is that only *fluid volume* is being replaced. Crystalloids contain nothing to replace the oxygen-carrying capacity of the lost RBCs or for the lost platelets that are necessary for clotting and bleeding control. Since it is difficult to keep up with the patient's fluid replacement needs in the field, delays in the field to initiate IV therapy should be kept to a minimum and the time on the scene kept as short as possible. Intravenous lines should be started while en route to the hospital unless the patient is entrapped at the scene or for some other reason cannot be moved.

SECONDARY SURVEY (FOCUSED HISTORY AND PHYSICAL EXAM)

The secondary assessment is a head-to-toe evaluation of the patient. Its objective is to identify injuries or problems that were not identified during the primary survey. Since a well-performed primary survey will identify all life-threatening conditions, the secondary assessment, by definition, deals with less serious problems. Therefore, the critical trauma patient should be transported as soon as possible following conclusion of the primary assessment and should not be held in the field for a secondary assessment.

Once transportation is underway and after life-threatening conditions are managed, the EMT should look for an opportunity to complete a more detailed examination of the patient. This more detailed examination is called a secondary assessment or a "focused history and physical exam/rapid trauma assessment" in the EMT curricula. Before the secondary survey can begin, all the patient's clothing must be removed. This is most easily accomplished by cutting the anterior part of the sleeves, pants, and chest and abdominal portions of the clothing and letting them fall away (see Figure 2-3 on page 44). The complete removal of clothes should be delayed until the patient is inside the ambulance (or the emergency department if transport time is short) for warmth and for modesty.

In the secondary survey, the "look, listen, and feel" approach is used to evaluate the skin and everything it contains. Rather than looking at the entire body at one time, then returning to listen to all areas, and finally returning to palpate all areas, the body is "searched"—injuries are identified and physical findings are correlated region-by-region, beginning at the head and proceeding through the neck, chest, and abdomen to the extremities, concluding with a detailed neurologic examination. The national standard EMT curricula suggest the use of the mnemonic device DCAP-BTLS to assist the EMT in remembering what is being sought in this detailed assessment. It stands for _deformities, contusions, abrasions, punctures and penetrations, burns, tenderness, lacerations, and swelling._

The following phrases capture the essence of the entire assessment process:

See, don't just look
Hear, don't just listen
Feel, don't just touch

The dictionary defines the word _see_ as "to perceive with the eye" or "to discover," whereas _look_ is defined as "to exercise the power of vision." _Listen_ is defined as "monitor without participation," and _hear_ is defined as "listen with attention." While examining the patient, the EMT should use all the information available to formulate a patient care plan. An EMT should do more than just provide the patient with hospital transport; an EMT should do all that can be done to assure survival.

SEE

Examine all the skin of each region. Be attentive for ecchymosis (bruising), deformation, hemorrhage, or anything else that is unusual. Are there any masses or swelling that should not be there? Does the skin have abnormal indentations? What is the skin color? Does anything just not "look right"?

HEAR

Are any unusual sounds coming from the patient? Use the stethoscope to listen to the bones while percussing at a distance. For example, place the stethoscope on the symphysis pubis and percuss the patella on both knees. If the sound waves are not transmitted equally there is probably a fracture of the femur that does not transmit the

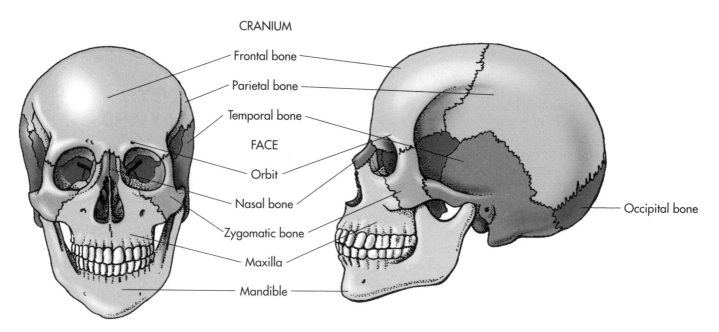

CRANIUM
— Frontal bone —
— Parietal bone —
— Temporal bone —
FACE
— Orbit —
— Nasal bone —
— Zygomatic bone —
— Maxilla —
— Mandible —
Occipital bone

Figure 2-4 Normal anatomical structure of the face and head.

sound or that transmits a weak sound wave. The same is true of the humerus or clavicle when the stethoscope is placed on the sternum, although this is more difficult to discern. Are there any unusual sounds (bruits) over the vessels that would indicate vascular damage? Are the breath sounds equal in both lung fields?

FEEL

Carefully move each bone in the region. Does this produce crepitus, pain, or unusual movement? Firmly palpate all parts of the region. Does anything move that should not? Does anything feel "squishy?" Where are pulses felt? Are there any pulsations that should not be there? Are the pulses all present?

REGIONAL EXAMINATION (RAPID TRAUMA ASSESSMENT)

Head

Visual examination of the head and face will reveal contusions, abrasions, lacerations, bone asymmetry, hemor-

rhage, bony defects of the face and supportive skull, and/or abnormalities of the eye, eyelid, external ear, mouth, and mandible.

Careful palpation of the bones of the face and skull to identify crepitus, deviation, depression, or abnormal mobility is extremely important in the nonradiographic evaluation for head injury. Also search thoroughly through the victim's hair (Figure 2-4).

Neck

Visual examination of the neck for contusions, abrasions, lacerations, and deformities of the larynx will alert the EMT to the possibility of underlying injuries. Palpation may reveal subcutaneous emphysema (of a tracheal, pulmonary, or laryngeal origin) or deviation of the trachea from the midline. Crepitus of the larynx, hoarseness, and subcutaneous emphysema compose the triad classically indicative of laryngeal fracture. Palpation of the cervical spine for tenderness certainly does not rule out cervical spine fractures but may frequently help to identify their presence. Such palpation should be performed carefully, making sure that the neck remains in a neutral in-line position. Figure 2-5 shows the anatomy of the respiratory system, including the normal anatomy of the neck.

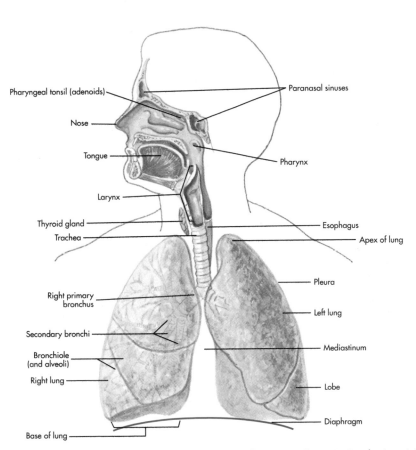

Figure 2-5 Respiratory system anatomy. (From LeFleur Brooks, M. *Exploring Medical Language.* 4th ed. St. Louis: Mosby, Inc., 1998.)

Chest

The thorax is very strong, resilient, and elastic. For that reason, it can absorb a significant amount of trauma. Close visual examination for minor deformities, small areas of paradoxical movement, contusions, and abrasions is necessary to identify underlying injuries. Other signs for which the EMT must be especially vigilant are splinting and guarding, unequal bilateral chest excursion, and intercostal, suprasternal, or supraclavicular bulging or retraction.

A contusion over the sternum, for example, may be the only indication of a myocardial contusion. A stab wound near the sternum may be the initial sign of a cardiac tamponade. A line traced from the fourth intercostal space anteriorly to the sixth intercostal space laterally to the eighth intercostal space posteriorly defines the upward excursion of the diaphragm at full expiration (Figure 2-6). A penetrating injury that occurs below this line or whose pathway may have taken it below this line should be considered to have traversed both the thoracic and abdominal cavities.

Except for the eyes and hands, the stethoscope is the most important instrument the EMT can use for the chest examination. The patient will most often be in a supine position, so that only the anterior and lateral chest is available for auscultation. The EMT should learn to recognize normal and decreased breath sounds with the patient in this position. A small area of rib injury may indicate a severe underlying pulmonary contusion. A fractured rib may even be deflected into the heart. Any type of compression injury to the chest can result in a pneumothorax (Figure 2-7).

Abdomen

The abdominal examination is initiated by visual evaluation, as with the other parts of the body. Abrasions and ecchymosis indicate the possibility of underlying injury. The abdominal area near the umbilicus should be examined carefully for a telltale contusion about 4 cm wide lying transversely across the abdomen, which indicates that an incorrectly worn seat belt has caused underlying soft-tissue injury. Almost 50% of patients with this sign will have hollow-organ injury in the abdomen. A high incidence of lumbar spine fractures is also associated with the "seat belt sign."

Examination of the abdomen also includes palpation of each quadrant to check for pain, abdominal muscle guarding, and masses. When palpating, note whether the abdomen is soft and whether rigidity or guarding are present. There is no need to continue palpating after abdominal tenderness or pain has been discovered. No additional information that will alter prehospital management can be learned, and the only outcome of continued abdominal examination is to cause the patient further discomfort and delay in transportation to the trauma center.

Identifying the specific abdominal injury is not a part of the prehospital evaluation as it will not alter the field care. The presence or absence of specific intra-abdominal injuries does not change the prehospital management unless there is a possibility of significant blood loss.

Pelvis

The pelvis is evaluated by observation and palpation. If the mechanism of injury and the history indicate possible injury to the pelvic region, the EMT should visually examine for abrasions, contusions, lacerations, open fractures, and signs of distention. Pelvic fractures can produce massive internal hemorrhage, resulting in rapid deterioration of the patient's condition.

The pelvis should be palpated once for instability as part of the secondary assessment. Since palpation can aggravate hemorrhage, this examination step should not be repeated. Palpation is accomplished by gently applying first lateral and then medial pressure to the iliac crests bilaterally. The hand is then moved to the symphysis pubis and gentle posterior pressure is exerted, again evaluating for pain and abnormal movement. Hemorrhage should be suspected if any evidence of instability is found.

Extremities

Examination of the extremities should begin with the clavicle in the upper extremity and the pelvis in the lower extremity and proceed toward the most distal portion of each extremity. Each individual bone and joint should be evaluated by visual examination for deformity, surrounding hematoma, or ecchymosis and by palpation to determine whether crepitus, pain, tenderness, or unusual movement are present. As discussed earlier, a stethoscope placed on the symphysis pubis with percussion on the patella is a good test for a fractured femur. Any suspected fracture should be immobilized until radiographic confirmation of its presence or absence is possible. A check of motor and sensory nerve function at the distal end of each extremity should also be accomplished.

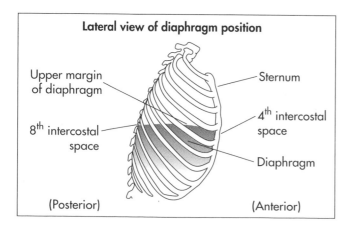

Lateral view of diaphragm position

Upper margin of diaphragm

Sternum

8th intercostal space

4th intercostal space

Diaphragm

(Posterior)

(Anterior)

Figure 2-6 Lateral view of diaphragm position.

Neurologic Exam

The neurologic examination in the secondary assessment, like the other regional examinations just described, is conducted in much greater detail than in the primary survey. Calculation of the Glasgow Coma Score (Figure 2-8), evaluation of motor and sensory function, and observation of pupillary response should all be included.

Pupillary Response

When examining a patient's pupils, the EMT should check for equality of response as much as for equality of size. A significant portion of the population has pupils of differing sizes as a normal condition. However, even in this situation, the pupils should react to light in a similar manner. Pupils that react at differing speeds to the introduction of light are considered to be unequal. Unequal pupils in an unconscious trauma patient may indicate increased intracranial pressure or pressure on the third cranial nerve, caused by either cerebral edema or a rapidly expanding intracranial hematoma (Figure 2-9). Direct eye injury can also cause unequal pupils.

Sensory Response

A gross examination of sensory capability and response will determine the presence or absence of weakness or loss of sensation in the extremities and will identify areas requiring further examination.

DEFINITIVE CARE

Included in assessment and management are the skills of packaging, transportation, and communication. Defin-

itive care is the end phase of patient care. For a patient with cardiac arrest, definitive care is defibrillation with resultant normal rhythm; CPR is just a holding pattern until the defibrillation can be accomplished. For a patient in a diabetic hypoglycemic coma, definitive care is intravenous glucose and a return to normal blood glucose levels; for the patient with an obstructed airway, part of the definitive care is the jaw thrust and assisted ventilation. For the patient with severe bleeding, definitive care is hemorrhage control. The definitive care was different in each of these examples, but all could be provided for the patient in the field, except for the trauma patient. Definitive care for this injury can be provided only in the operating room. Anything that delays the administration of that definitive care will lessen the patient's chance for survival. The care given to the trauma patient in the field is like CPR for the cardiac arrest patient: it is a holding action. It keeps the patient alive until something definitive can be done. For the trauma patient, the care given in the field is only definitive *field* care. It is not true definitive care. Anything that delays the arrival of the patient to the operating room and definitive care will lessen the chance of survival. This includes delivery of the patient to a hospital not dedicated to trauma management.

PACKAGING

As discussed earlier, spinal injury should be suspected in all trauma patients. Therefore, stabilization of the spine should be an integral component of packaging the trauma patient. If there is time, fractures should be carefully stabilized using specific splints. However, if the patient is in critical condition, all fractures should be immobilized as the patient is stabilized on a long backboard. Wounds should be bandaged as necessary and appropriate.

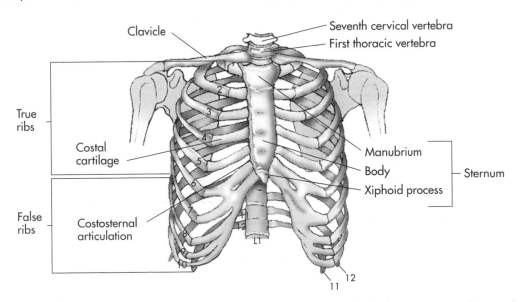

Figure 2-7 Normal anatomical structure of the chest. (From Thibodeau, G.A., and Patton, K.T. *Anatomy and Physiology.* 2d ed. St. Louis: Mosby–Yearbook, Inc., 1993.)

TRANSPORTATION

Transport should begin as soon as the patient is loaded and stabilized for the ride to the hospital. As discussed earlier in this chapter, delay at the scene to start an intravenous line or to complete the secondary assessment only extends the period of time before hemorrhage control can be accomplished and administration of blood can begin. Continued evaluation and further resuscitation should instead be completed en route to the hospital.

Trauma Score

The Trauma Score is a numerical grading system for estimating the severity of injury.[1] The score is composed of the Glasgow Coma Scale (reduced to approximately one third total value) and measurements of cardiopulmonary function. Each parameter is given a number (high for normal and low for impaired function). Severity of injury is estimated by summing the numbers. The lowest score is 1, and the highest score is 16.

Respiratory Rate	10-24/min	4
	24-35/min	3
	36/min or greater	2
	1-9/min	1
	None	0
Respiratory Expansion	Normal	1
	Retractive	0
Systolic Blood Pressure	90 mm Hg or greater	4
	70-89 mm Hg	3
	50-69 mm Hg	2
	0-49 mm Hg	1
	No Pulse	0
Capillary Refill	Normal	2
	Delayed	1
	None	0

Glasgow Coma Scale

Eye Opening	Spontaneous	4
	To Voice	3
	To Pain	2
	None	1
Verbal Response	Oriented	5
	Confused	4
	Inappropriate Words	3
	Incomprehensible Words	2
	None	1
Motor Response	Obeys Command	6
	Localizes Pain	5
	Withdraw (pain)	4
	Flexion (pain)	3
	Extension (pain)	2
	None	1

Total Glasgow Coma Scale Points

14-15	=	5
11-13	=	4
8-10	=	3
5-7	=	2
3-4	=	1

Total Trauma Score   **1-16**

Figure 2-8 A trauma score can be numerically calculated en route to the hospital. Such information is extremely helpful in preparing to manage a patient. (From Champion, H.R.; Sacco, W.J.; Carnazzo, A. J.; et al. "Trauma Score." *Crit Care Med* 9(9) (1981): 672-76.)

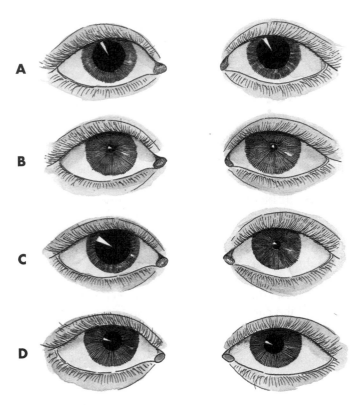

Figure 2-9 A, Pupil dilation. B, Pupil constriction.
C, Unequal pupils. D, Normal pupils.

trauma team. The operating room is staffed and ready. After 10 minutes in the emergency department for resuscitation and necessary radiographs and blood work for type and screen, the patient is taken into the operating room. The total time is 38 minutes. In comparison, the closest hospital has an available emergency physician, but the surgeon and the operating room crew are at home. The patient's 10 minutes in the emergency department for resuscitation would have stretched to 45 minutes by the time the surgeon came in from home and examined the patient. Another 30 minutes would have elapsed while waiting for the operating room team to arrive after the surgeon examined the patient and decided to call them in. The total time is 94 minutes, or 2.5 times as long. The 9 minutes saved by the shorter ambulance ride actually cost 57 minutes, during which operative management could have begun and hemorrhage control achieved.

Obviously, in a rural community the transport time to an awaiting trauma team may be 45 to 60 minutes or even longer. In this situation, the closest hospital with an on-call trauma team is the appropriate hospital.

Another aspect of the transportation equation is the transportation method. Some systems offer the option of air transportation as an alternative. Air medical services may offer a higher level of medical care than with ground units. Air transportation may also be quicker and smoother than ground transportation in some circumstances. As mentioned early in this chapter, if air transportation is available in a community, its use should be anticipated early in the assessment process so that it actually achieves a benefit for the patient.

The trauma triage scheme (see Figure 2-10) divides triage into three prioritized steps that will assist in the decision as to when it is best to transport a patient to the trauma center, if available. First is physiologic criteria, then anatomic criteria, and finally mechanism of injury (kinematics). Following this scheme will result in overtriage (not all patients taken to the trauma center will actually need trauma center level of care), but this outcome is better than undertriage (patients needing trauma center level of care are taken to nontrauma centers).

A patient whose condition is not critical can receive attention for individual injuries before transport, but even this patient should be transported rapidly, before a hidden condition becomes critical.

The facility to which the patient is transported should be chosen according to the severity of the patient's injury. In simple terms, the patient should be transported to the closest appropriate hospital—that is, the closest hospital best able to manage the patient's particular mix of problems. If the patient's injuries are severe or indicate the possibility of continuing hemorrhage, he or she should be taken to the hospital that will provide definitive care as quickly as possible. For example, adding 10 to 15 minutes of transport time to bring the patient to a facility with a trauma team ready to take him or her immediately to the operating room results in a shorter overall time from incident to definitive care than taking the patient to a hospital where the trauma team must come in from home (see the Introduction).

Consider a situation in which the ambulance responds in 8 minutes, and the EMS team spends 6 minutes on the scene to package the patient properly and load him into the unit. Fourteen minutes of the golden hour have passed. The closest hospital is 5 minutes away, and the trauma center is 14 minutes away. On arrival at the trauma center the surgeon is in the emergency department along with the emergency physician and the entire

COMMUNICATION

Communication with medical direction and the emergency department should begin as soon as possible. The information transmitted about the patient's condition, how he or she is being managed, and the ambulance's expected time of arrival will give the receiving hospital time to prepare. The EMS team should also transmit information about the mechanism of injury, the characteristics of the scene, the number of patients, and other pertinent facts that will allow the hospital staff to best coordinate its resources to meet each patient's needs.

Equally important is the written Prehospital Care Report (PCR). A good PCR is valuable for two reasons. First, it gives the hospital staff a thorough understanding of the events that occurred and of the patient's condition should any questions arise after the EMT leaves the hospital. Second, it helps to ensure quality control throughout the EMS system by making case review possible. For these reasons, the PCR should be accurately and completely filled out and provided to the hospital that is providing care for the patient. The report should stay with the patient; it does little good if the report does not arrive until hours or days after the patient arrives.

The PCR often becomes a part of the patient's medical record. It is a legal record of what was found and what was done and can be used as part of a legal action. The report is considered to be a complete record of the injuries found and the action taken by the EMTs. "If it is not on the report, it was not done" is a good adage to remember. All that the EMT knows, has seen, and has done to the patient should be recorded in the report.

The EMT must also verbally transfer responsibility for the patient ("sign off," "report off," or "transfer over") to the physician or nurse who takes over the patient's care in the emergency department. This verbal report is typically more detailed than the radio report and less detailed than the written record but does provide an overview of the significant history of the incident, the action taken by the EMTs, and the patient's response to this action. It is especially important at this point to highlight any significant changes in the patient's condition that may have taken place since the radio report was transmitted. Transfer of important prehospital information further emphasizes the team concept of patient care.

MONITORING AND REASSESSMENT (ONGOING ASSESSMENT)

Continue to monitor the patient, reassess the vital signs, and repeat the primary survey several times while en route. Continual reassessment of the points in the primary survey will help to ensure that the continuing progression of the patient's pathology does not compromise his vital functions. Particular attention should be paid to any significant change in the patient's condition. It may be necessary to reevaluate management if the patient's condition changes. Furthermore, the continued monitoring of the patient will help reveal conditions or problems that may have been overlooked during the primary survey. Often the patient's condition will be obvious, and much of the information will be gathered by looking at and listening to him or her. *How* the information is gathered is not as important as making sure that *all* the information is gathered. The re-

assessment should be conducted as quickly as possible, but no sacrifice in thoroughness should be made.

TRAUMA TRIAGE

The Trauma Score, originally developed by Drs. Champion, Sacco, and Carnazzo and since revised and updated, is a predictor of the survival of blunt trauma patients. The 1989 Revised Trauma Score (RTS) uses the Glasgow Coma Scale, systolic blood pressure, and respiratory rate to grade numerically or "score" different elements of the patient's condition. Each of these three components is assigned a value from 4 (best) to 0 (worst). The combined score indicates the patient's condition. The lowest possible combined score, 0, is obviously the most critical; the highest, 12, is the least critical. The combined score is valuable for analysis of the care given to the patient, but it is not necessarily a prehospital triage tool. In many EMS systems, the score is calculated and recorded at the hospital based on information provided in the radio report, but the EMTs are neither required nor expected to compute it before arriving at the hospital (see Figure 2-8).

The Triage Decision Scheme, developed by Dr. Champion, is more useful than the RTS in making prehospital patient triage evaluations (Figure 2-10). In some systems, it is used in the process of determining the most appropriate receiving facility for a trauma patient. Like any schematic tool, however, it should be used as a guideline and not as a replacement for the EMT's best judgment. There are three phases to this scheme. In priority order:

- physiologic condition
- anatomical location of injury(ies)
- mechanism of injury

TRIAGE

Triage is a French word meaning "to sort." In EMS, triage is used in two different contexts. In the first, there are sufficient resources to manage all patients. In this case, the most severe patients are treated and transported first while those with lesser injuries are transported later. In a second context, triage is used as a method to deal with multiple casualty incidents (MCIs) in which the number of patients exceeds the immediate capacity of on-scene EMS resources. The objective in triage is to ensure the survival of the largest possible number of injured patients. Patients are sorted into categories for patient care. In an MCI, patient care must be rationed. Relatively few EMTs will ever experience an MCI with 80 to 120 simultaneously injured persons, but many will be involved in MCIs with 10 to 20 victims, and rare is the EMT veteran who hasn't seen the multiple victim incident (2 to 10 victims).

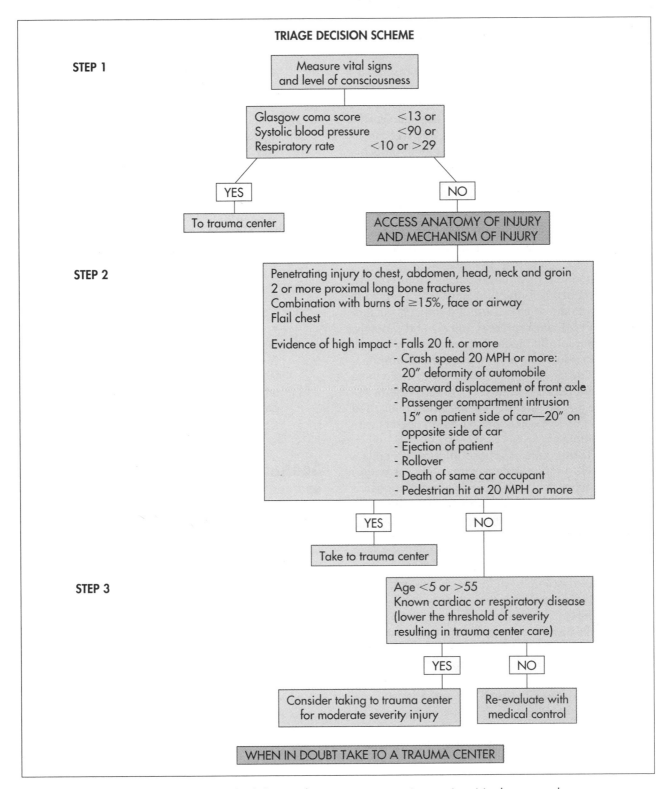

Figure 2-10 Deciding which hospital to transport a patient to is critical, as noted earlier. Those situations that will most likely require the in-house trauma team are detailed in the Triage Decision Scheme of the American College of Surgeons, which was developed by Dr. Howard Champion.

The purpose of triage is to salvage the greatest possible number of patients given the circumstances and resources available. Decisions must be made about who will be managed first, if at all. The usual rules about saving lives on a daily basis do not apply in an MCI.

In a choice between a patient with a catastrophic injury, such as severe open head trauma, and a patient with an acute intra-abdominal hemorrhage, the proper course of action in an MCI is to manage first the salvageable patient—the one with the abdominal hemorrhage. Treating the severe head trauma patient first will probably cause the loss of both patients: the head trauma patient because he is not salvageable and the abdominal hemorrhage patient because time, equipment, and personnel spent managing the unsalvageable patient keep the salvageable patient from getting simple care that will almost certainly keep her alive long enough to reach definitive surgical care.

In a triage situation, the catastrophically injured must be considered second priority; they must wait until there is more help and equipment. These are difficult circumstances, but the EMT must respond quickly and properly. It is inappropriate for the medical care team to waste all its effort trying to resuscitate a traumatic cardiac arrest patient who has little or no chance of survival while three other patients die because of airway compromise or external hemorrhage. The "sorting scheme" most often used divides patients into five categories based on need of care and chance of survival.

Immediate: Those patients whose injuries are critical but who will require only minimal time or equipment to manage and who have a good prognosis for survival. Patients with a compromised airway or massive external hemorrhage are examples.

Delayed: Those patients whose injuries are debilitating but who do not require immediate management to salvage life or limb. Patients with long bone fractures are good examples of those who belong in this category.

Expectant: Those patients whose injuries are so severe that they have only a minimal chance of survival. A patient with a 90% full-thickness burn and thermal pulmonary injury is an example.

Minimal: Those patients who have minor injuries that can wait for treatment or who may even assist in the interim by comforting other patients or helping out as litter bearers.

Dead: Any patient who is unresponsive, pulseless, and breathless. In a disaster, resources rarely allow for attempted resuscitation of arrested patients.

• Summary •

1. Patient assessment is the foundation upon which the rest of the trauma management system is based. The ability to rapidly and accurately assess a trauma patient is an essential skill for prehospital providers.
2. Scene-time is a critical issue in the management of the trauma patient. Assessment and management time should be kept to a minimum—in no circumstances more than 10 minutes—to avoid unnecessary delay in the patient's delivery to definitive care (within the golden hour following injury). Only those factors critical to survival should be done initially.
3. The three goals of assessment are:
   • rapid identification and management of shock and hypoxia
   • rapid assessment and management of life-threatening conditions
   • rapid transport
4. One of the most important questions that an EMT can ask in patient assessment is "Why?" Why are the patient's conditions or actions what they are? What physiologic change has produced this condition?

Scenario Solution

As you move quickly toward the patient, you note that there are no electrical wires down. There is a gasoline leak from the motorcycle under the car, but it is 50 feet away from where the patient is lying. You detect no other hazards and see no other patients. You confirm this from the bystanders as you reach the patient's side.

As you kneel down next to the patient, you place a hand on his helmet to stabilize his head. As you lean over him, his eyes open and he looks at you. He immediately describes intense back pain, as if it is on fire. He also describes pelvic pain, but no chest, belly, or extremity pain. Based on his ability to speak effectively, you assume that he does not have an airway problem and that he is breathing appropriately. You see no signs of obvious external hemorrhage. Your general impression of this patient is that he is not in immediate danger of dying, although you are concerned about the back pain and the pelvic pain.

As your partner arrives with the backboard and additional equipment, you suddenly realize that the patient is experiencing burning back pain for the same reason that your knees are suddenly burning—the asphalt is well over 100° in temperature, more than enough to provide second degree burns or worse. You stabilize the patient's head as your partner quickly assesses the pelvis. It seems that a fracture there is likely. The PASG are quickly laid out on the backboard, and the patient is log-rolled into place. You decide to leave the helmet in place since there is no evidence of an airway problem or an injury beneath it. The PASG patient is quickly immobilized to the board and loaded into the ambulance. Scene time, 7 minutes.

You ask your partner to make the radio report to the trauma center as you get the PASG inflated and set up your equipment to start an IV. Once the IV is in, a rapid secondary survey is conducted with no additional injuries found other than numerous abrasions and a major case of first and second degree burns on all of the posterior surfaces that were in contact with the hot asphalt. As the ambulance doors are opened at the hospital, you are able to provide an update on the patient's status and let everyone know that he appears stable

Review Questions

Answers provided on p. 333.

1 Which of the following statements best describes the importance of the patient assessment process in the overall management of the trauma patient?
A An effective patient assessment is necessary to reduce legal liability.
B The Prehospital Care Report (PCR) cannot be accurately completed unless a patient assessment is done.
C An effective patient assessment is the foundation upon which all patient care is based. It identifies life-threatening injuries and guides all subsequent activities.
D Selection of the appropriate protocol cannot be accomplished without patient assessment.

2 List the four major components of the patient assessment process, in the order in which they are completed.

3 As the EMT approaches the location of an incident, there is much information to be gained before reaching the patient's side. All of the following should be evaluated by the EMT as he or she approaches the patient, *except:*
A situation
B kinematics
C resources
D safety
E scene

4 The initial, global evaluation that enables the EMT to obtain a quick, overall impression of the patient's condition should be completed in what length of time?
A 15 seconds
B 30 seconds
C 60 seconds
D 1 minute
E 5 minutes

5 All of the following are life-threatening conditions that require immediate attention, *except:*
A lack of respiration
B full-thickness burns to the abdomen
C arterial bleeding from the thigh
D absence of a pulse
E massive facial injuries creating airway obstruction

6 The secondary survey is best completed by starting at the ends of the extremities and working toward the center of the body, concluding in the center of the abdomen.
A True
B False

CHAPTER OBJECTIVES

CHAPTER 3

Airway Management and Ventilation

At the completion of this course the student will be able to:

- Identify patients who require airway control.

- Define adequate minute volume and oxygenation and explain their importance as they relate to trauma patients.

- Define reduced perfusion and describe its implications for trauma patients.

- Explain the need for increased oxygenation and tidal volume exchange in trauma patients.

- List methods of manual and mechanical airway management and how to implement them while maintaining in-line cervical spine immobilization

- List methods of ventilation and how to implement them while maintaining in-line cervical spine immobilization.

- List common errors encountered with bag-valve-mask ventilation.

- List the indications, methods, and common errors of percutaneous transtracheal ventilation, endotracheal intubation, and needle thoracostomy.

- Describe techniques for initial and subsequent assessment of airway and ventilation interventions in trauma patients.

Scenario

You are dispatched to a motorcycle versus automobile crash. On your arrival, you observe that the cyclist has struck the rear of the automobile on the passenger side. Both the motorcycle and car are substantially damaged.

The driver of the car, an 18-year-old female, is visibly upset but shows no apparent injury. The motorcycle driver, a 30-year-old male, is lying in the grass approximately 30 feet from the incident site. Fire department First Responders have log rolled the patient onto a long backboard, and a cervical collar has been applied. They report that the patient has been unresponsive since their arrival. The heavily damaged helmet is lying beside the patient.

Periorbital ecchymosis (raccoon eyes) is already present. You observe bleeding from both nares and the right ear. Frequent suctioning is required to maintain a patent airway. Ventilations are irregular and snoring sounds are heard. The patient's skin is pale, and early cyanosis is observable around the lips. During your initial assessment, a police sergeant politely but firmly "advises" you that it is rush hour, and traffic needs to be reopened as quickly as possible.

- What indicators of airway compromise are evident in this patient?
- What other information, if any, would you seek from witnesses or the First Responders?
- How do you address the police sergeant's concern for returning traffic flow to normal?
- Describe the sequence of actions you would take to manage this patient before and during transport.

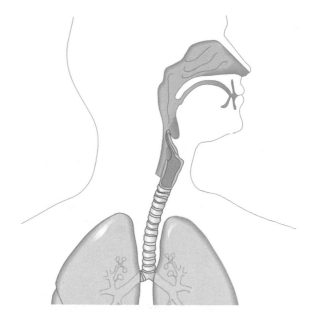

Figure 3-1 The respiratory system is composed of an upper and lower airway. Some of the air that passes into the nose is contained within the pharynx, larynx, trachea, and bronchi and thus does not reach the alveoli. This is known as dead space.

Airway management necessarily occupies a prominent place in the management of trauma patients. Its importance is recognized even more now than in years past. Studies carried out during the Championship Auto Racing Team (CART) auto racing circuit have demonstrated that patients with head injuries undergo a period of apnea within the first 5 minutes after impact. Although this apnea lasts only a short time and spontaneous respiration usually resumes quickly, it has a major influence on patient outcome. In one 3-year period after the CART introduced an emergency response team that included a paramedic, no major complications from head injuries occurred because the patient was ventilated during this period of apnea.

Cerebral oxygenation and oxygenation of other parts of the body provided by adequate airway management and ventilation remain the most important components of prehospital patient care. Because techniques and adjunct devices are changing and will continue to change, the well-informed prehospital provider must continually keep abreast of these changes.

The respiratory system serves two primary functions. First, the system provides oxygen to the red blood cells,

which then carry the oxygen to all the cells in the body. In aerobic metabolism, the cells use this oxygen as fuel and produce carbon dioxide as a byproduct. Removal of this carbon dioxide is the second job of the respiratory system. Inability of the respiratory system to provide oxygen to the cells or to eliminate carbon dioxide precipitates anaerobic metabolism, which can quickly lead to death.

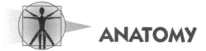

ANATOMY

The **respiratory system** is composed of the upper airway, the lower airway, and the lungs (Figure 3-1). Each part of the system plays an important role in ensuring that gas exchange—the process by which oxygen enters the bloodstream and carbon dioxide is removed—occurs.

UPPER AIRWAY

The airway system is an open path that leads atmospheric air through the nose, mouth, and bronchi to the alveoli. With each breath, the ventilatory system of an average adult takes in 1.2 liters (L) of air. The airway system holds up to 150 cubic centimeters (cc) of air that never actually reach the lungs to participate in the critical gas exchange

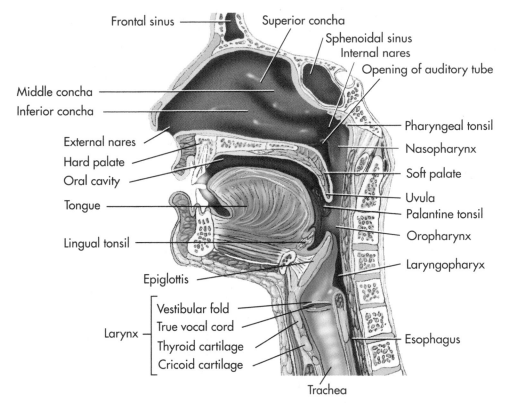

Figure 3-2 Sagittal section through the nasal cavity and pharynx viewed from the medial side. (From Seeley, R.R.; Stephens, T.D.; and Tate, P. *Essentials of Anatomy and Physiology.* St. Louis: Mosby–Year Book, Inc., 1991.)

process. The space in which this air is held is known as dead space. The air inside the space is not available to the body to be used for oxygenation.

The **upper airway** consists of the nasal cavity and the oral cavity (Figure 3-2). Air entering the nasal cavity is warmed, humidified, and filtered to remove all impurities. Beyond these cavities is the area known as the **pharynx,** which runs from the back of the soft palate to the upper end of the esophagus. The pharynx is composed of muscle lined with mucous membranes. The pharynx is divided into three discrete sections known as the **nasopharynx** (the upper portion), the **oropharynx** (the middle portion), and the **hypopharynx** (the distal end of the pharynx).

Below the pharynx lies the **esophagus,** which leads to the stomach, and the trachea, at which the lower airway begins. The first portion of the trachea is the **larynx** (Figure 3-3), which contains the vocal cords and the muscles that make them work, housed in a strong cartilaginous box. The **vocal cords** are folds of tissue that meet in the midline. The false cords, or vestibular fold, block the free passage of air and force the air flow through the vocal cords. Supporting the cords posteriorly is the **arytenoid cartilage.** Directly above the larynx is a leaf-shaped structure called the **epiglottis.** Acting like a gate,

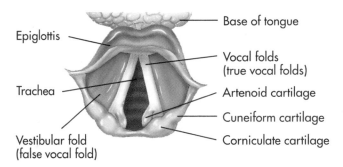

Figure 3-3 The vocal cords viewed from above, showing their relationship to the paired cartilages of the larynx and the epiglottis. (From Seeley, R.R.; Stephens, T.D.; and Tate, P. *Essentials of Anatomy and Physiology.* St. Louis: Mosby–Year Book, Inc., 1991.)

it directs air into the trachea and solids and liquids into the esophagus.

LOWER AIRWAY

The **lower airway** consists of the trachea, its branches, and the lungs. On inspiration, air travels through the upper airway and into the lower airway before reaching the **lungs,** where the actual gas exchange occurs (Figure 3-4). The **trachea** divides into a right and left mainstem bronchus. Each of the mainstem bronchi subdivides into several primary bronchi and then into bronchioles. **Bronchioles** (very small bronchial tubes) terminate at the **alveoli,** which are tiny air sacs surrounded by capillaries. It is at the alveoli where the respiratory system meets the circulatory system and gas exchange occurs.

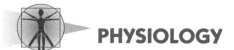

PHYSIOLOGY

With each breath, air is drawn into the respiratory system. The mechanics of normal ventilation are described in Chapter 5: Thoracic Trauma. When atmospheric air reaches the alveoli, oxygen moves from the alveoli, across the alveolar-capillary (A-C) membrane, and into the red blood cells. The circulatory system then delivers the oxygen-carrying red blood cells to the body tissues, where oxygen is used as fuel for metabolism.

As oxygen is transferred from inside the alveoli to the red blood cells, carbon dioxide is exchanged in the opposite direction, from the plasma to the alveoli. Carbon dioxide, which is carried in the plasma, not in the red blood cells, moves from the bloodstream, across the A-C membrane, and into the alveoli, where it can be eliminated during exhalation (Figure 3-5).

This exchange of oxygen with carbon dioxide at the A-C membrane is known as **pulmonary diffusion.** Upon completion of this exchange, the oxygenated red blood cells and plasma with a low carbon dioxide level return to the left side of the heart, to be pumped to all the cells in the body.

Once at the cell, the oxygenated red blood cells deliver their oxygen, which the cells then use as fuel for aerobic metabolism. Carbon dioxide, a byproduct of aerobic metabolism, is released into the blood plasma. This process, which is the opposite of what occurs during pulmonary diffusion, is called **cellular perfusion.** The oxygen-depleted red blood cells and the carbon dioxide–filled plasma return to the right side of the heart. The blood is pumped to the lungs, where it is resupplied with oxygen and the carbon dioxide is eliminated by diffusion.

It is critical to the process that the alveoli be constantly replenished with a fresh supply of air that contains an adequate amount of oxygen. This replenishment of air, known as ventilation, is essential for the elimination of carbon dioxide. Ventilation is measurable. The size of each breath, called the **tidal volume,** multiplied by the ventilatory rate for 1 minute equals the **minute volume.** During normal resting ventilation, about 500 cc of air is taken into the respiratory system. As mentioned earlier, part of this volume, 150 cc, remains in the airway system as dead space and does not participate in gas exchange.

If the tidal volume of each breath $= 500$ cc
and the respiratory rate per minute $= 14$,
then minute volume (500 cc $\times$ 14) $= 7000$ cc/min,
which converts to $= 7$ L/min.

Therefore, at rest, about 7 L of air must move in and out of the lungs each minute to maintain proper carbon dioxide elimination and oxygenation. If the minute volume should fall below normal, the patient has inadequate ventilation, a condition called **hypoventilation.** Hypoventila-

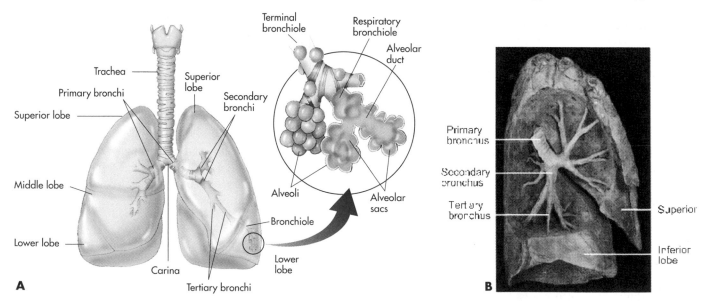

Figure 3-4 A, Drawing of the trachea and lungs. Inset shows enlargement of a terminal bronchiole and its associated alveoli. B, Branching of the bronchi in the left lung. (From Seeley, R.R.; Stephens, T.D.; and Tate, P. *Essentials of Anatomy and Physiology.* St. Louis: Mosby–Year Book, Inc., 1991.)

tion leads to a buildup of carbon dioxide in the body and promotes anaerobic metabolism, both of which are lethal. Hypoventilation is common when head or chest trauma causes an altered breathing pattern or an inability to move the chest wall adequately. For example, a patient with rib fractures who is breathing quickly and shallowly because of the pain of the injury may have the following minute volume, which indicates hypoventilation:

> tidal volume = 100 cc
> respiratory rate = 40
> minute volume = 100 cc × 40
> minute volume = 4000 cc/min or 4 L/min

If 7 L/min is necessary to allow adequate gas exchange in a nontraumatized person at rest, 4 L/min is far below what the body requires to eliminate carbon dioxide effectively. Furthermore, 150 cc of air is necessary to overcome dead space. If tidal volume is 100 cc, oxygenated air will never reach the alveoli. If untreated, this hypoventilation will quickly lead to severe distress.

Note that this patient is hypoventilating even though her respiratory rate is 40. Both rate and depth must be considered when evaluating a patient's ability to exchange air. A common mistake is to assume that any patient with a fast respiratory rate is hyperventilating. A much better judge of respiratory status is the amount of carbon dioxide elimination. The effect of carbon dioxide elimination on metabolism is discussed with the Fick principle and aerobic and anaerobic metabolism in Chapter 6: Shock and Fluid Resuscitation.

Prehospital assessment of respiratory function must include an evaluation of how well the patient is taking in, diffusing, and perfusing oxygen. Without proper intake and processing of oxygen, anaerobic metabolism will begin. In addition, effective ventilation must also be accomplished. The patient may accomplish ventilation completely, partially, or not at all. Prehospital providers must act aggressively to assess and manage inadequacies in oxygenation and ventilation.

PATHOPHYSIOLOGY

Trauma can affect the respiratory system's ability to adequately provide oxygen and eliminate carbon dioxide in seven ways:

1. Hypoventilation can result from loss of ventilatory drive, usually because of decreased neurologic function.
2. Hypoventilation can result from obstruction of air flow through the upper and lower airways.
3. Hypoventilation can be caused by decreased expansion of the lungs.
4. Hypoxia can result from decreased absorption of oxygen across the alveolar-capillary membrane.

5. Hypoxia can be caused by decreased blood flow to the alveoli.
6. Hypoxia can result from the inability of the air to reach the alveoli, usually because they are filled with fluid or debris.
7. Hypoxia can be caused at the cellular level by decreased blood flow to the tissue cells.

The first three components involve hypoventilation as a result of the reduction of minute volume. If untreated, hypoventilation results in carbon dioxide buildup, acidosis, anaerobic metabolism, and eventually death. Management involves improving the patient's ventilatory rate and depth by correcting any existing airway problems

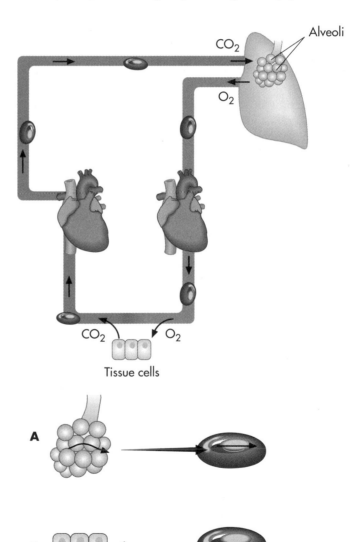

Figure 3-5 A and B, Oxygen moves into the red blood cells from the alveoli. They are transferred to the tissue cell on the hemoglobin molecule. After leaving the hemoglobin molecule, the oxygen travels into the tissue cell. Carbon dioxide travels in the reverse direction but not on the hemoglobin molecule. It travels in the plasma as carbon dioxide.

and assisting ventilation, which are discussed in this chapter.

The following sections discuss the first two components involved in inadequate ventilation: decreased neurologic function and mechanical obstruction. The third component, a reduction in minute volume as a result of decreased pulmonary expansion, is discussed in more detail in Chapter 5: Thoracic Trauma. The latter three components are discussed in Chapter 6: Shock and Fluid Resuscitation.

DECREASED NEUROLOGIC FUNCTION

Decreased minute volume can be caused by two clinical conditions related to decreased neurologic function: flaccidity of the tongue and decreased level of consciousness.

Flaccidity of the tongue associated with a reduced level of consciousness allows the tongue to fall into a dependent (toward the lowest area of the body) position. If the patient is supine, the base of the tongue will fall backward and occlude the hypopharynx. To prevent the tongue from occluding the hypopharynx, the EMT must manage the airway of any supine patient with a diminished level of consciousness, regardless of whether any signs of ventilatory compromise exist. Such patients also require periodic suctioning.

A decreased level of consciousness will also affect respiratory drive and will reduce the rate of ventilation, the volume of ventilation, or both. This reduction in minute volume may be temporary or permanent.

The CART medical staff identified one crucial aspect of neurologically based temporary loss of respiratory drive as a prehospital care concern. Ventilatory drive temporarily ceases within the first 4 or 5 minutes after a head injury occurs. The hypoxic injury to the brain that results can, in some cases, lead to permanent brain damage. If treated rapidly and aggressively, permanent brain injury may be avoided. Recognizing and treating hypoxia may be the most important factor in the prevention of permanent brain damage.

MECHANICAL OBSTRUCTION

Another cause of decreased minute volume is mechanical airway obstruction. The source of these obstructions may be neurologically influenced or purely mechanical in nature. Neurologic insults that alter the level of consciousness may disrupt the "controls" that normally hold the tongue in an anatomically neutral (nonobstructing) position. If these "controls" are compromised, the tongue falls rearward, occluding the hypopharynx.

Management of purely mechanical airway obstructions may also challenge prehospital personnel. Foreign bodies in the oral cavity may become lodged and create occlusions in the hypopharynx or the larynx. Crush injuries to the larynx and edema of the vocal cords are conditions that also warrant due consideration. Foreign bodies may originate from either the external environment or from within the patient's body.

Foreign bodies in the airway can be objects that were in the patient's mouth at the time of the injury, such as false teeth, chewing gum, tobacco, real teeth, and bone. Outside materials, such as glass from a broken windshield or any object that is near the patient's mouth at the time of injury can potentially threaten airway patency.

Upper and lower airway obstructions can also be caused by bone or cartilage collapse as a result of a fractured larynx or trachea, by a mucous membrane avulsed from the hypopharynx or tongue, or by facial damage in which blood and fragments of bone and tissue create an obstruction.

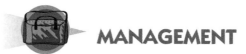

MANAGEMENT

AIRWAY CONTROL

Methods of airway control can be divided into three categories:
1. manual
2. mechanical
3. transtracheal

Any injury that directly affects the respiratory tract or its neurologic drive will ultimately lead to some level of respiratory insufficiency. Regardless of cause, decreases in tidal volume, and ultimately minute volume, will eventually result in retention of carbon dioxide and eventual acidosis.

Physiologically, the vascular system may be generally divided into three compartments. As one might expect, the heart and lungs receive the highest priority. Other organs/organ systems, such as the brain, thoracic organs, and extremities, may have their blood supply "reallocated" in the event of injury. As the pathologic process of shock proceeds, areas of diminished blood flow will "convert" to anaerobic metabolism to survive. Unfortunately, this process lacks the efficiencies of "normal" or aerobic metabolism and produces significantly more byproducts, which can lead to a state of metabolic acidosis.

Unchecked, shock can proceed to the so-called "washout" phase, in which these toxic metabolic byproducts are "washed" into the systemic circulation. At this point, the perfusion of tissue is severely compromised due to the heart's decreasing ability to overcome

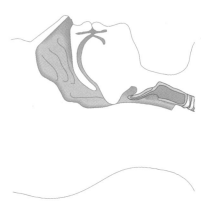

Figure 3-6 In an unconscious patient the tongue has lost its muscle tone and falls back into the hypopharynx, occluding the airway and preventing passage of oxygen into the trachea and lungs.

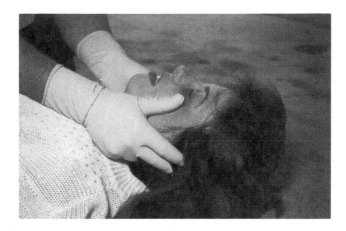

Figure 3-7 Trauma jaw thrust. The thumb is placed on each zygoma with the index and long fingers at the angle of the mandible. (Lift the mandible superiorly.)

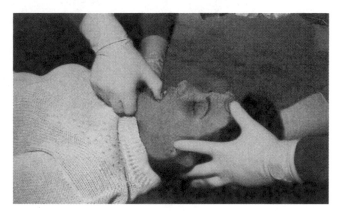

Figure 3-8 Trauma chin lift. The chin lift performs a function similar to that of the trauma jaw thrust: it moves the mandible forward by moving the tongue.

increased vascular resistance, decreased oxygenation, and a lack of circulating fluid volume.

Admittedly, prehospital personnel are at a marked disadvantage when the ultimate goal is to actually repair physiologic insults that precipitate shock. However, short-term restoration of circulating volume and respiratory support can be effectively accomplished out-of-hospital, and they should be viewed as priorities in the early care of trauma victims. By establishing near normal ventilation with enhanced FiO_2 levels and restoring intravascular volume, adequate minute volume and body cell oxygenation may be maintained.

The use of any of these methods of airway control requires simultaneous immobilization of the cervical spine. Emphasis is on maintaining the cervical spine (C-spine) in the neutral position. Refer to Chapter 9: Spinal Trauma, for more information about C-spine immobilization.

Manual Techniques

In unresponsive patients, the tongue becomes flaccid, falling back and blocking the hypopharynx. The tongue is the most common cause of airway obstruction. Manual methods may be used to clear this type of obstruction and are easily accomplished because the tongue is attached to the mandible and moves forward with it (Figure 3-6).

Trauma Mandible Lift

Any maneuver that moves the mandible forward will pull the tongue out of the hypopharynx. These maneuvers are called the trauma jaw thrust and trauma chin lift.

Trauma jaw thrust In cases of suspected head, neck, or facial trauma, the cervical spine must be maintained in a neutral in-line position. The trauma jaw thrust maneuver will enable the EMT to open the airway with little or no movement of the head and cervical spine (Figure 3-7).

The jaw is thrust forward by placing the thumbs on each zygoma (cheekbone), placing the index and long fingers on the mandible and at the same angle, pushing the mandible forward. In an unconscious patient, this maneuver may dislocate the jaw.

Trauma chin lift The trauma chin lift maneuver is another way to open the airway of a patient with suspected cervical spine compromise. This method is ideally used to relieve a variety of anatomic airway obstructions in patients who are breathing spontaneously (Figure 3-8). The mandible is pulled forward by grasping the chin and lower incisors and then lifting. The EMT must be careful that his or her thumbs are protected from body fluid contamination by the use of gloves.

Both of these techniques result in movement of the lower jaw anteriorly and slightly caudad, pulling the tongue forward, away from the airway, and opening the mouth. One technique—the trauma jaw thrust—pushes the mandible forward, whereas the other—the trauma

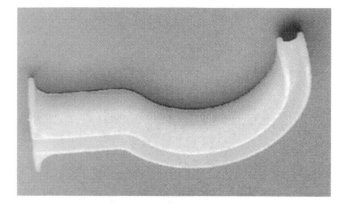

A

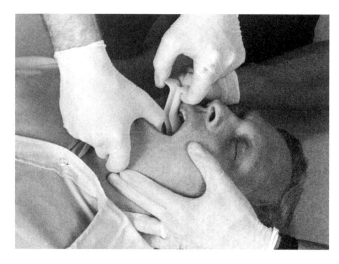

B

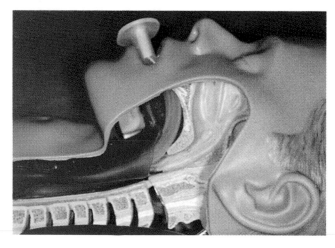

C

Figure 3-9 A, The oropharyngeal airway (OPA) is inserted into the mouth along the hard and soft palates. B, The airway is then slid into a position behind the tongue to support it and maintain an open airway. C, Once the airway is in place, the tongue is held forward and the patient can be adequately ventilated.

chin lift—pulls the mandible. The trauma jaw thrust and the trauma chin lift are modifications of the conventional jaw thrust and chin lift. The modifications allow the EMT to protect the cervical spine while opening the airway by removing the tongue from the posterior pharynx.

Mechanical Techniques: Artificial Airways

Assuring a patent airway is the first priority of trauma management and resuscitation, and nothing is more crucial in prehospital airway management than the appropriate assessment of the airway. When manual airway maneuvers are inadequate for correcting an anatomic airway obstruction, the use of artificial airways should be considered.

Basic Airways

Oropharyngeal airway The most commonly used artificial airway is the oropharyngeal airway (OPA) (Figure 3-9, A). The OPA may be inserted in either a "direct" or "inverted" fashion. Using the direct insertion approach, the OPA is inserted along the tongue until the teeth or gingiva obstruct further insertion (Figure 3-9, B). It then is positioned between the posterior pharynx and the root of the tongue, thus maintaining airway patency (Figure 3-9, C).

An alternate approach, "inverted" OPA insertion, is sometimes more easily accomplished. In this technique, the OPA is positioned so that the tip is inserted with the "point" of the device facing the roof of the patient's mouth. The EMT then slides the OPA along the roof, past the uvula or until resistance is encountered against the soft palate. The OPA is then rotated 180° to its position of function. As with all airway maneuvers, great care must be taken to avoid undue movement of the patient's neck. When using this technique, the EMT must take care to ensure that the tongue is not inadvertently pushed back into the throat. In some patients, this procedure is more easily accomplished when performed using a tongue blade to hold the tongue in position while the airway is inserted.

Regardless of the approach selected, prehospital personnel must always be mindful that the OPA often stimulates the oropharynx, and it will activate the gag reflex in conscious patients. Consequently, while the OPA usually will be well tolerated in unconscious patients, its use in conscious trauma patients may lead to gagging, vomiting, and laryngospasm.

Nasopharyngeal airway The primary advantage that the nasopharyngeal airway (NPA) has over the oropharyngeal airway (OPA) is that the NPA is better tolerated in fully conscious trauma patients or in those with an altered mental state. The NPA is a soft rubber (latex) device that is inserted through one of the nares and then along the curvature of the posterior wall of the nasopharynx and oropharynx (Figure 3-10). Bleeding may be a complication from insertion.

Advanced Airway: Endotracheal Intubation

Of all of the emergency and trauma care intervention skills performed by EMTs, endotracheal intubation is one of the most important because it can have a dramatic impact on a trauma patient's outcome (Figure 3-11). In most cases, the level of urgency will dictate the method of choice (i.e., orotracheal vs. nasotracheal).

The most important indication for electing to perform endotracheal intubation should be the EMT's inability to adequately ventilate the trauma patient with a standard bag-valve-mask (BVM) device or mouth-to-mask method. Another key determinant is the inability of the trauma patient to protect his or her own airway.

Endotracheal intubation is the most desirable method for achieving maximal control of the airway in trauma patients who are either apneic or require assisted ventilation. The head and neck must be immobilized in a neutral position. The nontrauma patient is often placed in a "sniffing" position to facilitate placement of the endotracheal tube (Figure 3-12). Because this position hyperextends the cervical spine at C1-C2, the second most common site for cervical spine fractures in the trauma patient, and hyperflexes it at C5-C6, the most common site for cervical spine fractures in the trauma patient, it cannot be used for trauma patients. The neck must be in the neutral position when the endotracheal tube is inserted.

In conscious trauma patients or in those with an intact gag reflex, endotracheal intubation may be difficult to accomplish and should only be attempted as a last resort. If spontaneous respirations are present, the EMT may choose to attempt a blind nasotracheal intubation. However, the patient must be breathing to ensure that the tube is positioned correctly through the vocal cords.

The EMT should decide whether to use this technique based on the patient's needs and on his or her ability to perform the skill. During the past few years, digital intubation and intubation with the aid of a lighted stylet and rapid sequence intubation using appropriate modification have been used by some EMS systems after they received the approval of local medical control committees.

Endotracheal intubation is the preferred method because it:

- isolates the airway
- allows for ventilation with 100% oxygen ($FiO_2 = 1.0$)
- eliminates the need to maintain an adequate mask-to-face seal
- prevents aspiration of vomitus, foreign material, or blood
- facilitates deep tracheal suctioning
- prevents gastric insufflation
- provides an additional route for medication administration
- provides positive ventilation control

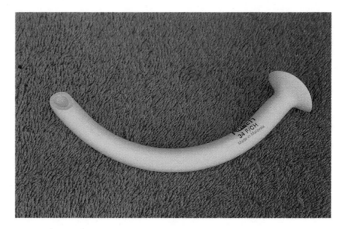

Figure 3-10 The nasopharyngeal airway goes through the nose but is placed far enough posterior to support the tongue and allow ventilation.

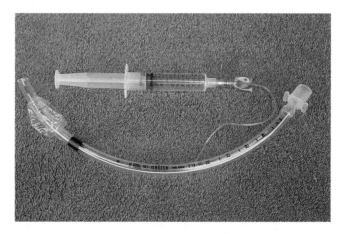

Figure 3-11 Endotracheal intubation allows direct control of the airway by placing a tube into the trachea.

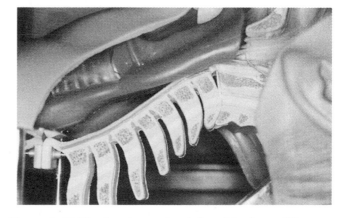

Figure 3-12 Placing the patient's head in the sniffing position provides ideal visualization of the larynx through the mouth. However, such positioning hyperextends the patient's neck at C1 and C2 and hyperflexes it at C5 and C6. These are the two most common points of fracture of the cervical spine.

As with any advanced life support skill, EMTs must have the proper equipment to accomplish this procedure. The standard components of an endotracheal airway kit should include the following:

- laryngoscope
- adult- and pediatric-size straight and curved blades
- adult- and pediatric-size endotracheal tubes
- stylet
- 10 ml syringe
- water-soluble lubricant
- Magill forceps
- adhesive tape or tube-securing device

The size and style of blade will depend on the type of patient and on the preference of the EMT who is performing the intubation.

The following is a brief overview of the endotracheal intubation technique; more detailed information is provided in Chapter 4: Airway Management and Ventilation Skills. The first step in performing endotracheal intubation is to ensure adequate ventilation with a bag-valve mask, using 100% oxygen. The patient should be hyperventilated for at least 15 to 30 seconds. It may be necessary to suction the airway before attempting the intubation. During these procedures, neutral in-line immobilization of the head and neck must be maintained.

The patient's mouth is opened with the fingers of the right hand. With the laryngoscope in the left hand, the blade is inserted into the right side of the patient's mouth, displacing the tongue to the left side. When the blade has reached the midline position, any additional pressure on the lips or teeth should be avoided. If the EMT is using a curved (MacIntosh) blade, the tip of the blade should be positioned in the space between the base of the tongue and the epiglottis (known as the vallecula). The tip of the straight (Miller or Flagg) blade directly covers the epiglottis. In either case, the glottic opening is exposed by lifting (not rotating) the laryngoscope handle. The mandible should be lifted anteriorly. An easy reminder is to lift in the direction the handle is pointing. Do not use any prying motion on the handle, and do not use the teeth as a fulcrum.

When the epiglottis and vocal cords are visible (see Figure 3-3), with the right hand, gently insert the endotracheal tube until the tube is at least 1 inch past the vocal cords. If a stylet has been used, it should now be withdrawn from the tube. The cuff must be inflated with enough air (<10 cc) to provide an adequate seal. Next, the chest should be auscultated over the lateral aspects of both lung fields and the epigastrium while the patient is ventilated by a bag-valve with 100% oxygen. Auscultation will identify correct or incorrect placement of the endotracheal tube. The presence of moisture or "fogging" in the endotracheal tube provides additional indication that a tube is properly placed. Gurgling sounds may indicate an esophageal intubation. If the esophagus has been intubated, the balloon cuff should be immediately deflated, the endotracheal tube removed, and the patient reoxy-

genated before another attempt is made. Another tool available to ensure proper placement and oxygenation is a CO_2 indicator. Throughout this procedure, the time from discontinuation of ventilation before intubation until resumption of ventilation after intubation should be no longer than 30 seconds.

Complications that may be encountered when performing endotracheal intubation include:

- hypoxemia from prolonged intubation attempts
- trauma to the airway
- right mainstem intubation
- esophageal intubation
- vomiting leading to aspiration
- loose or broken teeth
- avulsion of the vocal cords
- conversion of a cervical spine injury without neurologic deficit to a cervical spine injury with neurologic deficit

Verification of Endotracheal Tube Placement

Out-of-hospital endotracheal intubation (ETI) is often performed under adverse conditions and circumstances. For example, there are significant differences between attempting to intubate a 300-pound, head-injured vomiting male hanging upside-down in a cave and intubating the same patient in the comparatively controlled environment of an operating room. Yet, the importance of obtaining and maintaining a patent airway is equally critical in both situations.

Many options are available to verify endotracheal tube placement in the prehospital setting. Some are very simple and require only basic equipment and fundamental skills to accomplish. Others require more sophisticated equipment and/or advanced skills to be of value. Common examples include:

1. direct visualization of tube passing through the vocal cords
2. visualization of chest rising and falling during ventilation
3. fogging (water vapor condensation) in the ET tube on expiration
4. presence of bilateral breath sounds (auscultate laterally below the axilla)
5. absence of air sounds over the epigastrium
6. bulb or syringe aspiration
7. pulse oximetry
8. end-tidal capnometry
9. lighted stylette

Regardless of the methods selected and because none are 100% accurate, a minimum of two and preferably more devices/techniques should be used when the initial intubation occurs and following any movement of the patient. Findings from each technique/device used should be reflected in the patient's medical record. In any instance, if there is **any** question of proper placement, the endotracheal tube should be immediately removed and reinserted, with placement reverified.

Alternative Airway Maneuvers

Esophageal-Tracheal Tube (ETC) and Pharyngotracheal Lumen (PTL) Airways

The ETC and PTL airways are similar in structure in that both are double-lumen devices that are inserted blindly into the esophagus. After an assessment of proper placement has been made, the patient is ventilated through the appropriate opening. The primary reasons for developing these devices were to remedy the difficulty of effecting a proper face seal and to prevent the inadvertent tracheal intubations that have occurred with esophageal obturator and esophageal gastric tube airways. Obtaining and maintaining an adequate seal are problematic with PTL or similar airways, as well. In addition, there are no studies that have compared the effectiveness of the PTL with that of basic airway techniques. However, the complication rates for both the ETC and the PTL are low. Yet none of these devices afford the level of airway safety and control that is afforded by endotracheal intubation. For the most part, they are useful as interim measures for short-term airway support until endotracheal or surgical airway access can be obtained.

Laryngeal Mask Airway

The laryngeal mask airway (LMA) affords another alternative for unconscious or seriously obtunded adult and pediatric patients. The device consists of an inflatable silicone ring attached diagonally to a silicone tube. When inserted, the ring creates a low pressure seal between the LMA and the trachea without direct insertion of the device into the larynx.

Advantages of the LMA include the following:

- The device is designed for blind insertion. Direct visualization of the trachea/vocal cords is unnecessary.
- With proper cleaning and storage, the LMA may be reused multiple (generally up to 40–50) times.
- The device is only minimally stimulating to the upper airway and may be tolerated more easily by patients who are unduly stimulated by direct laryngoscopy.
- The LMA, unlike other devices of this type, is available in a range of sizes to accommodate both pediatric and adult patient groups.

Prehospital use of the LMA has thus far been more prevalent in Europe than in the United States. As the device is more widely accepted, its use will likely increase significantly. Limitations of the LMA include high initial acquisition cost, potential for laryngeal spasm, and an inability to completely prevent regurgitation and subsequent aspiration.

Esophageal Tracheal Double Lumen Airways (ETDLA)

Esophageal tracheal double lumen airways (ETDLA) provide EMTs with a functional alternative airway, particularly in instances where endotracheal intubation attempts are unsuccessful or as a "back-up" airway for rapid sequence intubation. The device may be used by EMT basic–level personnel and typically requires minimal training to achieve competency. The airway's greatest single advantage is that it may be inserted independent of the patient's position (i.e., "blindly" inserted), which may be especially important in trauma patients with high suspicion of cervical injury.

Indications The ETDLA may be considered when the following conditions are present in a patient:

1. unconscious with no purposeful response
2. age 16 years or older
3. absent gag reflex
4. height at least 5 feet
5. apnea or respiratory rate less than six per minute

Contraindications ETDLA should not be used when the following conditions exist in a patient:

1. intact gag reflex
2. age less than 16 years
3. height under 5 feet
4. known esophageal disease
5. caustic substances recently ingested

Insertion procedures

1. Provide respiratory support as needed. Use usual personal protective equipment (PPE) appropriate for intubation.
2. Inspect and prepare equipment.
3. Insert the ETDLA between ventilations.
4. If the patient is supine, lift the tongue and lower jaw upward with one hand. Be cautious to avoid tearing the ETDLA cuff when inserting past broken teeth or dental appliances.
5. Watch for the marker rings on the ETDLA to measure depth of insertion. The rings should be aligned with the teeth or alveolar rings.
6. Using the large syringe, inflate the pharyngeal cuff with 100 cc of air. The device should seat itself in the posterior pharynx just behind the hard palate.
7. Using the small syringe, inflate the distal cuff with 15 cc of air.
8. Typically the device will be placed in the patient's esophagus. Begin ventilation through the esophageal tube. If auscultation of breath sounds is positive and gastric insufflation is negative, continue ventilation.
9. If auscultation of breath sounds is negative, and gastric insufflation is positive, immediately ventilate via the shorter tracheal connector (generally marked with a #2). Reauscultate to affirm proper tube placement.

All esophageal airways are dependent on the patient having no gag reflex. If the patient regains consciousness, these devices must be removed immediately. Extubation of esophageal airways nearly always causes vomiting or regurgitation. Consequently, it is essential that suction equipment be readily available at the time the device is removed. Proper PPE should also be worn to avoid exposure/contamination of personnel.

Percutaneous Transtracheal Catheter Ventilation

In some rare instances, a trauma patient's airway obstruction is not relieved by the methods already discussed. In this situation, a needle tracheostomy may be performed using a percutaneous transtracheal catheter ventilation (PTV) procedure.

One of the advantages of the PTV is that the landmarks are easily accessible, and a needle can be inserted directly through the skin into the trachea. The needle is inserted caudally while negative pressure is maintained on the syringe. After the catheter is inserted correctly (air should be easily aspirated into the syringe), the metal stylette (needle) is removed, leaving the plastic catheter in place. An oxygen connecting tube fitted with two female connections from a 40 to 50 lbs/inch^2 gas source is then attached to the catheter for ventilation. A hole is cut in the side of the tubing. The caregiver's thumb occludes this opening for 1 second to provide lung inflation, and then he or she should remove the thumb for 4 seconds to allow passive deflation of the lungs. The ventilation ratio (measured in seconds) of inflation to deflation is 1:4. A gradual increase in the $PaCO_2$ may occur after 30 to 45 minutes of ventilating a trauma patient using this method. The types of equipment and procedures for the performance of this skill are detailed in Chapter 4: Airway Management and Ventilation Skills.

Advantages of PTV include:
- ease of access
- ease of insertion
- minimal equipment required
- no surgical procedures necessary
- minimal education required

Digital Intubation

Digital, or blind, intubation generally was a precursor to the current use of laryngoscopes for endotracheal intubation. Essentially, the intubator's fingers act in a fashion very similar to a laryngoscope blade by manipulating the epiglottis and acting as a guide for placement of the endotracheal tube. The technique can be used effectively when intubation equipment is in short supply, when the airway is obscured or blocked due to large volumes of blood or vomitus, when the laryngoscope fails, or when the patient is entrapped.

Complications/contraindications for digital intubation differ very little from those inherent to "normal" endotracheal intubation procedures. The most significant difference is in the level of attention which must be given to protecting the intubator's fingers from biting or laceration. This procedure should not be attempted without use of a dental clamp or bite stick to hold the patient's mouth open. As with any type of intubation

procedure, emergency personnel should wear appropriate PPE.

Retrograde Intubation

In the prehospital setting, retrograde tracheal intubation (RTI) is potentially useful because it is not impeded by blood or secretions that may hinder more common intubation methods. RTI, although comparatively time consuming, is a less invasive (and less risky) procedure than surgical cricothyrotomy when the neck is properly immobilized and naso- or orotracheal intubation attempts have failed.

RTI is actually a fairly straightforward procedure. Following administration of local anesthesia, an 18-gauge needle is inserted into the caudal aspect of the cricothyroid membrane. A guide wire is advanced through the needle into the oropharynx. The guide wire is then attached through the distal side hole of the ET tube. The neck end of the guide wire is then withdrawn to advance the tube into the trachea. Because it is often difficult to perform these procedures expediently, RTI is generally **not** recommended for use in apneic patients.

Surgical Cricothyrotomy

Surgical cricothyrotomy is a procedure that should be considered a "last resort" in prehospital airway management. Indications for this procedure include ongoing tracheobronchial hemorrhage, massive midface trauma, and inability to control the airway using less invasive maneuvers. Contraindications to the procedure include any patient who can be safely intubated either orally or nasally, patients with laryngotracheal injuries, small children under 10 years of age, and patients with acute laryngeal disease of traumatic or infectious origin. Common complications include prolonged execution time, hemorrhage, aspiration, misplacement or false passage of the endotracheal tube, injury to neck structures or vessels, and perforation of the esophagus. The use of this surgical airway in the prehospital arena is controversial. Excellent endotracheal intubation skills should minimize the need to even consider its use. Surgical cricothyrotomy should **never** be the initial airway control method utilized. Use of this procedure should only be considered when all other methods of airway control have been unsuccessful. There is insufficient data at this time to support a recommendation that surgical cricothyrotomy be established as a national standard for routine use for prehospital airway control. Local protocols should govern the implementation of surgical cricothyrotomy.

USING PARALYTIC AGENTS

Rapid sequence intubation (RSI) using paralytic agents may occasionally be required to facilitate endotracheal intubation of injured patients. In skilled hands, this technique can facilitate effective airway control when other methods fail or are otherwise not acceptable. To maximize the effectiveness of this procedure and to ensure patient safety, personnel using RSI must be familiar with all applicable local protocols, medications, and indications for use of the technique.

Indications for Rapid Sequence Intubation

Use of RSI is not without risk. Consequently, personnel trained in this technique must apply its use judiciously. RSI is a procedure of necessity, **not** convenience. Any patient who requires a stable airway and is difficult to intubate because of uncooperative behavior (as induced by hypoxia, closed head injury, hypotension, or intoxication) is a candidate for this procedure. The major complication with this procedure is a paralyzed patient and inability to insert the ET tube.

Contraindications for RSI

As with any medical procedure there are circumstances where utilization of RSI may be inadvisable or inappropriate.

Relative contraindications:

1. alternative (i.e.: multi-lumen blind insertion) airway is available
2. severe facial trauma that would impair or preclude successful intubation
3. neck deformity or swelling that complicates or precludes placement of a surgical airway
4. known allergies to RSI medications
5. medical problems that would preclude use of RSI medications

Sample Protocol

1. Assure availability of required equipment.
   a. oxygen supply
   b. bag-valve-mask of appropriate size/type
   c. non-rebreather mask
   d. laryngoscope with blades
   e. endotracheal tubes
   f. surgical/alternative airway equipment
   g. RSI medications
   h. materials or devices to secure the ET tube following placement
2. A minimum of one, but preferably two patent IV lines must be present.
3. Hyperoxygenate the patient via the non-rebreathing bag-mask (NRBM) or by mask with 100% O_2. Hyperoxygenation for 3 to 4 minutes is preferred.
4. Apply cardiac and pulse oximetry monitors.
5. If patient is conscious, use of sedative agents should be strongly considered.

6. Administration of sedative agents and lidocaine should be considered in the presence of potential or confirmed closed head injury.
7. Following administration of paralytic agents, the Sellig (cricoid pressure) maneuver should be used to decrease the potential for aspiration.
8. Tube placement must be confirmed immediately following intubation. Continuous electrocardiogram (ECG) and pulse oximeter monitoring is required following RSI. Tube placement should be reconfirmed periodically throughout transport and each time the patient is moved.
9. Repeat doses of paralytic agents may be used as needed to maintain paralysis.

Procedure

1. Assemble required equipment.
2. Assure patency of IV lines(s).
3. Hyperoxygenate the patient (3 to 4 minutes).
4. Place patient on ECG, pulse oximeter monitors.
5. Administer sedative if appropriate. Versed 0.05 mg/kg, 2 to 3 minutes prior to paralytic.
6. In presence of confirmed or potential CHI, administer Lidocaine 1 mg/kg, 2 to 3 minutes prior to paralytic agent.
7. Atropine 0.01 mg/kg may be given to pediatric patients 1 to 3 minutes prior to paralytic administration to preclude muscular fasciculation.
8. Administer Succinylcholine IV

   adult:　　　1 to 1.5 mg/kg
   pediatric:　1.5 to 2 mg/kg
   (Paralysis and relaxation should occur within 30 seconds.)

9. Place ET tube. If initial attempts are unsuccessful, repeat attempts should be preceded by hyperoxygenation.
10. Confirm tube placement.
11. If repetitive attempts to achieve ET intubation fail, placement of an alternative or surgical airway should be considered.
12. Additional doses of vecuronium may be used to continue paralysis.

    initial dose:　　　　0.05 mg/kg IV push
    subsequent doses:　0.01 mg/kg/15 min.

Drugs

Succinylcholine

Succinylcholine (Anectine) is a depolarizing agent that is rapidly metabolized by the body and has a very short duration of action, thus making it ideal for rapid sequence intubation. When the drug is administered, muscular fasciculation will occur, and there will be an increase in intra-abdominal pressure (leading to the possibility of regurgitation). Often intracranial pressure increases, too.

Primary indication is endotracheal intubation when paralysis is required.

1. Contraindications:
   a. patients who could be difficult to ventilate after paralysis
      1. patients with epiglottitis
      2. patients with upper airway obstruction
   b. patients with known cholinesterase deficiencies
   c. patients with hyperkalemia from any cause
   d. patients with penetrating injuries to the globe (A rise in intraocular pressure often occurs after administration of Succinylcholine.)
   e. patients with a history of malignant hyperthermia
2. Relative contraindications:
   a. massive burns (These patients may experience an increase in potassium two to three days **after** the burn.)
   b. massive crush injuries
   c. chronic neurologic or muscular illnesses such as muscular dystrophy, paralysis, etc.
3. Adverse reactions secondary to the administration of the Succinylcholine include:
   a. tachycardia or bradycardia
   b. nausea and vomiting
   c. muscle pain and spasm

Dosage of Succinylcholine is 1.5 milligrams per kilogram IV push. An adequate dose for a normal sized adult is usually 100 milligrams. Pediatric dosage is 1.5 to 2 milligrams per kilogram IV push. If a repeat dosage of Succinylcholine is required, the dose is 1 to 1.5 milligrams per kilogram. There is a higher incidence of hyperkalemia and bradycardia with repeat usage of Succinylcholine. Paralysis occurs within 30 seconds to 1 minute after the IV dose. Duration of paralysis is 4 to 6 minutes after the initial dose.

Vecuronium (Norcuron)

Vecuronium (Norcuron) is a non-depolarizing agent that is useful to maintain paralysis after intubation and can also be used for rapid sequence intubation if there is a contraindication for Succinylcholine. The onset of action is somewhat slower than that of Succinylcholine with paralysis beginning 1 to 2 minutes after the IV dose. The duration of action for this drug is much longer than for Succinylcholine.

Contraindication—patients who are difficult to intubate after paralysis due to the following:
1. epiglottitis
2. upper airway obstruction
3. myasthenia gravis

Dosage of Vecuronium when used as a primary paralytic is 0.10 milligrams per kilogram IV push. The dose for children is the same as the dose for adults. Paralysis oc-

curs within 1 to 2 minutes after initiation of the IV dosage. Paralysis generally lasts 25 to 35 minutes after IV administration. The only complication known with Vecuronium is the inability to intubate the patient.

Continuous Quality Improvement

All out-of-hospital uses of RSI medications and/or techniques should be individually reviewed by the service medical director or his or her designate. Specific points should include:

1. adherence to protocol/procedures
2. proper indications for use of paralytic medications
3. proper documentation of drug dosage routes and monitoring of patient during and after RSI
4. confirmation of tube placement procedures
5. outcome/complications

Medical directors should closely monitor each use of RSI, including indication and success rate. Refresher training for RSI should not exceed intervals of 6 months.

SUCTIONING

A trauma patient with or without an artificial airway may not be capable of effectively removing the buildup of secretions, vomitus, blood, or foreign objects from his trachea. Providing suction for this patient is as important as stabilizing the airway with one of the artificial devices already discussed.

The most significant complication is that suctioning for prolonged periods of time will produce hypoxemia that may manifest as a cardiac abnormality, such as initial tachycardia without dysrhythmia. Preoxygenating the trauma patient will help to prevent hypoxemia. In addition, during an extended period of suctioning, cardiac dysrhythmia may occur from arterial hypoxemia leading to myocardial hypoxemia and vagal stimulation secondary to tracheal irritation. True vagal stimulation may lead to profound bradycardia and hypotension.

The suction catheter should be made of soft material to limit trauma to the tracheal mucosa and to minimize frictional resistance. It must be long enough to pass the tip of the artificial airway (20 to 22 inches) and should have smooth ends to prevent mucosal trauma. The soft catheter will probably not be effective in suctioning copious amounts of foreign material or fluid from a trauma patient, and in this case the device of choice will be one with a tonsil-tip design.

While suctioning a patient, sterile procedure is vital, and the following basic technique should be implemented. First, the EMT should ensure that the trauma patient is adequately preoxygenated with 100% oxygen. Next, the catheter is inserted without suction. Aspiration is continued for 15 to 30 seconds. Finally, the patient is reoxygenated and ventilated for at least 5 assisted ventilations.

OXYGENATION AND VENTILATION OF THE TRAUMA PATIENT

By this point, it should be very clear that aggressive airway management and supplemental oxygen delivery are vitally important to obtaining desirable patient outcomes following injury. At the same time, it is helpful to review the pharmacokinetic implications of excess cellular oxygenation (**hyperoxia**) and more importantly, inadequate cellular oxygenation, or **hypoxia.**

Under normal circumstances, oxygen is quite possibly the safest drug to administer to most medical and trauma patients. Patients with severe chronic obstructive pulmonary disease (COPD) are a notable exception, however. These patients may stop breathing if abnormally high (from their baseline) FiO_2 levels are present. Although certainly an issue of concern, cessation of breathing is manageable through use of a variety of airway maneuvers and devices. In the injured patient, increasing FiO_2 is a more vital concern than maintaining an already suspect respiratory drive. Consequently, supplemental oxygen should not be withheld from these patients because respiratory arrest could result.

The **oxygenation process** within the human body involves three phases: external respiration, blood oxygen transport, and internal respiration. **External respiration** is the transfer of oxygen molecules from the atmosphere to the blood. All alveolar oxygen exists as free gas. Therefore, each oxygen molecule exerts pressure. Increasing the percentage of oxygen in the inspired atmosphere will obviously increase alveolar oxygen tension. Oxygen available from ventilation at the alveolar level is a factor of inspired volume multiplied by the respiratory rate per minute multiplied by the percentage of inspired air.

Blood oxygen transport is the result of an oxygen transfer from the atmosphere to the red blood cell during ventilation and the transportation of these RBCs to the tissues via the vascular system. This process primarily involves cardiac output, hemoglobin concentration, and hemoglobin oxygen affinity. The volume of oxygen consumed by the body in 1 minute is known as **oxygen consumption.** In a sense, one could describe the RBCs as the body's "oxygen tankers." These tankers move along the vascular system "highways" to "off-load" their supply of oxygen at the body's distribution points, the capillary beds. Because the actual exchange of oxygen between the red blood cells and the tissues occurs in these thin-walled structures, oxygen available for consumption will be decreased if FiO_2 is low (interruption in supply) or if circulation to the capillary beds is compromised (road blocked). The tissues simply cannot consume adequate amounts of oxygen if adequate amounts of oxygen are not available. This movement, or diffusion, of oxygen between the RBCs into the tissue cells is known as **internal respiration.**

Adequate oxygenation depends on external respiration, oxygen blood transport, and internal respiration. While the ability to assess tissue oxygenation in prehospital situations is improving rapidly, it is still vitally important that all trauma patients receive appropriate ventilatory support with supplemental oxygen to try and insure that hypoxia is corrected or averted entirely. In deciding which method or equipment to use, prehospital personnel should consider the following devices and their respective oxygen concentrations (Table 3-1).

Pulse Oximetry

Over the past few years, pulse oximetry has become regarded as a "fourth vital sign." Appropriate use of pulse oximetry devices allows prehospital caregivers to detect early pulmonary compromise or cardiovascular deterioration before overt physical signs are detectable. Pulse oximeters are particularly useful for prehospital applications due to their high reliability, portability, ease of application, and applicability across all age ranges and races.

Table 3-1 Ventilatory devices and oxygen concentration

Device procedure	Liter flow (LPM)	Oxygen concentration*
Without Supplemental Oxygen		
Mouth-to-mouth	N/A	16%
Mouth-to-mask	N/A	16%
Bag-valve-mask	N/A	21%
With Supplemental Oxygen		
Nasal cannula	1–6	24%–26%
Mouth-to-mask	10	50%
Simple face mask	8–10	40%–60%
BVM without reservoir	8–10	40%–60%
Partial rebreather mask	6	60%
Simple mask with reservoir	6	60%
BVM with reservoir	10–15	90%–100%
Non-rebreather mask with reservoir	10–15	90%–100%
Demand valve	Source	90%–100%

*Percentages indicated are approximate.

Pulse oximeters provide spot measurements of arterial oxyhemoglobin saturation (SpO_2) and pulse rate. SpO_2 is determined by measuring the absorption ratio of red and infrared light passed through tissue. Changes in light absorption caused by the pulsation of blood through vascular beds are correlated by a small microprocessor to determine arterial saturation and pulse rate. Normal SpO_2 is between 93% and 95%. When SpO_2 falls below 90%, severe compromise of oxygen delivery to the tissues is most likely present.

To ensure accurate pulse oximetry readings, it is important that caregivers follow these general guidelines:

1. Use the appropriate size and type of sensor.
2. Ensure proper alignment of sensor light.
3. Ensure that sources and photodetectors are clean, dry, and in good repair.
4. Avoid sensor placement on grossly edematous sites.
5. Cover the sensor sites with an opaque material in the presence of bright sunlight or room lighting.

Common problems that can produce inaccurate SpO_2 measurement include:

1. excessive motion
2. moisture in SpO_2 sensors
3. improper sensor application/placement
4. poor patient perfusion
5. anemia
6. venous pulsations

It has been noted that pulse oximetry is a "spot," or point in time, measurement of SpO_2. In this respect, it is similar to the monitoring of other so-called vital signs. While no significant findings may be detected at a given point, the trend of measurements may portend upcoming catastrophe. To this end, pulse oximetry can be a valuable addition to the prehospital responder's "tool box," when combined/integrated with a thorough knowledge of trauma pathophysiology and strong assessment and intervention skills.

Ventilatory Devices

Masks

Regardless of which mask is chosen to support ventilation of the trauma patient, several issues must be considered. The ideal mask has a good fit; is equipped with a one-way valve; is made of a transparent material; has an oxygen insufflation port (15 to 22 mm); and is available in infant, pediatric, and adult sizes.

Mouth-to-mask ventilation most satisfactorily delivers adequate tidal volumes by ensuring a tight face seal even when performed by those who do not use the skill very often. Mouth-to-mouth ventilation is the technique of choice for the EMT who is acting without additional support.

Bag-Valve-Mask

The bag-valve-mask (BVM) consists of a self-inflating bag and a non-rebreathing device; it can be used in conjunction with basic or advanced artificial airways. Most of the BVM devices currently on the market have a volume of 1600 cc and can deliver up to approximately 90% to 100% oxygen concentration. However, a single EMT attempting to ventilate with a BVM will create only poor tidal volumes because it is difficult to create a tight face seal and squeeze the bag adequately. An EMT must continually practice this skill to ensure that his or her technique is effective so that the trauma patient receives adequate ventilatory support.

Manually Triggered (Oxygen-Powered) Devices

Manually triggered devices are easy to use and can deliver oxygen concentrations of 90% to 100%. Because the EMT cannot feel compliance of the chest during the ventilation process, he or she must take care not to overinflate the lung. Maintaining a tight face seal with this device is easy because the trigger mechanism requires only one hand to operate. Problems may include gastric distension, lack of tactile feel for inflation, overinflation of the lung, barotrauma, and lung rupture. These devices should not be used in the field except in very unusual circumstances.

• Summary •

1. Recognition of respiratory insufficiency and airway instability are of prime importance in the prehospital care of injured patients.
2. Regardless of the techniques or devices used, aggressive airway management must always be the highest care priority for the EMT.
3. The quality and timeliness of airway care administered in the field directly affects long-term outcome and length of stay at the hospital.
4. Prehospital care providers must continuously practice airway intervention techniques and stay abreast of new techniques and airway control devices.

Scenario Solution

Physical evidence at the scene (impact damage to the car, motorcycle, and helmet) suggest that the rider has likely been subjected to kinetic forces capable of creating life-threatening injuries. The position of the patient suggests that multiple impacts have occurred. It is also important that the female driver be medically assessed and treated as required, even though no injury is readily apparent.

The motorcycle driver exhibits several signs of airway compromise and ventilatory insufficiency. His respirations are sonorous and irregular, he has an altered level of consciousness, and he requires frequent suctioning. Bleeding from the nares and ears, coupled with early presence of "raccoon eyes," strongly suggest the presence of a basilar skull fracture. The initial assessment indicates a rapidly deteriorating patient who requires aggressive airway care and rapid transport.

It is understandable that law enforcement authorities are concerned with reestablishing normal traffic patterns quickly, particularly considering the time of day. This desire cannot override patient care considerations, however. Assure the officer that the necessary interventions should proceed quickly and that all efforts will be made to clear the scene as rapidly as possible.

First Responder personnel should already be administering oxygen in conjunction with respiratory assistance via BVM. If this has not been done, oxygen therapy should begin immediately. Ventilatory support and cervical spine immobilization should continue while preparations for endotracheal intubation are made. EMS personnel must be careful to assure that the airway remains clear and that manual ventilations are effective.

The patient should be orally intubated with an appropriately sized endotracheal tube. Cervical spine immobilization must continue before, during, and after the intubation attempt. Once placed, it is important to assure proper positioning of the endotracheal tube via auscultation of breath sounds, the use of an esophageal intubation detector, or end tidal capnometry (if available). The patient should be throughly suctioned before transport and as often as needed thereafter.

After the patient is completely immobilized and the tracheal tube secured, transport should be initiated without delay. Intravenous (IV) access may be established while the patient is en route to a trauma receiving facility. Care must be taken to maintain the effectiveness of immobilization efforts and to frequently reassess the patient's condition. To insure proper activation of the hospital's trauma response, early notification from the scene or during transport is necessary. Upon arrival at the trauma center, it is important that all pertinent information regarding the incident, the patient, and your medical interventions are concisely conveyed to the receiving physician or other appropriate trauma team member.

Review Questions

Answers provided on page 333.

1 The most common cause of airway obstruction in unconscious patients is:
A flaccid tongue blocking the hypopharynx
B crush injury to trachea
C foreign body obstruction
D edema of the vocal cords

2 Which of the following manual airway maneuvers is **not** recommended for use on trauma patients?
A trauma mandible lift
B trauma jaw thrust
C head tilt, chin lift
D trauma chin lift

3 The first priority of trauma management and resuscitation is:
A assuring scene safety
B rapid completion of primary patient survey
C ensuring a patent airway
D control of external hemorrhage

4 _____ is the most desirable method of achieving maximum control of the airway for trauma patients who are apneic or require assisted ventilation.
A The pharyngeal lumen (PTL) airway
B Endotracheal intubation
C An oral airway
D Percutaneous transtracheal catheter ventilation (PTLV)

5 Potential complications of endotracheal intubation include:
A esophageal intubation
B hypoxemia from prolonged intubation attempts
C conversion of cervical injury without neurologic deficit to a cervical spine injury with neurologic deficits
D all of the above

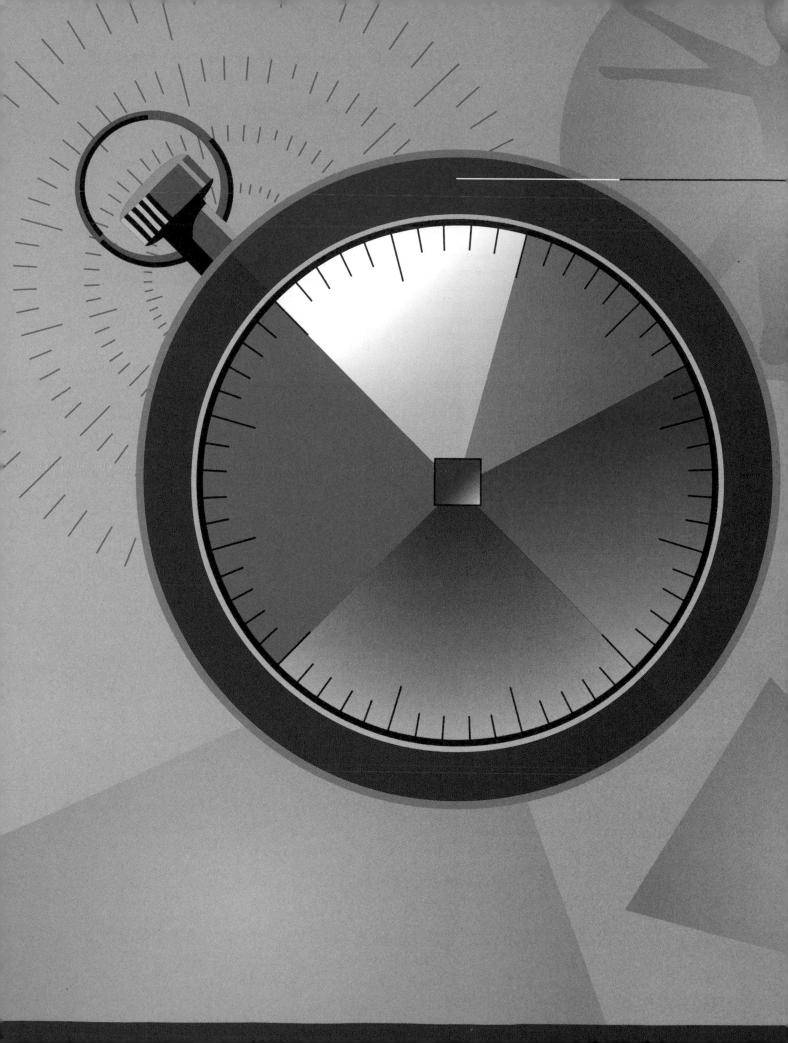

CHAPTER 4

Airway Management and Ventilation Skills

irway management and ventilation are the highest priorities in the management of both trauma and medical patients. Mastery of individual airway and ventilation skills, including selecting the best method(s) to meet the patient's needs, is a paramount responsibility for any EMT in providing proper patient care. This chapter presents a wide variety of skills and techniques oriented to the care of the trauma patient. Detailed discussions of airway management, ventilation, oxygenation, and respiratory and ventilatory anatomy, physiology, and pathophysiology are contained in Chapter 3: Airway Management and Ventilation and Chapter 5: Thoracic Trauma.

The most common airway and ventilation methods (chin lift, bag-valve-mask ventilation, endotracheal intubation, etc.) involve moving the patient's head and/or neck. Moving the patient's head usually requires hyperextension and anterior movement of the head into a "sniffing" position. In trauma patients, these methods must be modified in two ways. First, since hyperextension are contraindicated, the EMT must be able to perform airway management and ventilation with the patient's head maintained in a neutral in-line position. Second, manual immobilization must be provided and maintained throughout to avoid movement of the patient's spine. Therefore, recognizing the possibility of an unstable spine in a trauma patient and providing proper spine protection are key ingredients in providing proper airway management and ventilatory care for trauma patients. When ventilation and airway management are required after the patient has been mechanically immobilized to the longboard or other rigid immobilization device, manual immobilization should be provided to protect against the movement that naturally occurs during manual airway maneuvers such as inserting an airway or maintaining a mask seal.

Airway management and ventilation skills for trauma patients are best done with two EMTs: one to maintain the neutral in-line immobilization of the neck and head and one to actually perform the airway or ventilation skill. The techniques and skills in this chapter are first presented showing the positions and roles for each of the two EMTs. Some of the skills shown can be modified to allow a single EMT to maintain in-line immobilization and simultaneously manage the airway and/or provide ventilation. These modifications are noted at the end of the presentation of the two-EMT method. When these skills are performed by one EMT, however, the risk of moving the head and neck is increased, and the effectiveness of the ventilation is limited. Therefore, use of single-operator techniques should be limited to those maneuvers that can be properly done by a single EMT. In addition, single-EMT maneuvers should be used only when required by limited resources or unusual circumstances.

MANUAL IMMOBILIZATION

Manual in-line immobilization of the spine patient during airway and ventilation maneuvers can best be provided by the EMT from one of two positions: (1) kneeling or lying beyond the patient's head (facing down along the patient's body) or (2) from a kneeling position next to the patient's midtorso (facing the patient's head). The EMT providing the manual immobilization should be positioned to provide the least interference or the best assistance to the EMT who is managing the airway or ventilating the patient.

MANUAL IMMOBILIZATION FROM ABOVE THE PATIENT'S HEAD ————

When providing manual immobilization to a patient who is on the ground, the EMT lies beyond the patient's head as shown in Figure 4-1. When necessary, immobilization can also be done in a kneeling position; however, more stable immobilization can be provided when lying down with both elbows on the ground.

The patient's head is held between the EMT's hands and brought into an in-line position. The thumbs are placed in the maxillary notch on each side of the nose, and the little finger or last two fingers are placed under the posterior lower head. The remaining fingers are spread (pointing in a generally caudad direction) on the flat lateral planes at each side of the head.

Pressure between the thumbs and the finger(s) under the posterior lower head prevents flexion or hyperextension of the neck, and pressure between the remaining fingers at the sides of the head prevents lateral movement or sideway rotation. Once the head is immobilized in this manner, the second EMT can perform a trauma chin lift or

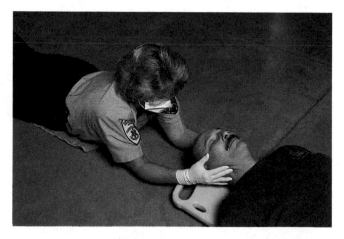

Figure 4-1 EMT provides manual immobilization by lying above the patient's head.

ventilate the patient without producing unwanted movement of the head and neck.

When ventilation is to be done with any resuscitator that involves a mask, a slight change in hand position will allow the EMT providing the immobilization from above the patient's head to also hold the mask. In this way, the EMT can ensure a good mask seal, properly elevate the chin, and maintain the head immobilization at the same time. The second EMT is then free to ensure that adequate ventilations are provided. Figure 4-2 shows a variation using three EMTs. This technique is covered in more detail in the following section on specific skills.

In those patients in whom neutral in-line positioning produces a significant space between the back of the head and the ground, suitable padding should be inserted as early as possible. Padding this space makes the task of the EMT at the head easier and reduces the chance that obtaining a mask seal will cause movement of the head.

When the patient is elevated on a cot, the same method of immobilization can be used by standing above the head end of the cot.

MANUAL IMMOBILIZATION FROM BESIDE THE PATIENT

Manual immobilization of the spine from alongside the patient is similar to immobilization from above the patient's head. When done from the patient's side, however, the fingers point cephalad instead of caudally. The EMT positions himself or herself at the patient's midtorso, angled so that he or she faces the patient's head with one knee almost touching the patient.

The thumbs are placed on each cheek below the zygoma in the maxillary notch. The little fingers (or last two fingers) are placed under the back of the lower one-third

of the head. The remaining fingers are spread on the flat lateral planes at the sides of the head (Figure 4-3). Forearms resting on the clavicle provide unit immobilization of the head, neck, and upper torso.

If padding is needed behind the head, it should be inserted as soon as possible. Providing immobilization from this position leaves the area above the patient's head free for airway management and ventilation.

BODY SUBSTANCE ISOLATION PRECAUTIONS

It is almost impossible for the EMT to avoid contact with blood and other body fluids while examining and treating a trauma patient. Rubber gloves, eye protection, and other protective clothing suitable to the particular situation should be applied prior to any patient contact. It is particularly important while providing airway management, suctioning, and ventilation to make sure that rubber gloves do not become torn and that proper eye protection is worn.

Given present-day standards and conditions, it is an unnecessary risk for on-duty EMTs to provide mouth-to-mouth or mouth-to-nose ventilation. Airway kits or personal equipment should include either a mask with a one-way valve or a bag-valve-mask device. (All references to mouth-to-mask ventilation in this text mean "mouth to a one-way valve connected to a mask." A one-way valve is required as an infection control precaution.) These devices should be used in place of methods that do not provide proper protection against contact with exhaled sputum, blood, or other body fluids.

Although the question is still under study of whether absolute protection can be provided by the valves in this equipment, the current literature clearly indicates that the

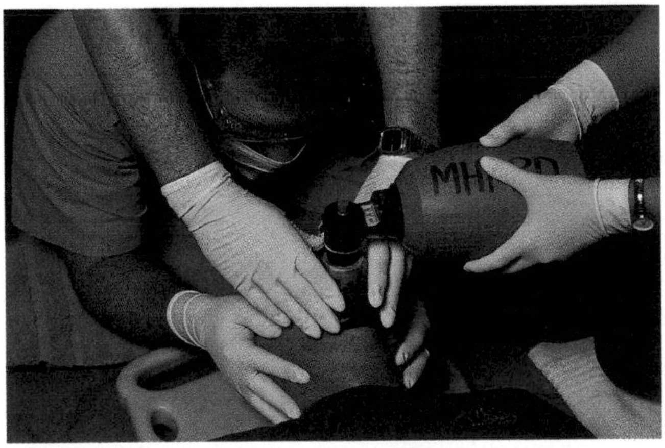

Figure 4-2 One EMT provides mask and seal and jaw elevation while the second EMT maintains head immobilization. A third EMT bags with both hands.

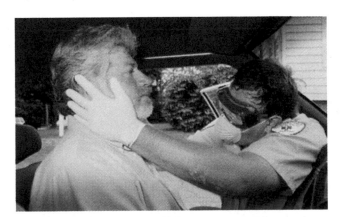

Figure 4-3 EMT holding manual in-line immobilization from the side.

inclusion of such a valve is essential in contributing to the EMT's safety. At present, insufficient scientific proof exists to conclude that thin shield or filter membranes constitute a safe infection control practice when providing mouth-to-mouth ventilation. Therefore, their use at this time is not recommended.

GENERAL SEQUENCE OF MANAGEMENT

The sequence in which the EMT selects and applies different skills or techniques to manage the patient's airway and ensure adequate ventilation varies from patient to patient based on the patient's needs.

An alert, talking, trauma patient with a patent airway and adequate spontaneous ventilation can usually be managed with the provision of a high FiO_2 by a non-rebreather reservoir mask. A nonbreathing, unconscious patient requires insertion of an airway adjunct and artificial ventilation. A conscious patient with inadequate ventilation needs assisted ventilation and supplemental oxygen.

The overall sequence for an unresponsive, nonbreathing patient appears simple: open the airway, provide ventilation, and then address other priorities. The variety of different techniques and equipment available—each with different specific advantages and disadvantages—requires the EMT to understand a more detailed general sequence for ventilatory resuscitation.

- First, provide manual in-line immobilization of the head and neck when head or spine trauma is suspected, manually open the airway and, as needed, provide hyperventilation with mouth-to-mask or a bag-valve-mask (BVM). Do not delay for oxygen hookup or more complex equipment.
- Second, identify and resolve any airway obstruction, abdominal distention, or thoracic condition(s) that may interfere with adequate ventilation. Suction as needed.
- Third, once the patient is being hyperventilated, insert an oropharyngeal (OPA) or nasopharyngeal airway (NPA) and add high-flow oxygen and a reservoir, or switch to other equipment that ventilates with a high FiO_2.
- Fourth, if indicated and when properly trained personnel are present, perform endotracheal intubation using an accepted trauma technique.
- Lastly, every 3 to 4 minutes, reevaluate the quality of ventilation, check the level of oxygenation (by pulse, skin, and changes in level of consciousness), and watch for return of adequate spontaneous ventilation.

The need for additional assessment, bleeding control, chest compressions, pneumatic antishock garment usage, and other activities have purposely not been included in this sequence. The urgent initial patient management is a team effort involving several EMTs. This discussion focuses on the priorities of the EMT(s) responsible for airway and ventilation; another EMT should simultaneously meet the patient's other needs.

The individual skills presented in the following pages need to be applied using this general sequence, in the context of the patient's other priorities and the resources available to the EMT.

TRAUMA JAW THRUST

In both the trauma jaw thrust and the trauma chin lift, while manual neutral in-line immobilization of the head is maintained, the mandible is moved anteriorly and slightly caudad (pushed in the case of the trauma jaw thrust and pulled in the case of the trauma chin lift). This maneuver moves the tongue forward, away from the airway, and holds the mouth slightly open.

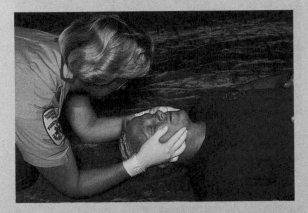

Figure 4-4A

1 From a position above the patient's head, the EMT moves the patient's neck and head into a neutral in-line position (Figure 4-4A). When a single EMT maintains neutral head immobilization from behind the patient, the fourth and fifth digits of both hands are positioned to perform a trauma jaw thrust.

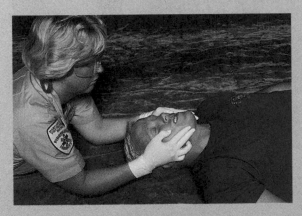

Figure 4-4B

2 While maintaining immobilization, the angle of the mandible at each side is pushed anteriorly by the fourth and fifth fingers until the lower jaw is extended (Figure 4-4B). The mandible is then lifted while maintaining head support.

OR

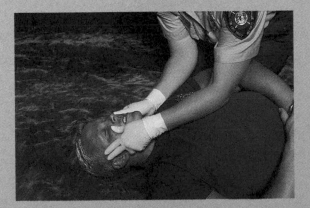

Figure 4-4C

The trauma jaw thrust can also be performed from alongside the patient. The EMT's fingers point cephalad rather than caudad (Figure 4-4C). The alternate position is to perform the trauma jaw thrust from the side of the patient's chest.

Note: The trauma jaw thrust represents the most practical way for a single EMT to simultaneously maintain an open airway and head immobilization without the use of an airway adjunct.

TRAUMA CHIN LIFT

1 One EMT (from above the head) moves the patient's head into a neutral in-line position and maintains manual immobilization (Figure 4-5A). EMT #1 maintains neutral head support of an unconscious trauma patient, while EMT #2 prepares to perform a trauma chin lift.

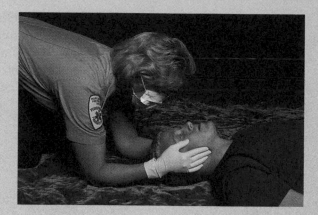

Figure 4-5A

2 The second EMT grasps the chin at the midline between her thumb and first two fingers. The first two fingers hook under the mandible (Figure 4-5B). EMT #2 inserts her index finger and thumb to perform a trauma chin lift. While the first EMT keeps the head from moving, the second EMT pulls the chin anteriorly and slightly caudad, elevating the mandible and opening the mouth as shown.

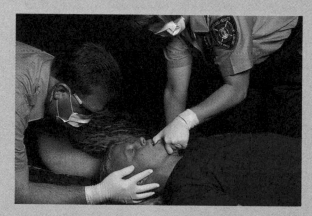

Figure 4-5B

OROPHARYNGEAL AIRWAY: TONGUE-JAW LIFT INSERTION METHOD

The oropharyngeal airway (OPA) is placed superior to the tongue, holding it anteriorly out of the pharynx. Airways come in a variety of sizes. The proper size should be selected to ensure that a patent airway is provided. *Use of an oropharyngeal airway is contraindicated in patients who have an intact gag reflex.*

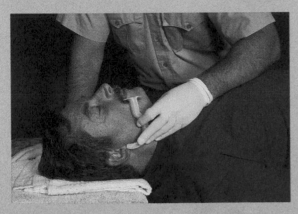

Figure 4-6A

1 One EMT maintains neutral in-line immobilization of the patient's head and maintains the open airway with a jaw thrust. The second EMT selects and measures an OPA. The acceptable method for measuring the size of the airway is shown in Figure 4-6A. The distance from the lower ear to the corner of the mouth is a good estimate. EMT #1 holds the patient's head, while EMT #2 measures the OPA from the corner of the mouth to the lower ear.

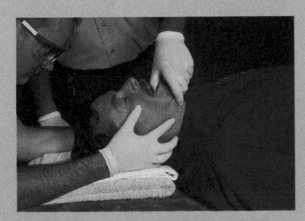

Figure 4-6B

2 After confirming that the patient is unconscious, the second EMT inserts his or her thumb into the patient's mouth and holds the tongue against the lower palate (Figure 4-6B). The lower jaw is elevated simultaneously, keeping the tongue out of the way. This maneuver is called a tongue-jaw lift. The tongue-jaw lift is helpful when inserting any airway into the mouth as it ensures that the device passes superior to the tongue. Otherwise, the device could push the tongue into the pharynx and obstruct the airway. EMT #1 holds the patient's head, while EMT #2 does the tongue-jaw lift with his left hand.

3 The oropharyngeal airway is held at a right angle to the long axis of the body, with the distal tip pointing posteriorly and slightly laterally. The distal tip should not "catch" the tongue as it is inserted (Figure 4-6C). The EMT performs the initial insertion at 90° from midline.

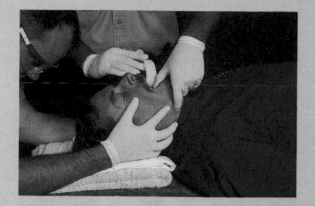

Figure 4-6C

4 The airway is advanced into the oropharynx, allowing it to turn medially toward the midline of the patient's body (Figure 4-6D). As it is inserted further, the OPA tends to follow the normal anatomical curve of the patient's airway. If the patient gags at any time during insertion of an OPA, stop at that point and immediately withdraw it. When halfway in, the OPA is almost in-line with the midline of the patient's body.

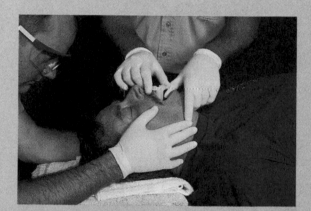

Figure 4-6D

5 Continue inserting the airway until the flanged end lies just anterior to the lips. The EMT providing manual immobilization moves his or her ring and index fingers (second and third fingers) under the curve of the mandible (Figure 4-6E). This modified chin lift used after an OPA has been inserted maintains the proper mouth position and helps to keep the airway in place. It also supports the mandible in the slightly elevated position needed to obtain a proper mask seal.

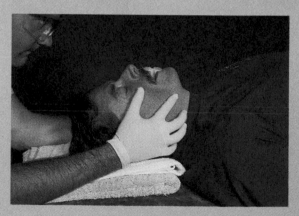

Figure 4-6E

OROPHARYNGEAL AIRWAY: TONGUE BLADE INSERTION METHOD

An OPA can be inserted using a tongue blade instead of using the previously described method employing the tongue-jaw lift. The tongue blade insertion method is safer for the EMT because it eliminates the possibility of accidental tearing or puncturing of gloves or the skin by sharp, pointed, or broken teeth. It also eliminates the possibility of being bitten if the patient's level of unconsciousness is not as deep as previously assessed or if any seizure activity occurs.

Note: Keep tongue blades in the airway kit to avoid any additional delay in locating a tongue blade for this option.

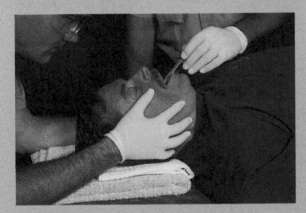

Figure 4-7A

1 While the head is immobilized in a neutral position and a trauma jaw thrust is maintained by EMT #1, EMT #2 kneels at the side of the patient's head, facing caudally. EMT #2 firmly grasps a tongue blade in one hand and a correctly sized OPA in the other hand. While visualizing the mouth, EMT #2 carefully inserts the tongue blade at an angle (the distal end being more cephalad than the held proximal end), superior to the tongue until it is at a depth just beyond half the tongue's length. In Figure 4-7A, EMT #1 continues to hold the head with the trauma jaw thrust. EMT #2 is preparing to insert the tongue blade (distal tip is slightly cephalad).

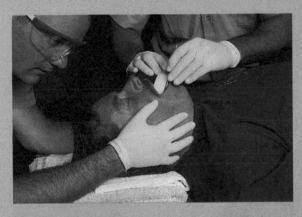

Figure 4-7B

2 The tongue blade is then rotated so that the distal tip is more caudad than the held proximal end, which elevates the tongue against the lower palate (Figure 4-7B). Next, EMT #2 slightly extends and lifts the arm holding the tongue blade to elevate the mandible and open the mouth more. The OPA is held just below the flange and in alignment with the midline of the patient's body; its distal end points posteriorly into the open mouth. In the photo, the tongue blade has been inserted, and the OPA is held as described with the distal tip just at the mouth opening and the flange end clearly caudad.

3 When a tongue blade is used, the OPA is inserted and turned sideways (pointing laterally) as in the previously described tongue-jaw lift method (Figure 4-7C). Insert it in alignment with the midline. As it is inserted, the distal tip should be turned slowly from pointing posteriorly as it passes over the tongue to a caudad-facing position when fully inserted; the curve of the device will naturally follow the anatomical curvature of the upper airway. In the photo, the OPA is shown fully inserted and turned as described.

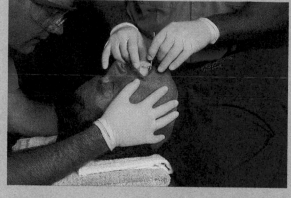

Figure 4-7C

4 Once the airway is fully inserted (the flange is just anterior to the upper lip), release the tension on the tongue blade and remove it. EMT #1 (who is immobilizing the head) then hooks the index and ring finger of each hand under the curve of the mandible at each side, and with mild pressure, elevates the mandible and secures the device.

NASOPHARYNGEAL AIRWAY

The nasopharyngeal airway (NPA) is a simple airway adjunct that provides an effective way to maintain a patent airway in patients who still have an intact gag reflex. When properly sized, the NPA will be tolerated by most patients. NPAs come in a range of diameters (internal diameters of 5 millimeters [mm] to 9 mm), and the length varies appropriately with the size of the diameter. They are available in a flexible rubberlike material or a rigid hard plastic. Because insertion of the flexible style is easier and safer, it is generally preferred for prehospital use. Because it is easy to damage the tissue at the septum, use of the rigid style is generally limited to cases where the NPA's rigidity will prevent shutting of the nostril when maxillofacial swelling is expected.

1 While one EMT maintains manual in-line immobilization and a trauma jaw thrust, the second EMT kneels at the upper thorax, slightly facing the patient's head. EMT #2 examines the nostrils with a light, and he or she selects the one that is largest and least deviated or obstructed (usually the right nostril). EMT #2 then measures the outer diameter of several of the sizes of NPAs available against the size of the anterior nostril or against the diameter of the patient's little finger (Figure 4-8A). The diameters of the

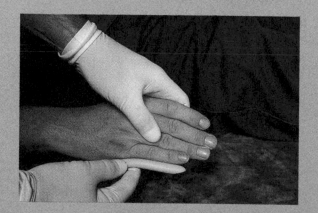

Figure 4-8A

anterior nostril and little finger are the same in most people. The NPA selected should be just smaller than the size of the nostril. The distal tip of the NPA is then liberally lubricated with water-soluble jelly.

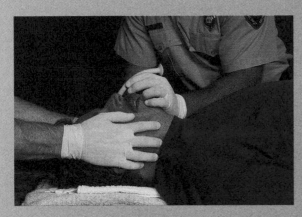

Figure 4-8B

Holding the airway between the thumb and **2** first two fingers with the airway near the patient's midline, EMT #2 slowly inserts it into the nostril of choice (Figure 4-8B). Insertion should be in an anterior-to-posterior direction along the floor of the nasal cavity toward the posterior pharynx and not in a superior direction. If resistance is met at the posterior end of the nostril, a gentle back-and-forth rotation of the airway between the fingers will usually aid in passing beyond the turbinate bones without damage. Should the NPA continue to meet an obstruction, do not use force. Instead, withdraw the airway, re-lubricate the distal tip, and attempt to insert it through the other nostril.

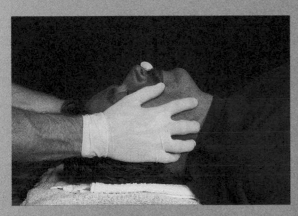

Figure 4-8C

Continue insertion until the flange is next to **3** the anterior naris or until the patient gags. To avoid the possibility of obstruction if the tongue should fall back, the distal tip of the NPA should pass slightly into the posterior pharynx behind the posterior tongue (Figure 4-8C). If the patient gags as the last 1/2 inch is inserted, it may be too long and should be withdrawn slightly to be tolerated.

SPECIFIC SKILLS

ESOPHAGEAL TRACHEAL DOUBLE LUMEN AIRWAYS (ETDLA)

Esophageal tracheal double lumen airways (ETDLA) provide prehospital providers with a functional alternative airway. The device is an acceptable field device for EMT use and typically requires minimal training to achieve competency. The airway's greatest single advantage is that it may be inserted independent of the patient's position (i.e., "blindly" inserted), which may be especially important in trauma patients with high suspicion of cervical injury. The indications for placement of an ETDLA are the same as for the placement of any airway: the necessity of obtaining a patent airway in a patient (see Chapter 3: Airway Management and Ventilation). The following conditions, however, must be met for consideration of ETDLA insertion: unconscious patient with no purposeful response, older than 16 years, absent gag reflex, height over 5 feet tall, and presence of apnea or respiratory rate less than six per minute. Insertion of an ETDLA should not be attempted if any of the following are present: intact gag reflex, patient under 16 years old, height less than 5 feet, known esophageal disease, or known ingestion of a caustic substance.

ETDLA INSERTION PROCEDURES

1 Provide respiratory support as needed. Attempts must be made to hyperventilate the patient with high FiO_2 using a simple airway adjunct or manual airway maneuver. Use the usual personal protective equipment (PPE) appropriate for intubation.

2 Inspect and prepare the equipment (Figure 4-9A). For the insertion of the ETDLA the equipment required is minimal: the device itself and two syringes for inflating the balloons (a large 60 cc and smaller 20 cc).

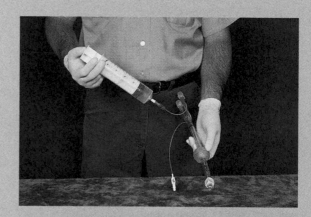

Figure 4-9A

3 Insert the ETDLA between ventilations being provided by the method chosen in step 1.

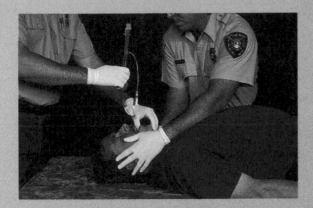

Figure 4-9B

If the patient is supine, lift the tongue and **4** lower jaw upward with one hand. Be cautious to avoid tearing the ETDLA cuff when inserting it past broken teeth or dental appliances (Figure 4-9B).

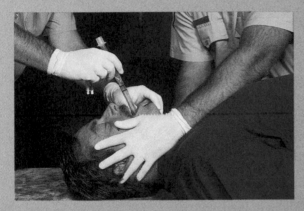

Figure 4-9C

Watch for the marker rings on the ETDLA to **5** measure depth of insertion. The rings should be aligned with the teeth or alveolar rings (Figure 4-9C).

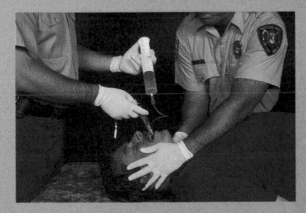

Figure 4-9D

Using the large syringe, inflate the pharyngeal cuff with 100 cc of air. The device **6** should seat itself in the posterior pharynx just behind the hard palate (Figure 4-9D).

7 Using the small syringe, inflate the distal cuff with 15 cc of air (Figure 4-9E).

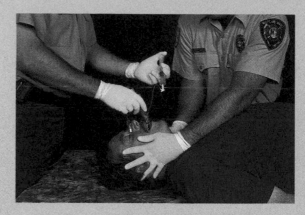

Figure 4-9E

8 Typically the device will be placed in the patient's esophagus. Begin ventilation through the esophageal tube (Figure 4-9F). If auscultation of breath sounds is positive and gastric insufflation is negative, continue ventilation.

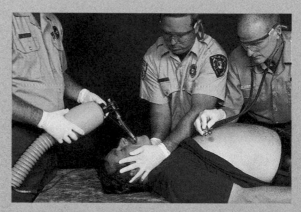

Figure 4-9F

9 If auscultation of breath sounds is negative, and gastric insufflation is positive, immediately ventilate via the shortened tracheal connector (generally marked with a #2). Re-auscultate to affirm proper tube placement (Figure 4-9G).

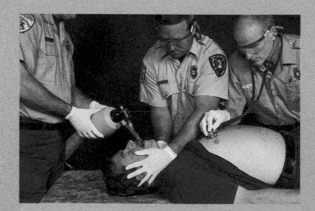

Figure 4-9G

All esophageal airways are dependent on the patient having no gag reflex. If the patient regains consciousness, these devices must be removed immediately. Extubation of esophageal airways nearly always causes vomiting or regurgitation. Consequently, it is essential that suction equipment be readily available at the time the device is removed. Proper PPE should also be worn to avoid exposure/contamination of personnel.

VISUALIZED OROTRACHEAL INTUBATION OF THE TRAUMA PATIENT (WITH NEUTRAL IN-LINE IMMOBILIZATION)

Visualized orotracheal intubation of trauma patients is performed with the patient's head immobilized in a neutral in-line position. Intubation while maintaining the manual immobilization requires additional training and practice beyond that for intubation of nontrauma patients. It should only be attempted by personnel trained and qualified in endotracheal intubation and who have demonstrated their ability to their medical director or his or her designate.

In hypoxic trauma patients who are not in cardiac arrest, intubation should not be the initial airway maneuver. It should only be performed after the patient has first been hyperventilated with a high FiO_2, using a simple airway adjunct or manual airway maneuver. *Contact with the deep pharynx when intubating a severely hypoxic patient without previous hyperoxygenation can easily produce vagal stimulation, resulting in dangerous bradycardia.*

The EMT should interrupt ventilation for 20 seconds or less when intubating the patient. Ventilation should not be interrupted for more than 30 seconds for any reason.

Visualized orotracheal intubation is contraindicated in conscious patients or patients with a gag reflex present. Prehospital use of topical anesthesia in such patients is not recommended.

Use of a straight blade tends to produce less rotary force (pull toward a "sniffing" position) than that produced by the shape and method when using a curved blade. However, since the success rate of intubation is often related to the EMT's comfort with a given design, the style of blade selected must remain a matter of individual preference.

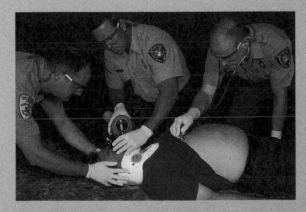

Figure 4-10A

1 While manual in-line immobilization, airway control using a simple airway adjunct, and ventilation with a high FiO_2 are being provided, auscultate the left and right mid-lung fields for the presence or absence of bilateral breath sounds to establish a baseline. In Figure 4-10A, EMT #1 ventilates the patient with a BVM, while EMT #2 auscultates the lung fields.

2 Without interrupting manual immobilization or ventilation, one EMT takes over the manual immobilization from the patient's side (as previously described). If the neutral in-line positioning results in a void between the back of the patient's head and the ground, a towel or other padding should be placed under the head at this time (Figure 4-10B). This additional support will be an important aid in maintaining neutral alignment during intubation.

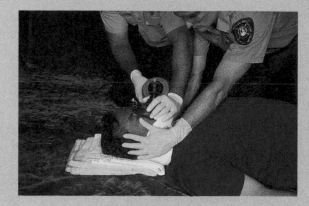

Figure 4-10B

3 The correct size endotracheal tube is selected and all of the additional equipment required is assembled. Use of a stylet has proven to be helpful but remains a matter of personal preference. The laryngoscope and endotracheal tube should be tested in the usual manner. When ready, the EMT who will intubate (EMT #2) instructs the EMT providing ventilation (EMT #1) to move to the patient's side opposite from the EMT providing the immobilization, and then instructs him or her to hyperventilate the patient (Figure 4-10C).

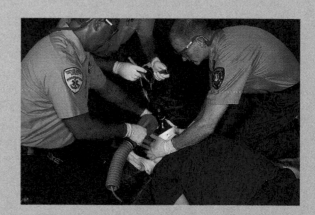

Figure 4-10C

4 EMT #2 sits on the ground with one leg over each of the patient's arms and gently moves forward until the patient's head can be secured between his or her thighs. Firm pressure is applied with the thighs to the side of the head. The grip of both EMTs will keep the head from moving about or rotating to hyperextension during intubation. In Figure 4-10D, EMT #1 maintains head support while EMT #2 supports the patient's head with his thighs and begins to position the laryngoscope.

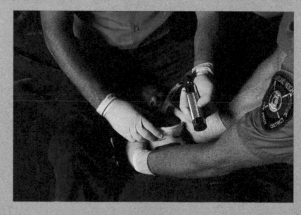

Figure 4-10D

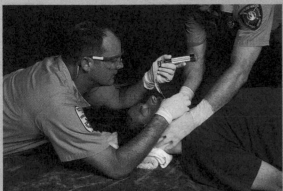
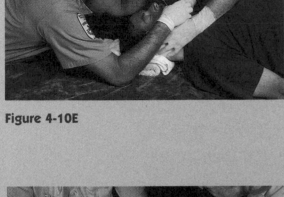

Figure 4-10E

OR

An alternative method is for EMT #2 to lie prone at the patient's head. When using this technique, EMT #1 alone has the task of maintaining the head in a neutral in-line position during intubation. Figure 4-10E shows this alternate method. EMT #1 maintains head support while EMT #2 attempts an intubation while lying at the patient's head.

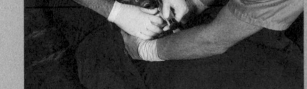

Figure 4-10F

5 When ready, EMT #2 instructs EMT #1 to stop hyperventilating the patient (Figure 4-10F). If suctioning is necessary, it should be provided and ventilation reinstated for a short period before the instruction to stop is repeated. If an orotracheal airway is in place, remove it. While visualizing the mouth, insert the laryngoscope into the mouth in the usual manner.

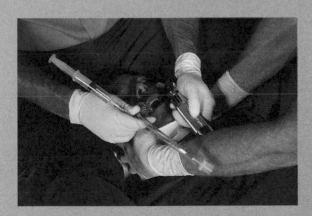

Figure 4-10G

6 Once the blade is properly placed, elevate the tongue and apply gentle traction in a caudad and upward direction (about a 45° angle to the floor of the mouth) by extending the left arm. Care must be taken to avoid touching the upper incisors or using them as a fulcrum. In Figure 4-10G, EMT #2 has inserted the laryngoscope and endotracheal tube halfway in.

In the sitting position, it may be necessary for EMT #2 to tilt his or her upper torso back in order to visualize the vocal cords. Once the vocal cords are clearly visualized, slightly advance the endotracheal tube between the cords.

7 After EMT #2 has seen the cuff pass through the vocal cords, he or she should advance the tube slightly farther (not more than 1 inch), remove the stylet (if used), inflate the cuff, and remove the syringe from the one-way valve. Attach the bag-valve device to the adapter on the endotracheal tube and reinstitute ventilation, hyperventilating the patient (Figure 4-10H).

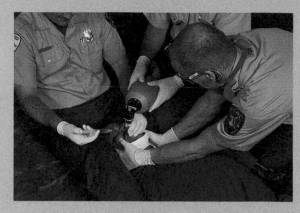

Figure 4-10H

8 Before securing the tube, visually check for adequate chest rise and auscultate for good breath sounds at the midlung field on each side (Figure 4-10I). Should sounds be present on the right side but absent on the left (unless a left pneumothorax was present upon auscultation when establishing the initial baseline prior to intubation), the endotracheal tube has been inserted too far, intubating the right mainstem bronchus. To correct this situation, withdraw the endotracheal tube 1 cm and reauscultate both midlung fields. Repeat the process until breath sounds are heard equally in both lungs. The EMT at the patient's head is bagging. The EMT at the patient's side is responsible for immobilization.

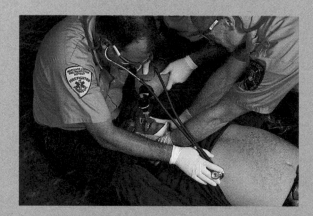

Figure 4-10I

Note: To further confirm proper placement, auscultate over the epigastrium. No "rushing air" or "bubbling" sounds should be heard. If air sounds are heard over the epigastrium when the bag is squeezed, or if chest rise and distinct breath sounds over the midlung fields are not observed, the EMT must assume misplacement of the endotracheal tube has occurred. Immediately deflate the cuff and remove the endotracheal tube. Hyperventilate the patient for 2 to 3 minutes and then attempt to intubate again, following the preceding steps. Observation of "fogging" inside the tube and a color change CO_2 detector are additional findings of proper placement.

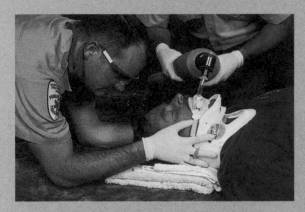

Figure 4-10J

Once proper placement has been con-**9** firmed, secure the endotracheal tube using a commercial endotracheal tube holder. Tape anchored to the tube at the level of the teeth can also be used (Figure 4-10J).

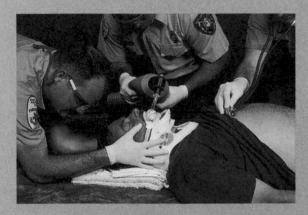

Figure 4-10K

Continue ventilations (Figure 4-10K) and **10** periodically reauscultate for good breath sounds over each midlung field to confirm that the endotracheal tube remains properly placed and that good alveolar ventilation is occurring bilaterally.

BLIND NASOTRACHEAL INTUBATION

This technique depends on the patient's spontaneous respiration to ensure proper alignment when passing the tube through the vocal cords into the trachea. It is therefore limited to use in breathing patients and to use in an environment that allows for the hearing and feeling of air exchange at the external end of the endotracheal tube.

Blind nasotracheal intubation should be used as the initial method of intubation for breathing trauma patients who have an intact gag reflex. It should also be used in patients who have injuries that preclude or make undesirable the use of an orotracheal method for insertion. In other trauma patients, it is only elected after attempting visualized orotracheal intubation, either when visualization has proven a problem (necessitating a "blind" method) or after several visualized attempts have been unsuccessful.

Contraindications for the use of blind nasotracheal intubation are apnea; injury to the maxilla, zygoma, inferior orbit, nose, or cribriform plate; or the presence of an anterior basilar skull fracture.

This technique should only be attempted by personnel qualified in endotracheal intubation and who, after practice, have demonstrated their ability to their medical director or his or her designate.

1 While manual in-line immobilization is maintained by EMT #1, the patient is provided with a high FiO_2 using a non-rebreather reservoir mask or a BVM (with collector and high-liter flow O_2) to assist ventilations. The EMT who will intubate (EMT #2) kneels at the upper torso, turned slightly toward the patient's face. Auscultate the lungs bilaterally to establish a baseline. In Figure 4-11A, EMT #2 auscultates the midlung field, and an O_2 mask and non-rebreather are on the patient.

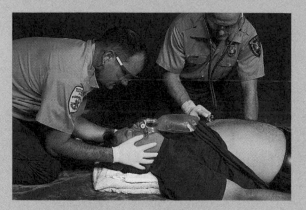

Figure 4-11A

2 Briefly interrupt oxygenation. Inspect the nostrils with a light. Select the largest and least deviated or obstructed naris, usually the right one. Compare several sizes of endotracheal tubes to the size of the anterior nostril and select the one with an outside diameter slightly smaller than the diameter of the nostril selected. While oxygenation is continued, gather and check the equipment needed. A stylet is not usually used when performing nasotracheal intubation since it can impair proper insertion and could possibly cause additional significant injury. When ready to proceed, lubricate the distal tip and cuff of the endotracheal tube liberally with lubricating jelly. In Figure 4-11B, EMT #2 inspects the nostril, while above the patient's head, EMT #1 provides immobilization.

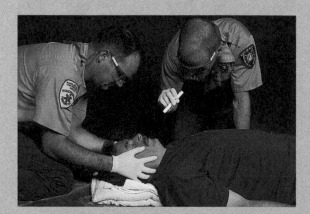

Figure 4-11B

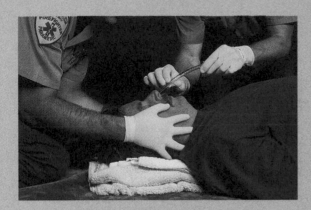

Figure 4-11C

Hold the endotracheal tube between the thumb and first two fingers with the distal tip pointing posteriorly into the selected nostril and the other end (with the adapter) pointing caudally. Advance the tube into the nostril, guiding it in an anterior-to-posterior direction. Be sure not to advance it superiorly as this will commonly result in resistance and potential injury at the turbinate bones. Slight back-and-forth rotation of the tube between the fingers may be useful in aiding passage through the posterior nostril into the pharynx. In Figure 4-11C, EMT #1 maintains support, while EMT #2 prepares to insert the endotracheal tube into the naris. **3**

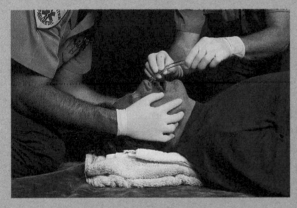

Figure 4-11D

At this point, EMT #1 should perform a jaw thrust. The jaw thrust will elevate the tongue, keeping it up anteriorly as the endotracheal tube is advanced further into the pharynx. As the tube is advanced, listen closely to the breath sounds at the external end of the tube. Slightly rotate the tube back and forth while listening. Stop further rotation when breath sounds are the loudest and the most misting of the tube occurs when the patient exhales. The distal end of the tube should be lined up with the opening in the vocal cords and the trachea beyond it when breath sounds and misting are at their greatest. If the patient is conscious, ask him or her to take a deep breath and gently pass the tube into the trachea (Figure 4-11D). **4**

5 Once the endotracheal tube is successfully in the trachea, advance it to the correct depth to ensure that the cuff is beyond the vocal cords. Inflate the cuff and confirm proper placement by observing chest rise, by feeling air exchange at the external tube (not around it), and by auscultation of good bilateral breath sounds over midlung fields. Further confirm proper placement by the absence of air sounds when auscultating over the epigastrium. Remedy any placement problems as previously described. Once proper placement has been ensured, secure the endotracheal tube, provide ventilations as needed, and periodically reauscultate for breath sounds. In Figure 4-11E, EMT #1 ventilates the patient while EMT #2 auscultates the lung fields and EMT #3 maintains immobilization.

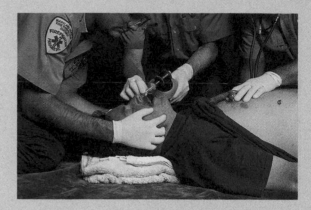

Figure 4-11E

MOUTH-TO-MASK VENTILATION

Several styles of mouth-to-mask units are available. Responders should only use units for mouth-to-mask ventilation with a one-way valve. Mouth-to-mask units selected for on-duty response should also include a nipple for connection to supplemental oxygen. Mouth-to-mask ventilation replaces mouth-to-mouth as a rapid interim ventilation method before other equipment can be readied. Since mouth-to-mask equipment with supplemental oxygen provides an FiO_2 of only 0.50, the EMT should switch to other equipment that can provide ventilations with an FiO_2 of 0.85 to 1.00 as soon as possible.

TWO-RESCUER METHOD

1 Once unresponsiveness has been determined, the initial EMT (EMT #1) provides manual in-line immobilization and performs a trauma jaw thrust. Alternatively, EMT #2 opens the airway using the chin lift method. EMT #2 evaluates the patient for air exchange. If the patient is apneic, ventilations should be provided without delay. While the manual immobilization is maintained by EMT #1, EMT #2 kneels alongside the patient, facing his or her mouth. EMT #1 maintains head support in the prone position while EMT #2 begins to position the pocket mask with a one-way valve to the mask (Figure 4-12A).

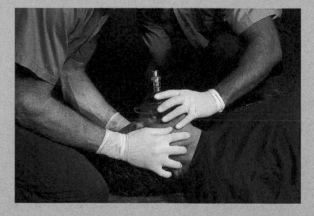

Figure 4-12A

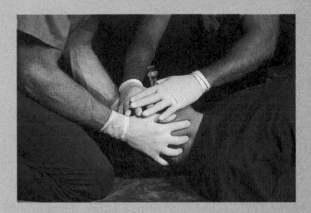

While sealing the mask with both hands and keeping the jaw elevated with several fingers, EMT #2 ventilates the patient. In Figure 4-12B, EMT #1 maintains neutral immobilization, jaw thrust, and the mask seal. EMT #2 is ready to ventilate the patient.

Figure 4-12B

After five or six ventilations, insertion of an OPA or NPA will provide easier, more stable airway management. Once ventilation is reinstituted, supplemental oxygen at 10 to 15 liters per minute (lpm) should be added. Mouth-to-mask ventilation should continue until another ventilating device capable of delivering an FiO_2 of 0.85 to 1.00 is readied.

SINGLE-RESCUER METHOD

When the number of EMTs available is limited, one EMT may have to simultaneously provide the initial immobilization, airway management, and ventilation. Mouth-to-mask ventilation represents the easiest and most stable single-rescuer method of ventilation prior to intubation. From a kneeling position above the patient's head, the EMT holds the head, maintains the mask seal, and with a trauma jaw thrust keeps the airway open and the jaw elevated against the mask. Breaths can be delivered by leaning forward over the patient's head. Insertion of an OPA or NPA makes it much easier to maintain the airway and should be done as soon as possible. Connection to supplemental oxygen should be initiated to increase the FiO_2 to at least 0.50.

BAG-VALVE-MASK RESUSCITATOR

Ventilation using a bag-valve-mask (BVM) is considered by most to be the preferred method of ventilation since it provides the rescuer with feedback by the feel of the bag. Positive feedback assures the operator of successful ventilations; changes in feedback indicate a loss of mask seal, the presence of a pathological airway, or a thoracic problem interfering with delivery of successful ventilations. This "feel" and the control it provides also make the BVM particularly suitable for providing assisted ventilations.

The BVM's portability and ability for immediate use when not attached to oxygen make it useful for the immediate delivery of ventilations upon identifying the need. Without supplemental oxygen, a BVM provides an FiO_2 of only 0.21; as soon as time allows, an oxygen collector and high-liter flow supplemental oxygen should be connected to it, raising the FiO_2 to 0.85 to 1.00. The attachment of supplemental oxygen should always include a collector. When oxygen is connected without a collector, the FiO_2 will be limited to 0.50 or less.

If a BVM is used to replace mouth-to-mask ventilation to raise the FiO_2, it is recommended that the BVM, collector, and supplemental oxygen be connected and turned on prior to making the switch. A wide variety of bag-valve-mask devices are available, including disposable single-patient-use models that are relatively inexpensive. Different brands have varying bag, valve, and collector designs. All of the parts used should be of the same model and brand since these parts are usually not safely interchangeable.

Bag-valve-mask units come in adult, pediatric, and neonatal sizes. Although an adult bag can be used with the proper size pediatric mask in an emergency, use of the right bag size is recommended as a safe practice.

When ventilating with any positive-pressure device, care must be taken not to continue inflation once the chest has risen maximally. When using the BVM, rescuers should visualize the chest and recognize the marked increased resistance in the bag when lung expansion is at its maximum. Care must also be taken to allow adequate time for exhalation (1:3 ratio between time for inhalation and time for exhalation). If not enough time is allowed, "stepped breaths" occur, providing a greater volume of inspiration than expiration. Stepped breaths produce poor air exchange and result in hyperinflation, increased pressure, opening of the esophagus, and gastric distention.

TWO- AND THREE-RESCUER METHOD

1 Once the patient is found unresponsive and apneic, one EMT (EMT #1) maintains in-line immobilization and keeps the airway open, while EMT #2 takes the BVM out of its case and attaches the proper size mask to the bag. While immobilization, jaw thrust, and a good mask seal are maintained by EMT #1 positioned above the patient's head, EMT #2, while kneeling at the side of the patient's head, squeezes the bag with both hands, providing ventilations greater than 800 cc/breath at a rate of 16 to 24 ventilations per minute. At this point, do not delay the start of ventilation to attach oxygen adjuncts. In Figure 4-13, EMT #1 maintains immobilization; EMT #2 kneels at the patient's side (at head) and is bagging with two hands. EMT #3 maintains the mask seal.

Often, an OPA can be inserted without delay when initiating the initial BVM ventilation, making airway management easier than with a manual method. If the EMT finds that

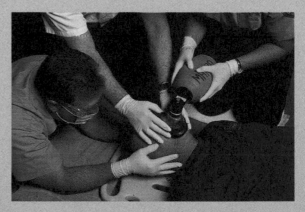

Figure 4-13

airway insertion would delay ventilation, then initial ventilations should be initiated with a jaw thrust. After 1 to 2 minutes of hyperventilation, ventilation should be interrupted (for less than 20 seconds) to measure and insert either an OPA or NPA. Once the airway is inserted, continue to hyperventilate the patient.

As rapidly as resources allow, the collector **2** and supplementary oxygen should be added to the BVM. While immobilization and hyperventilation are continued, a third EMT (or in between breaths, by EMT #2) attaches the collector by a universal oxygen connecting hose to the regulator of a portable oxygen unit. The tank is opened and the liter flow is set at the "high" setting or between 10 to 15 LPM. Lastly the collector (filling with oxygen) is attached to the bag.

Once ventilation with high FiO$_2$ has been **3** established, auscultate the patient's lungs to confirm good bilateral ventilation and to establish a baseline. After 1 or 2 minutes, if indicated, more definitive airway management can be achieved with endotracheal intubation.

SPECIFIC SKILLS

SINGLE-RESCUER METHOD

It is difficult for one EMT to both maintain a mask seal and provide ventilations by deflating the bag. Regardless of one's expertise, the ability to provide good ventilation is difficult when one EMT maintains the mask seal *and* deflates the bag while in the back of a moving ambulance. Having one EMT maintain immobilization and the mask seal while a second EMT deflates the bag with both hands provides for higher and more consistent volumes.

1 In the event that it is necessary for one EMT to provide both the mask seal and deflate the bag, a simple airway adjunct should be inserted first. The EMT providing ventilations positions himself or herself above the patient's head. The mask seal is held by encircling the mask with the thumb and first two or three fingers. The thumb is placed on the cephalad part of the mask and the first two or three fingers on the caudad part.

The little finger or ring and little finger hook under the posterior mandible to keep the mandible elevated, avoiding a loss of seal caused by any posterior movement of the chin. It is difficult for one person to consistently provide volumes exceeding the minimum standard of at least 800 cc/breath when simply squeezing the bag unsupported in the air with one hand. On the other hand, consistently high volumes (1,000 cc to 1,200 cc) were obtained by experienced personnel when the bag was squeezed between the free hand and a part of the EMT's body. Therefore, ventilations should be provided by squeezing the bag with the free hand against your other forearm, thigh, or thorax to ensure a consistently high volume with each breath (Figure 4-14).

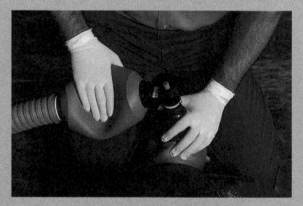

Figure 4-14

For short periods of time, one EMT may have **2** to provide both the manual immobilization and ventilations prior to mechanical immobilization on a longboard. Should this need arise, while one EMT (EMT #1) temporarily provides immobilization positioned beside the patient's thorax, the EMT providing ventilations (EMT #2), from a kneeling position beyond the patient's head, moves forward on his or her knees (caudally to the patient) until the knees are equal to the patient's midneck. Once in place, EMT #2 lowers himself or herself, kneeling with the upper leg resting on the lower leg and gently squeezing the head between the inside of the thighs.

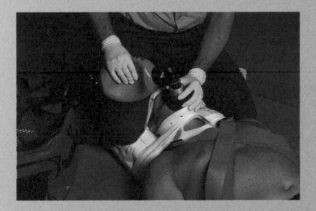

Figure 4-15

EMT #1 can now let go and is available to perform other priority care. Immobilization is maintained by holding the head between the thighs while ventilations are provided as described earlier (Figure 4-15). The EMT supports the patient's head in a neutral in-line position with his legs and thighs.

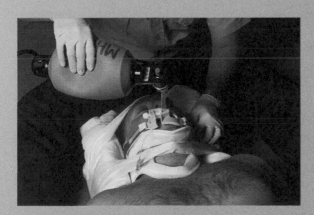

Figure 4-16

Single-rescuer BVM ventilation is more easily done once the patient has been intubated since the need to maintain a mask seal no longer exists. Similarly, single-rescuer ventilation is easier once the patient has been fully immobilized to the longboard since immobilization while ventilating is being provided mechanically by the head immobilizer (Figure 4-16).

ASSISTED VENTILATIONS USING A BAG-VALVE-MASK

When assisting ventilations using a BVM in an *unconscious* breathing patient with inadequate minute volume, the procedure is the same as when providing ventilation to an apneic patient. The selection of airway adjunct is based on the level of unconsciousness of the patient and the presence or absence of a gag reflex. Assisted ventilation with a BVM should include a collector and connection to high-liter flow oxygen. In such cases, the equipment can be assembled, attached, and turned on before starting.

When assisted ventilation is required in a *conscious* patient, the procedure must be modified to avoid resistance from the patient or combativeness caused by fear. The EMT should carefully explain to the patient what he or she will be doing. This explanation should include stating that it may be uncomfortable at first, but as more air is exchanged the patient will feel better. Honor the patient's anxieties by agreeing to remove the mask and pause if necessary. Removing the mask on request provides the patient with a feeling of some control, allaying some of his or her fears, and usually resulting in a more cooperative patient. Remember that anxiety and combativeness are by-products of cerebral hypoxia.

Use of a manual maneuver versus an NPA should depend on how altered the patient's level of consciousness is, how well the patient can maintain his or her airway, and what the patient will readily tolerate.

In a conscious patient, start by matching the volume and rate of the patient's ineffectual breathing. If the patient's breathing is very shallow and fast, use shallow deflations of the bag. "Puffs" of air will be delivered, allowing for the rapid refill of the bag to maintain the high rate per minute of the patient's ventilations. Without delay, increase the volume delivered after every 3 to 6 breaths, until you are providing over 800 cc/breath or until maximum chest rise has been reached. As you increase the volume every few breaths, the time needed to refill the bag will be greater, reducing the rate of ventilation. Once a proper volume is achieved, maintain a rate of between 16 and 24 ventilations per minute.

Should the conscious patient be breathing too slowly, once assisted ventilation has started at the patient's depth and rate, immediately increase the volume to deliver over 800 cc per breath or until maximum chest rise has been reached. Increase the rate every few breaths until a rate of between 16 and 24 breaths per minute is achieved.

In either case, continue talking to the patient. Ask the patient if he or she feels better. Once the patient realizes that the assisted ventilations are helping, the patient will be less anxious. As the patient's blood oxygen levels rise, his or her spontaneous rate will return to a more normal range. In conscious patients, the additional 30 to 60 seconds of delay caused by synchronizing ventilations to their rate and evolving to a proper rate and volume is time well spent. In most conscious patients it prevents conflicts, increased anxiety, and the need to repeatedly stop assisted ventilations to calm the patient. Use of a steady evolution to a proper rate and depth increases the patient's tolerance of the procedure.

DEMAND-VALVE RESUSCITATOR (MANUALLY ACTIVATED POSITIVE-PRESSURE OXYGEN RESUSCITATOR WITH A DEMAND VALVE)

Demand-valve resuscitators are connected to a threaded high-pressure connector on the regulator (not to the normal low-pressure supplemental oxygen nipple) by a flexible high-pressure oxygen hose. A standard mask attaches to the head of the device and positive-pressure oxygen flow for inhalation is activated when the EMT presses a button or handle on the unit's head. Exhalation through a one-way valve near the mask occurs when the button or handle is released.

Should spontaneous ventilation return, a demand-valve feature provides supplemental oxygen when the patient "demands" it by attempting to inhale. Negative pressure is produced against the demand valve and supplemental oxygen flows at normal low pressure (not with positive pressure). Sustained oxygenation using this demand feature should be avoided in patients with spontaneous respiration since it requires an unnecessary effort on the part of the patient. A normal non-rebreather reservoir mask connected to the low-pressure supplemental oxygen nipple should be substituted.

These units are equipped with a pressure-relief valve. If an excess ventilatory volume or an obstruction causes a dangerous rise in pressure in the lungs and/or pharynx, the valve will release before injury to the patient occurs. Due to the design of the unit's head and trigger, it is easier for one EMT to provide ventilations while maintaining a mask seal than when one EMT performs these functions with a BVM. However, since the demand-valve resuscitator does not give the EMT feedback by allowing him or her to feel the lung's compliance (unlike the BVM), it is more difficult to provide the correct volume at each breath. Thus, more complications, such as gastric distention, can occur. The lack of "feel" also makes it more difficult to recognize changes or problems in the patient's ventilation, which may result in hypoventilation or the need for other intervention. Use of a demand-valve resuscitator with an intubated patient may be dangerous and is therefore not recommended.

Oxygen flows to the demand head independently of the valve that regulates the liter flow to the supplemental oxygen nipple. To avoid wasting oxygen and the potential danger from its unnecessary release, the liter flow valve should be in the off position when using the device as a resuscitator.

TWO-RESCUER METHOD

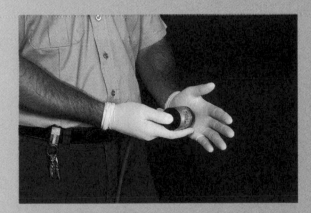

Figure 4-17A

The EMT who will provide ventilations with the demand-valve resuscitator (EMT #2) selects the correct size mask; attaches it to the head of the device; and presses the trigger to purge the line, filling it with oxygen. He or she then ensures that the unit is operating properly. In Figure 4-17A, EMT #2 is testing the pressure of the demand-valve resuscitator. To check that the high-pressure relief valve is operating, occlude the delivery hole in the unit's head while activating the trigger for a few seconds.

1

Next, bare the patient's chest fully or at least remove enough clothing to allow clear visualization of chest rise and fall. Ask the EMT ventilating by mouth-to-mask to hyperventilate the patient. Remove the mouth-to-mask device; if an airway adjunct has not been inserted, select, measure, and insert one now.

2

While the EMT at the head maintains immobilization (EMT #1), place the mask of the demand-valve resuscitator on the patient's face, obtain a good seal, and activate the trigger. In Figure 4-17B, EMT #1 provides immobilization. EMT #2 has obtained a mask seal, and the trigger is depressed. Carefully visualize the chest. When maximum chest rise is achieved, immediately release the trigger. Releasing it too early will result in hypoventilation and continued hypoxia. Releasing it too late will result in increased pressure in the lungs and pharynx. When this increased pressure exceeds the esophageal adhesion pressure, the esophagus will inflate and any excess volume will be delivered to the stomach. If the esophagus inflates repeatedly, it will cause gastric distention and possibly regurgitation and aspiration.

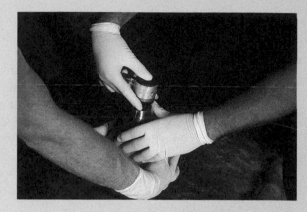

Figure 4-17B

3 Continue careful visualization of the chest. In Figure 4-17C, EMT #2 has taken his finger off the trigger. Once the trigger has been released, allow enough time for the patient to exhale. Inhalation is rapidly provided by the positive pressure. Exhalation, however, is a passive process requiring considerably more time. The ratio for positive pressure inhalation to exhalation is about 1:3. As with knowing when to stop inhalation, assuring that exhalation has fully occurred is based on the EMT's careful observation of the patient's chest. If insufficient time is allowed for exhalation, actual air exchange will be minimized, the FiO_2 will be reduced, and CO_2 retention will occur. Also, if inhalations are delivered too rapidly without enough volume being allowed to escape, "stepped breaths" occur, resulting in gastric distention

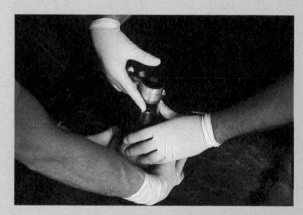

Figure 4-17C

by the same mechanism as described in step 2. Either positive pressure continued too long at each breath or inadequate exhalation time can easily result in delivery of excessive volume and inadvertent inflation of the stomach.

Continue ventilations as just described at a rate of 16 to 24 delivered breaths per minute, carefully visualizing the chest at all times. While the patient is being ventilated, the chest should be auscultated to ensure that good bilateral ventilation is occurring and to establish baselines. EMT #1, who is providing the immobilization, can also hold the mask seal. However, unlike ventilating the patient with a BVM, it is not absolutely necessary to free up both hands of the EMT providing the ventilations when using a demand-valve. When ventilating with a demand-valve resuscitator, a full "D" tank will only last between 16 and 30 minutes. Tanks that are less than completely full commonly continue in service as they are not replaced at the end of each call. Therefore, care must be taken to monitor tank pressure so that oxygen will not run out prior to switching to on-board oxygen in the ambulance.

SINGLE-RESCUER METHOD

The demand-valve resuscitator and mouth-to-mask device represent the easiest way for one EMT to continue immobilization, maintain a mask seal, and provide ventilations simultaneously. Unlike mouth-to-mask, the demand-valve resuscitator provides an FiO_2 of 0.85 to 1.00. The insertion of an OPA (or NPA if indicated) will make maintaining the airway much easier and should therefore be done before one-rescuer ventilation with a demand-valve resuscitator is initiated. When ready to evolve to one-rescuer ventilation, a second EMT prepares the resuscitator and places it next to the patient's side so that the equipment is ready to use (unless already done for two-rescuer use). When ready, the second EMT places the mask on the patient's face. The EMT immobilizing the patient's head from above moves his or her fingers so that he or she can maintain the immobilization and provide a mask seal. One finger is placed on the trigger, and the patient is ventilated in the manner described in steps 1, 2, and 3 of the previous section.

SPECIFIC SKILLS

PERCUTANEOUS TRANSTRACHEAL VENTILATION

Transtracheal procedures should only be performed by advanced level EMTs who have practiced the specific procedure and who have demonstrated their ability to properly perform it to the satisfaction of their medical director or his or her designate. Retraining and reverification are needed every 6 to 12 months to maintain proficiency. Percutaneous transtracheal ventilation (PTV) by such personnel should only be used in the prehospital environment when other methods of providing a patent airway and ventilation have been unsuccessful, or if extensive maxillofacial injury precludes the advisability of the use of other methods. Since the need for this procedure is rare, few individuals perform it regularly. Squads authorized to perform it should counteract decay of skills with periodic training and practice.

The procedure cannot be successfully done if the equipment parts, which are not usually commercially designed to connect together, do not fit together to form airtight joints. Therefore, squads authorized to perform this procedure should test the compatibility of all required equipment prior to being on a call that might need this technique.

It is highly recommended that all parts except the needle, tank, and regulator be modified as needed, preassembled, and then taken to the hospital for packaging and resterilization. This will ensure successful assembly. When this technique is needed, time is of the essence. The equipment should be ready to use, requiring only connection to the regulator and needle. The following equipment is required:

- several needles: either short 10-gauge emergency tracheal needles or large bore (12 to 14 gauge) over-the-needle intravenous catheters
- a syringe: 10 to 30 cc
- an oxygen delivery hose: a standard universal oxygen connecting hose with a hole cut into one side of the tubing (this length of tubing will connect to the oxygen source on one end and onto the needle on the other); alternatively, such a tube can be cut in two and the whistle-stop part of a suction catheter inserted using plastic connectors between the two halves (not recommended unless this has been assembled in advance, ready for immediate use)

OR

- a plastic T or Y connector of a size compatible with the oxygen tubing used and connected to the oxygen source with a length of standard universal oxygen tubing

AND

- a short piece of tubing that will fasten over the lower end of the T or Y and snugly fit onto the hub of the needle (this leaves one opening of the T or Y connector free with nothing attached to it)
- an oxygen tank with a regulator that has a 50 psi delivery pressure at its supplemental oxygen nipple
- strips of 1/2-inch adhesive tape

Studying a representation of the equipment, assembled as it would be in use, will aid in understanding the step-by-step procedure that follows.

In order for this procedure to be performed, the patient must be in the supine position, while manual in-line immobilization is maintained. To save time in a patient who cannot be adequately ventilated with other methods, one EMT will prepare and intubate the trachea, while a second connects the hosing and turns on the oxygen. If partial ventilation through the mouth is possible, it should be continued until ready to replace it with the PTV.

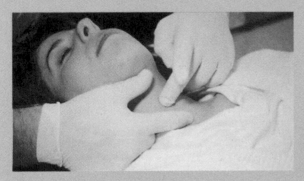

Figure 4-18A

The larynx is located and stabilized using **1** the thumb and middle finger of one hand, preventing the trachea from lateral movement. In Figure 4-18A, the EMT locates the larynx with the thumb and index finger. Then, with the index finger or with the other hand, the "Adam's apple" is located.

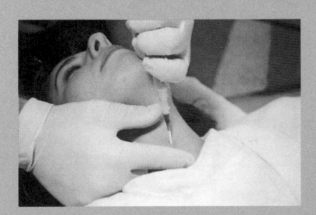

Figure 4-18B

The index finger is slid downward to locate **2** the cricothyroid membrane. The EMT positions the syringe and is ready for insertion of the needle (Figure 4-18B). Next, the needle attached to the syringe is inserted through the membrane or at another location through the anterior wall of the trachea near its midline, at a 60° angle caudally, while negative pressure is applied in the syringe.

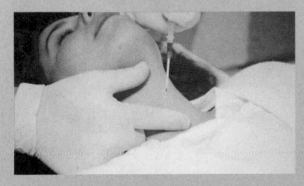

Figure 4-18C

Once the needle has entered the trachea, air **3** will be sucked into the syringe, confirming that the tip of the needle is properly located. The catheter is advanced into the trachea (Figure 4-18C) an additional centimeter or so. Remove the syringe from the needle. If an over-the-needle intravenous catheter has been used, remove the inner metal needle, leaving the plastic catheter in place. Care must be taken that the Teflon catheter does not kink upon removing the inner needle. Quickly form a loop with tape around the needle or hub of the catheter and place the ends of the tape on the patient's neck to secure it. Do not make this fastening too tight or bend the catheter.

4 Confirm that the tubing assembly is properly connected to the regulator and the oxygen is turned on and flowing at maximum liter flow. In Figure 4-18D, needle cricothyroidotomy is being connected to the oxygen tubing with the pre-cut side hole. Alternatively, connect the tubing from the T or Y connector to the hub of the needle or catheter.

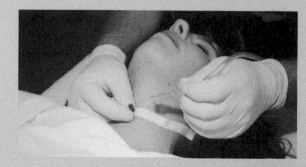

Figure 4-18D

5 To ventilate the patient, simultaneously occlude the whistle-stop (the hole in the oxygen feed tube) or the opening at one side of the T or Y connector with the operator's thumb while holding the tubing assembly steady with the other hand (Figure 4-18E). This maneuver closes the system to the outside, leaving only the needle in the trachea as a possible pathway for the oxygen. Watch the chest rise to indicate that inhalation is occurring.

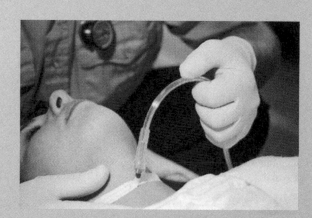

Figure 4-18E

6 To stop the flow of oxygen into the lungs, the operator's thumb is removed from the occluded opening (the whistle-stop or hole in the oxygen source tubing, or the opening in the T or Y connector) (Figure 4-18F). Keep supporting the tubing assembly with the other hand. Opening the hole in the oxygen source opens the flow of oxygen to the outside, causing it to exit rather than continuing to exert flow and pressure to the needle. The opening in the T or Y connector provides an easy pathway from the needle for the exhaled air. Remember that the passive process of exhalation normally takes three to four times as long as inhalation. In this method exhalation will require more time than other methods of ventilation due to the restricted minimal opening provided by the catheter or needle.

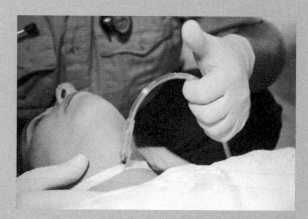

Figure 4-18F

Continue ventilating the patient by alternately closing the appropriate hole to provide the positive flow of oxygen for inhalation and opening the same hole to stop the oxygen flow and allow a ready route for exhalation. The proper time sequence for these maneuvers is 1 second of occlusion of the proper hole to allow oxygen flow into the lungs and 4 seconds of removing the thumb from the hole to stop oxygen flow into the lungs and allow for passive exhalation. This sequence of 1 second occlusion (oxygen flow into lungs) to 4 seconds nonocclusion (passive exhalation) is continued until the patient has a more definitive airway established or is delivered to the appropriate medical facility. This method is used when ET intubation and BVM ventilation are not effective. This is usually associated with an occluded or partially occluded larynx and provides only minimal ventilation. After 45 to 60 minutes, it can produce a high $PaCO_2$ level due to CO_2 retention as a result of the restricted expirations.

If air (oxygen) escapes through the patient's mouth and nose when providing inhalations, some airway patency still exists. In such cases, normal positive-pressure ventilation through the mouth and nose should again be attempted without removing the PTV equipment. Normal positive-pressure ventilation will provide more adequate volumes of air exchange and better oxygenation and should be used when possible. If this attempt proves unsuccessful, return to providing PTV. Should air continue to escape upon providing inhalations, a second EMT should place his or her hand over the patient's mouth, closing it while squeezing the nostrils shut between the thumb and first finger at each inhalation phase, in order to produce a closed system. During exhalation, the EMT should remove his or her hand. In such cases, leaving the mouth and nose open during exhalation will be beneficial by increasing the available pathway for the exhaled air.

Warning

Patients being ventilated using PTV may remain hypoxic and unstable. Transportation should be initiated to a suitable facility without delay since this patient is in urgent need of a more definitive surgical transtracheal procedure (cricothyroidotomy or tracheostomy) for adequate ventilation and oxygenation.

EMERGENCY NEEDLE THORACOSTOMY (DECOMPRESSION OF A TENSION PNEUMOTHORAX)

In patients with increasing intrathoracic pressure from a developing tension pneumothorax, the side of the thoracic cavity that has the increased pressure must be decompressed. If this pressure is not relieved, it will progressively limit the patient's ventilatory capacity and cause inadequate venous return and encumbered cardiac function, producing inadequate cardiac output and death. A detailed discussion of tension pneumothoraces is found in Chapter 5: Thoracic Trauma.

In cases in which an open pneumothorax has been treated by use of an occlusive dressing and a tension pneumothorax develops, decompression can usually be achieved through the wound, which provides an existing opening into the thorax. Open the occlusive dressing over the wound for a few seconds. A rush of air should be heard at the wound as the air rushes out, relieving the increased pressure in the thorax.

Once the pressure has been released, reseal the wound with the occlusive dressing to allow for proper alveolar ventilation and to stop air from "sucking" into the wound. The patient should be monitored carefully and if any signs of tension reoccur, the dressing should again be "burped" to release the pressure.

Decompression in closed tension pneumothoraces is achieved by providing a surgical opening—a thoracostomy—in the affected side of the chest. Different methods for performing a thoracostomy exist. Since needle thoracostomy is the most rapid method and does not require special equipment, it is the method selected for use in the field.

Indications for an emergency needle thoracostomy are the signs and symptoms of increased intrathoracic pressure associated with a closed tension pneumothorax. This procedure is not indicated by the presence of a simple pneumothorax or simple hemothorax alone without signs or symptoms of tension.

This procedure should only be performed by advanced EMTs who have practiced it in a suitable laboratory environment and who have proven their competence to the satisfaction of their medical director or his or her designate.

Necessary equipment includes a needle, 1/2-inch adhesive tape, alcohol swabs, and a one-way valve. The needle(s) should be large bore over-the-needle intravenous catheter(s) between 10 gauge and 14 gauge. A 16 gauge can be used if a larger bore is not available.

Although the finger cut from a sterile glove can be used as a one-way valve, use of a Heimlich-type valve or other one-way valve is easier. A #3 pediatric endotracheal tube, once the adapter (to fit a BVM) is removed, will fit over the intake nipple of the Heimlich valve. Once the catheter is placed, the distal tip of the endotracheal tube will fit snugly into the hub of the catheter. It is recommended that squads performing this procedure preconnect the endotracheal tube to such a valve and have it packaged and resterilized at the hospital so that it is ready for use. If the finger from a sterile glove is to be used instead, it should be cut from the glove and a small hole cut in the distal end so that it will fit over the catheter's hub. In order for it to work properly as a valve, the talcum powder packed inside the glove must be rinsed out of the finger, using sterile water or sterile saline, prior to use.

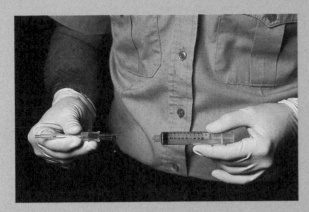

Figure 4-19A

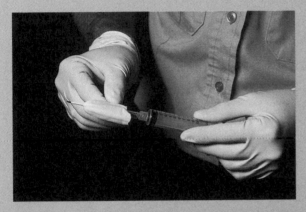

Figure 4-19B

Prepare the equipment you will need. In Figures 4-19A and 4-19B, the EMT assembles the needle and syringe. The EMT inserts the needle through the cut section of the thumb of a glove. Reauscultate the chest to confirm which side has the tension pneumothorax by the absent or diminished breath sounds on that side, or reconfirm signs of hyperinflation, such as intercostal bulging, on that side. Remember that if tracheal deviation has already occurred, the lower trachea will deviate contralaterally to (away from) the injured side.

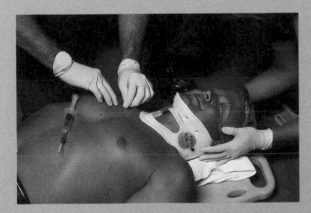

Figure 4-19C

With the fingers of one hand at the midclavicular line, locate the second or third intercostal space. In Figure 4-19C, the EMT determines the location of the third rib with his hand, and the skin is prepped. You should be able to clearly feel the ribs on each side of the intercostal space. With a firm rotary motion, clean the area with an alcohol swab. Again by feeling carefully, locate the upper margin of the third rib.

3 While keeping track of the location of the top of the third rib with several fingers of one hand, place the tip of the needle against the skin at the midclavicular line and hold it so that the hub is held just lower than the tip. Insert the needle, pointing posteriorly but slightly upward, sliding it over the top curve of the lower (third) rib. In Figure 4-19D, the needle is inserted into the chest. By inserting it over the top of the lower rib, the EMT is sure that the needle is not near the bottom of the upper rib where blood vessels are located.

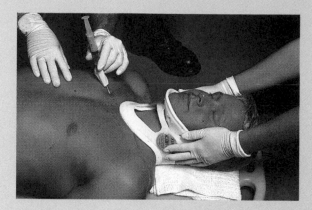

Figure 4-19D

4 Once inserted, hold the catheter (being careful not to kink the Teflon catheter) and remove the needle (Figure 4-19E). If chest decompression occurs, a rush of air will be heard.

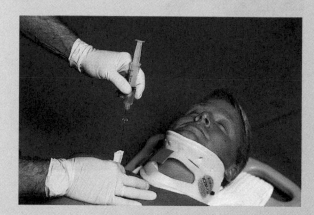

Figure 4-19E

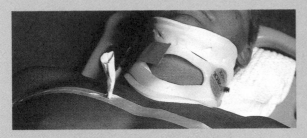

Figure 4-19F

Attach the one-way valve (Heimlich-type or finger from a sterile glove) to the hub of the catheter and secure the catheter to the chest with tape loops (Figure 4-19F). Tape should also be placed around the endotracheal tube at the hub to secure the valve. If a glove finger was used, place tape around the finger and hub. Auscultate the chest and recheck the patient's respiration and other vital signs. Initiate transport without delay.

When no EMT certified in this procedure is present and the assessment has shown that a closed tension pneumothorax exists, the EMTs present should rapidly initiate transport to the nearest suitable facility where chest decompression can be achieved.

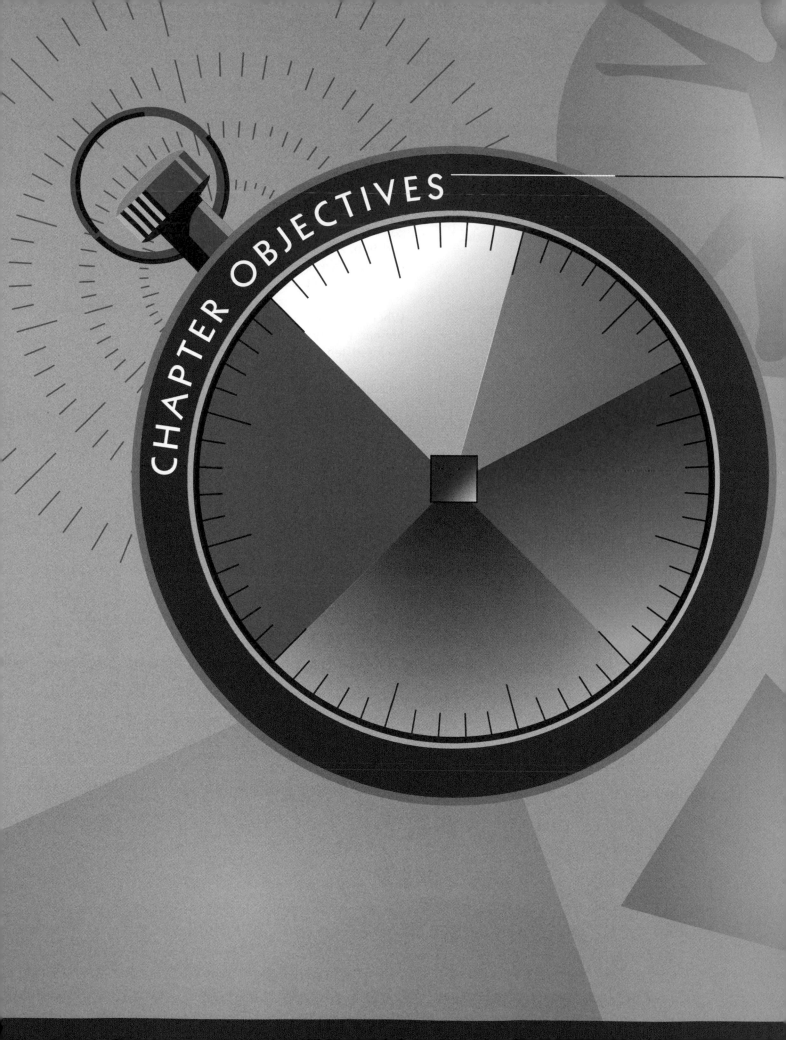

CHAPTER OBJECTIVES

CHAPTER 5

Thoracic Trauma

At the completion of this course the student will be able to:

- Identify the general anatomy of the chest.

- Describe the normal anatomy and physiology necessary for adequate ventilation.

- Define the associated pathology and pathophysiology pertinent to ventilation and circulation in the thorax.

- List the basic diagnostic signs and treatment of the following:
  a. rib fractures
  b. flail chest
  c. pulmonary contusion
  d. pneumothorax (open and closed)
  e. tension pneumothorax and hemothorax
  f. myocardial contusion
  g. pericardial tamponade
  h. aortic, tracheal, and bronchial rupture
  i. traumatic asphyxiation
  j. diaphragmatic rupture

- Define the relationship of kinematics to thoracic trauma.

- Identify the need for rapid stabilization and transportation to the hospital.

Scenario

You and your partner are dispatched on a report of a shooting to the chest. As you near the given address, you scan the scene to look for any signs of a possible assailant. The police are already on the scene and report that they have cleared it. As you approach the patient, you can hear him loudly decrying his current fate in life and threatening the well-being of his alleged assailant. As you prepare to evaluate the patient, you quickly assimilate the information already available to you and plan your next steps.

Before you even introduce yourself or perform an assessment, you already have obtained a lot of information. You know that the patient is awake, unhappy that he has been shot, and vocalizing that unhappiness. Thus you know that his airway is intact, he is conscious, and that his breath and circulation—while perhaps not completely normal—are at least reasonable enough to allow him to think through and voice his planned revenge. At his side you note that he is slightly diaphoretic. After you remove his shirt, you note that he has a single wound to his right chest in the third intercostal space in the mid-clavicular line. Rolling him does not reveal any other wound. Visually, the wound is not sucking any air or bubbling. Palpation of the area of the wound and the surrounding chest reveals a small amount of subcutaneous emphysema, and auscultation of his lungs reveals his breath sounds are diminished.

- What do you suspect are the most likely injuries?
- What is your treatment priority?
- How much time do you plan to spend on the scene?
- To what kind of facility will you transport the patient?

Chest injuries are the second leading cause of trauma deaths each year, although the vast majority of all thoracic injuries (90% of blunt trauma and 70% to 85% of penetrating trauma) can be managed without surgery. Chest injuries that are missed or go unrecognized due to an incomplete or inaccurate assessment can impair the ventilating or oxygen exchange systems and produce tissue hypoxia (decreased oxygen), hypercarbia (increased CO_2 in the blood), and acidosis (accumulation of acids and decreased pH of the blood). Tissue hypoxia results from inadequate delivery of oxygenated blood to the tissue cells, either from decreased perfusion or decreased oxygenation of the red blood cells. Hypercarbia is due to decreased ventilation. Acidosis is secondary to anaerobic metabolism by inadequately oxygenated cells.

Traumatic chest injuries can be caused by a variety of trauma mechanisms, including motor vehicle collisions, falls, sports injuries, crush injuries, stab wounds, and gunshot wounds.

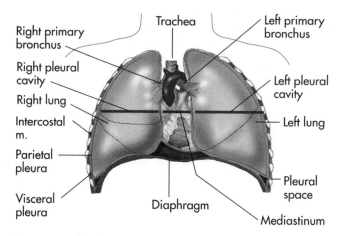

Figure 5-1 The thoracic cavity. (Includes ribs, intercostal muscles, diaphragm, mediastinum, lungs, heart, great vessels, bronchi, trachea, esophagus.) (From Thibodeau, G.A., and Patton, K.T. *Anatomy and Physiology.* 3rd ed. St. Louis: Mosby, 1996.)

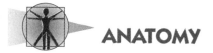 **ANATOMY**

The **thorax** is a hollow cylinder composed of twelve pairs of ribs that articulate posteriorly with the thoracic spine and anteriorly with the sternum via the costal cartilages. A nerve, an artery, and a vein are located along the underside of each rib. Intercostal muscles connect each rib to the one above. These muscles, along with the diaphragm, are the primary muscles of respiration (Figure 5-1).

The pleura is a thin membrane consisting of two distinct pleurae. The parietal pleura lines the inner side of the thoracic cavity. The visceral pleura covers the outer surface of each lung. A small amount of fluid is present between the pleural surfaces of the lung and the inner chest wall. Just as a drop of water between two panes of glass makes it difficult to pull the two panes apart, this pleural fluid creates surface tension between these two pleural membranes and causes them to cling together. In this way, the pleural membranes oppose the natural elasticity and tendency of the lung to collapse. Normally, no space is present between the two pleural membranes; adhesion keeps these layers together. Lack of connection to outside air also keeps them together. If a hole develops in the thoracic wall or the lung, this space fills with air and the lung collapses. This potential space can hold a volume of 3,000 cubic centimeters (cc) or more in an adult.

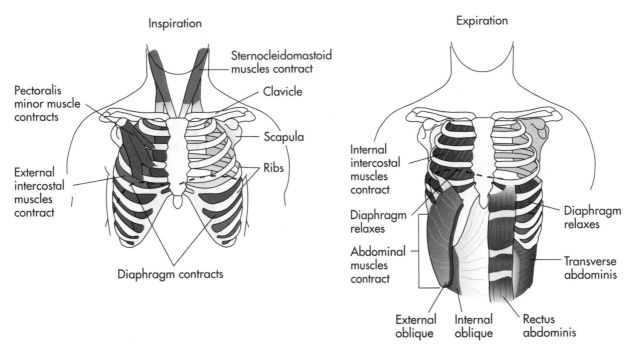

Figure 5-2 During inspiration, the diaphragm contracts and flattens. Muscles of inspiration, such as the external intercostals, pectoralis minor, and sternocleidomastoid muscles, lift the ribs and sternum, which together increases the diameter and volume of the thoracic cavity. In expiration during quiet breathing, the elasticity of the thoracic cavity causes the diaphragm and ribs to assume their resting positions, which decreases the volume of the thoracic cavity. In expiration during labored breathing, muscles of expiration such as the internal intercostals and abdominal muscles contract, causing the volume of the thoracic cavity to decrease more rapidly. (From Seeley, R. R.; Stephens, T. D.; and Tate, P. *Essentials of Anatomy and Physiology.* St. Louis: Mosby–Year Book, Inc., 1991.)

The lungs occupy the right and left halves of the thoracic cavity (see Figure 5-1). An area called the mediastinum is located in the middle of the thoracic cavity. Within the mediastinum lie all the other organs and structures of the chest cavity: the heart, the great vessels, the trachea, the mainstem bronchi, and the esophagus. Any or all of these structures may be injured by thoracic trauma.

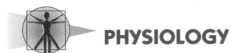

PHYSIOLOGY

THE MECHANICS OF VENTILATION ——

To fully appreciate the consequences and management of chest injuries, it is important to understand the mechanics of ventilation. **Ventilation** is the mechanical process by which air moves from the atmosphere outside the body into the mouth, nose, pharynx, trachea, bronchi, lungs,

and alveoli and then out again. **Respiration,** a biologic process, is the exchange of oxygen and carbon dioxide between the outside atmosphere and the cells of the body. Respiration includes ventilation. Although the terms ventilation and respiration are frequently used interchangeably, in reality they represent different levels of function. It is critical to understand that the patient's ability to get life-sustaining oxygen to the cells of the body depends on both processes: the mechanical one (ventilation) that brings air into the lungs as well as the biologic one (respiration) that allows the oxygen to reach the cells where it can be used as fuel for the body. This chapter is concerned primarily with ventilation; Chapter 6, which deals with shock, further discusses the importance of respiration.

During inspiration, the diaphragm and intercostal muscles contract, causing the diaphragm to move downward and the ribs to spread and lift (Figure 5-2). This motion increases the volume inside the thoracic cage. Because volume and pressure are inversely proportional in a closed system, the intrathoracic pressure decreases to a level lower than that of the air outside the body, causing air to be inhaled into the lungs through the mouth, nose, pharynx, trachea, and bronchi (Figure 5-3).

During exhalation, the diaphragm and intercostal muscles relax, causing the diaphragm to move upward and the ribs to return to their resting position. The intrathoracic volume decreases from that at peak inhalation, while the intrathoracic pressure increases to a level greater than that of the air outside the mouth, and the air in the lungs is forced out of the body through the bronchi, trachea, pharynx, nose, and mouth.

Within the lungs are the alveoli, minute sacs of tissue each intimately related to a network of capillaries (see Figure 3-4, page 60). Carbon dioxide and oxygen diffuse through the walls of the capillaries and alveoli (Figure 5-4).

NEUROCHEMICAL CONTROL OF RESPIRATION

The respiratory center, located in the brain stem, contains chemoreceptor cells that are sensitive to changes in cer-

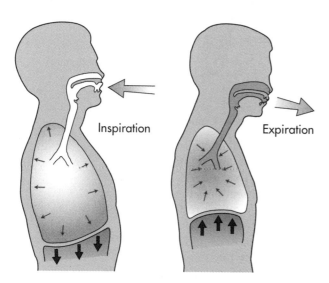

Figure 5-3 When the diaphragm is relaxed and the glottis is open there is equality between the pressure inside the lungs and that outside. When the chest cavity expands, the intrathoracic pressure decreases and air goes

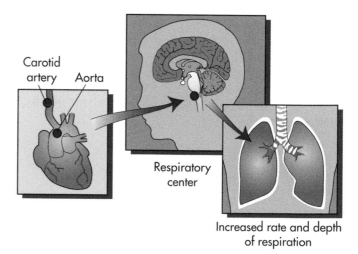

Figure 5-5 An increased level of carbon dioxide and pH is detected by nerve cells sensitive to this change, which stimulates the lung to increase both depth and rate of ventilation.

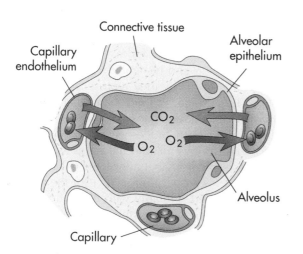

Figure 5-4 The capillaries and alveolus lie in close proximity; therefore oxygen can easily diffuse through the capillary, the alveolar walls, the capillary walls, and the red blood cells. Carbon dioxide can diffuse back in the opposite direction.

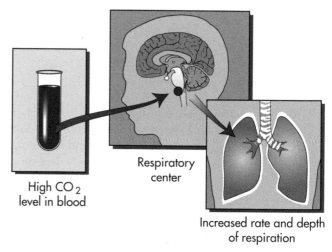

Figure 5-6 Receptors located in the aorta and carotid arteries are sensitive to the oxygen level and will stimulate the lungs to increase air movement into and out of the alveolar sacs.

tain chemical levels in the body. These cells in turn stimulate nerve impulses that control inspiration. The chemical to which the respiratory center's chemoreceptor cells normally respond is carbon dioxide (CO_2).

If the patient's respiration is inadequate for any reason, or if there is metabolic acidosis or anaerobic metabolism, the level of carbon dioxide ($PaCO_2$) will increase. The chemoreceptors will detect the change in the pH of the blood and stimulate the nerve cells to increase the rate and depth of breathing in order to remove the excess (Figure 5-5). The CO_2 stimulus can increase ventilation so effectively that the alveoli receive up to ten times more air than during a normal breath. Some chronic respiratory diseases inhibit the normal elimination of CO_2. The body compensates and becomes accustomed to the increased level of carbon dioxide in the blood ($PaCO_2$). In this situation, the dominant ventilatory control is the level of oxygen in the blood (PaO_2). Located in the aorta and carotid arteries are receptors that react to a PaO_2 below 60 mm Hg (Figure 5-6). These receptors alert the brain to cause the ventilatory muscles to increase their activity, which produces increased **minute volume** (the amount of air exchange that occurs in one minute).

During normal nonforced ventilation, about 500 cc of air is exchanged between the lungs and the atmosphere with each breath. This is called the **tidal volume.** After normal inhalation with nonforced inspiratory effort, a total of 3,000 cc of air may additionally be inhaled. This is called the **inspiratory reserve volume.** The total volume of air in the lungs after a forced inhalation is called the **total lung capacity.**

Some air always remains trapped in the alveoli and bronchi. This air, approximately 1,200 cc, cannot be forcibly exhaled. It is called the **residual volume.** The residual air in the alveoli normally permits the exchange of oxygen and carbon dioxide in the blood between breathing cycles.

The total ventilation volume expired per minute (VE) is equal to the volume of air moved per breath (VI) multiplied by the breaths per minute (f). Under normal resting conditions, the overall ventilation of the lung approximates 6 to 7 liters (L) per minute.

Therefore, if the volume of each breath (VI) equals 500 cc, and the rate per minute (f) equals 14, then

$$VE = VI \times f = 500 \times 14$$
$$= 7,000 \text{ cc/minute}$$
$$= 7 \text{ L/minute.}$$

Minute ventilation becomes significant when the patient has an altered breathing pattern for whatever reason. For example, a patient with rib fractures who is breathing fast and shallowly because of the pain and injury may have the following VE, which can soon lead to severe distress:

$$VI = 100 \text{ cc}$$
$$f = 40$$
$$VE = 100 \times 40$$
$$VE = 4,000 \text{ cc/minute}$$
$$= 4 \text{ L/minute}$$

Thus, the patient's ventilation has decreased significantly. This decrease in ventilation may therefore impair respiration and lead to severe distress.

PATHOPHYSIOLOGY

Chest injuries may be penetrating or blunt. Penetrating injuries are caused by forces distributed over a small area as in gunshot wounds, stabbing, or falls onto sharp objects. With penetrating trauma, any structure or organ in the chest cavity may be injured. Most often, the organs injured are those that lie along the path of the penetrating object.

In blunt trauma, the forces are distributed over a larger area, and many injuries occur from deceleration, bursting, and shearing forces. Conditions such as pneumothorax, pericardial tamponade, flail chest, pulmonary contusion, and aortic rupture should be suspected in blunt trauma or when the mechanism of injury involves rapid deceleration. Because of the large number and complexity of these conditions, the pathophysiology, assessment, and management of specific injuries are presented later in this chapter.

ASSESSMENT

SYMPTOMS

The symptoms of chest trauma related to the chest wall and lung are shortness of breath, tachypnea, and chest pain. The pain is usually pleuritic; that is, there is pain upon breathing. The pain may occur with motion and may be described as a chest tightness or discomfort. Conditions such as pneumothorax, major vascular injuries, or injuries to the esophagus might not produce any symptoms. The symptoms associated with chest injuries are like symptoms in other injured body areas: when they are present, pathology is indicated. However, the lack of symptoms does *not* indicate that there is no injury.

SIGNS

Because the organs of respiration and circulation are located in the chest, major chest injury can produce life-threatening physiologic disturbances of ventilation and circulation. The presence of shock must be rapidly correlated with the physical examination findings in order to appropriately intervene and treat that patient. Examination of the chest classically follows this sequence:

- observation
- palpation
- auscultation

A thorough visual examination of the chest can be done in less than 30 seconds. *Observation* of the neck and chest wall may reveal cyanosis, bruises, lacerations, distended neck veins, tracheal deviation, subcutaneous emphysema, open chest wounds, lack of bilaterally symmetrical chest rise, and paradoxical chest motion. The neck and chest should be *palpated* for the presence of tenderness, bony crepitus, subcutaneous emphysema, and an unstable chest wall segment. Because of pain, "splinting" or trying to limit chest motion on inspiration may be noted. The lungs should be *auscultated* for the presence or absence of breath sounds, the volume inspired, and bilateral symmetry of air movement. Diminished or absent breath sounds on one side of the chest in a trauma victim may indicate air or blood in the pleural space. Rapid evaluation, initiation of resuscitation, and transport are the keys to the survival of patients with chest injuries.

MANAGEMENT OF SPECIFIC INJURIES

RIB FRACTURES

Although any rib may be fractured, the most common location is the lateral aspect of ribs 3 through 8. These ribs are long, thin, and poorly protected (Figure 5-7). On the other hand, the uppermost ribs, particularly ribs 1 and 2, are short, broad, relatively thick, and well protected by the scapulae, clavicles, and upper chest muscles. It takes

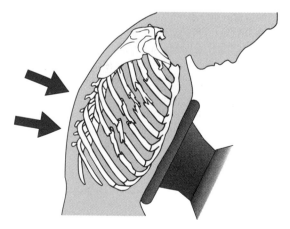

Figure 5-7 Ribs 3 through 8, which are long and thin, are usually fractured by external compression.

considerable force to break these ribs. An indication of the amount of force needed is reflected in the fact that up to 30% of patients with fractures of the first and second ribs die from associated injuries; as many as 5% of these patients have a ruptured aorta.

Pathophysiology

A single rib fracture occurs when pressure is applied to one specific rib with enough force to exceed the tensile strength of that rib. At the instant of release of the restraining force, the broken end of the rib can travel several centimeters into adjacent structures, such as the lung, and can damage them. This tissue can tear or contuse and result in rupturing of cells, capillaries, and perhaps major vessels. In the case of rib fractures, associated injuries include pulmonary contusion, laceration of the intercostal artery and/or vein, pneumothorax, and hemorrhage and hematoma formation in the chest wall or in the alveoli or surrounding tissue.

Assessment

Simple rib fractures by themselves are rarely life threatening in adults. The signs and symptoms of broken ribs are pain with movement, local tenderness, and perhaps bony crepitus. Of greater importance is the evaluation and recognition of associated injuries to underlying structures, which may be life threatening. Fracture of the lower ribs (R8 to R12) can be associated with spleen, kidney, or liver injuries.

Management

The initial management of patients with simple rib fractures is splinting, using the patient's arms and a sling and swath. Management should also include patient reassurance and an anticipation of potential complications such as open or closed pneumothorax and hypovolemia. Care must be taken to evaluate tidal volume and the presence of hypoxemia; should ventilation be significantly encumbered, ventilatory assistance is indicated. Deep, full ventilations and coughing should be encouraged despite the associated pain. Such actions prevent atelectasis (collapse of alveoli or part of the lung) leading to pneumonia. Fractured ribs should *not* be stabilized by taping or any other firm bandaging or binding that encircles the chest. Such attempts at management can inhibit chest movement and limit ventilation and can lead to atelectasis and pneumonia.

FLAIL CHEST

The cause of a **flail chest** is usually an impact into the sternum or the lateral side of the thoracic wall. In a frontal collision the sternum stops against the steering column. The continued forward motion of the posterior thoracic wall bends the ribs until they fracture (see Figure 1-17, page 10). In a T-bone type collision at an intersection, impact will be into the lateral thoracic wall.

Pathophysiology

Flail chest occurs when two or more adjacent ribs are each fractured in at least two places.

Paradoxical Movement

The segment of chest wall that is flailed has lost its bony support and attachment to the thoracic cage. This "free" segment will move in the opposite direction from the rest of the chest wall during inspiration and expiration. With inspiration, as the diaphragm moves downward and the ribs elevate and separate, intrathoracic pressure decreases. The combination of the lower pressure in the chest and higher atmospheric pressure outside the chest causes the flail segment to move inward, rather than outward, during inspiration. This motion of the chest is called **paradoxical motion** or **movement** (Figure 5-8).

During expiration, when the diaphragm moves upward and the ribs come together, intrathoracic pressure increases. The floating segment of the chest wall moves out rather than in. The result of both of these paradoxical movements of the chest wall is decreased ventilation producing hypoxia and hypercarbia.

Pain

The movement of several broken ends of the ribs against each other produces pain. The pain is similar to the pain produced by a single fractured rib, except that it is more severe. Therefore the patient has a greater tendency to splint and does not move air adequately into the lungs.

Pulmonary Contusion

The compression of the lung tears tissue, producing hemorrhage into the alveolar walls and the alveolar space, and producing a bruise or contusion of the lung. The result is decreased air into the lung and decreased transfer of oxygen across the alveolocapillary membrane to the red blood cells.

Assessment

Tenderness and/or bony crepitus elicited by palpation should lead to a closer inspection of that area of the chest wall for paradoxical motion. Initially, intercostal muscle spasm may prevent significant paradoxical motion, but as these muscles tire, the flail segment becomes more obvious.

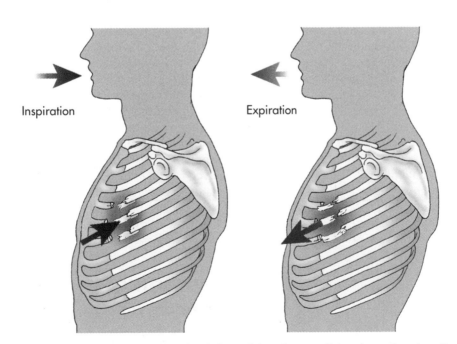

Inspiration   Expiration

Figure 5-8 Paradoxical motion. If stability of the chest wall has been lost by ribs fractured in two or more places, when intrathoracic pressure decreases during inspiration, the external air pressure forces the chest wall in. When intrathoracic pressure increases during expiration, the chest wall is forced out. (From American College of Emergency Physicians. *Paramedic Field Care: A Complaint Based Approach.* St. Louis: Mosby, 1997.)

Initial and ongoing evaluation of the respiratory rate is essential to recognize developing hypoxemia or respiratory failure. As the patient becomes increasingly hypoxic, the respiratory rate will gradually increase. Only by careful and repeated determinations of the respiratory rate will the EMT note subtle changes indicating that a patient is getting into trouble. When available, pulse oximetry can also be used to help recognize hypoxia; however, it is not a substitute for repeated evaluations of the respiratory rate.

Management

There are four consequences of flail chest: (1) a decrease in the vital capacity proportional to the size of the flail segment; (2) an increase in the labor of breathing; (3) pain produced by the fractured ribs, limiting the amount of thoracic cage expansion; and (4) most significant clinically, contusion of the lung beneath the flail segment. Several considerations are important in the management of this injury.

If the patient is in respiratory distress, two simple steps can be used in the field. The flail segment can be either splinted in the inward position with simple hand pressure or with bulky dressings or towels taped to the chest wall. These steps will reduce the motion of the flail segment, as well as the pain, but they will not remedy the reduced ventilation. The key step in management, therefore, is to assist the patient's ventilation with positive-pressure ventilation by the bag-valve-mask method.

Assisted ventilation expands the collapsed alveoli, both in the area of the flail segment as well as in the area involved when the patient splints. Blood passing through the capillaries lining the collapsed (nonventilated) alveoli leaves the lung still unoxygenated. Providing additional oxygen to the unaffected alveoli, combined with forced expansion of the collapsed alveoli, decreases the amount of oxygen-deprived blood entering the left side of the heart and the aorta.

A large percentage of patients with significant flail chest will progress to respiratory failure and require eventual and often prolonged ventilatory support in the hospital. Management of a severe flail injury includes intubation and positive-pressure ventilation. Some patients may require intubation in the field.

The use of sand bags to prevent movement in patients with a flail chest (described in earlier textbooks) has been found to decrease aeration of the lungs and to promote alveolar collapse. *This method should no longer be used.*

PULMONARY CONTUSION
Pathophysiology

A pulmonary contusion is an area of a lung that has been traumatized to the point where there is interstitial and alveolar bleeding. The amount of interstitial fluid increases in the area between the walls of the capillaries and alveoli. The result is decreased oxygen transport across the thickened membranes. Hemorrhage into the alveolar sac prevents any oxygenation of the affected segment. The EMT may have only the mechanism of injury and the presence of associated injuries to alert him or her to a potential pulmonary contusion during the initial assessment of the patient.

Pulmonary contusion can be the result of blunt trauma, as in flail chest. It can also result from penetrating trauma. In this scenario, an area of contusion surrounds the pathway that was produced by the cavitation effect of a missile. Whether caused by blunt or penetrating trauma, however, the clinical result is the same: areas of lung are no longer ventilated. When large areas of lung are no longer functioning properly, it compounds the significant mechanical problems of a flail chest. A pulmonary contusion produces significant compromise of oxygenation, and as such, is the most serious complication of a flail chest. Even without the associated presence of a flail chest, pulmonary contusion is the most common potentially lethal chest injury seen in the United States; the respiratory failure produced can develop rapidly in the first 8 to 24 hours.

Management

Patients with contused lungs do not tolerate excess fluid well. The extra fluid increases the amount of interstitial fluid and decreases oxygen transport even more. Therefore, these patients should be closely monitored. If they are hemodynamically normal, intravenous fluid administration should be limited to that needed for maintenance only. Hypotensive or tachycardic patients with multiple injuries should not have fluids restricted.

As with other traumatic conditions involving the lungs, appropriate management includes ensuring adequate ventilation and enriched oxygen administration. If pulse oximetry is available, it can help guide management. Supplemental oxygen should be provided to maintain oxygen saturation of about 90%. If the patient cannot maintain adequate ventilation or is suffering from preexisting chronic pulmonary disease, an altered level of consciousness, or other major injuries, the EMT should use bag-valve-mask ventilation and, if required, endotracheal intubation.

PNEUMOTHORAX
Pathophysiology

A **simple pneumothorax** is caused by the presence of air in the pleural space. This air can come from the outside through an opening in the chest wall, from the inside through a defect in the lung itself, or both. The air separates the two pleural surfaces (parietal and visceral), causing the lung on the involved side to collapse as the separation expands (Figure 5-9). As air continues to accumulate and pressure in the pleural space increases, the size of the lung on the affected side continues to decrease. The lung may then either partially or totally collapse.

The large reserve capacity of the ventilatory and circulatory systems usually prevents acute serious consequences from a simple pneumothorax in young and healthy patients. Individuals with decreased reserves due to advanced age or cardiopulmonary disease will be more adversely affected.

Assessment

The signs and symptoms of a pneumothorax may include pleuritic chest pain and difficult and rapid breathing. Decreased or absent breath sounds on the involved side are the classic signs. Although percussion for bell tympany is an excellent indicator, it may be difficult to detect in the field. In trauma patients in the prehospital setting, absent or decreased breath sounds plus ventilatory distress equals pneumothorax. When the lung collapse is partial, reduced or absent breath sounds may be heard over the apices and bases of the lung earlier than over the midlung fields. These patients require constant monitoring in anticipation of the development of a tension pneumothorax.

Management

The patient is placed in the position of comfort (usually a semisitting position) unless contraindicated by a possible spine injury, hypovolemia, or another injury. High-concentration oxygen (FiO_2 of 0.85–1.0) should be administered. Bag-valve-mask assisted breathing may be necessary for patients whose respiratory rate is less than 12 or greater than 20 breaths per minute or who display signs of hypoxia. However, positive-pressure ventilation may increase the possibility of a tension pneumothorax. The patient must be transported rapidly and carefully monitored for signs of a tension pneumothorax while en route. Steps must be taken to alleviate the tension pneumothorax if it develops.

When working at the EMT-basic level, it is especially important that rapid transportation occurs as soon as practical in anticipation of the possibility of a developing tension pneumothorax in the patient.

OPEN PNEUMOTHORAX (SUCKING CHEST WOUND)

Pathophysiology

Penetrating wounds to the chest can produce open chest wall injuries **(open pneumothorax).** These injuries are most often the result of gunshot or knife wounds, but they can also occur from impaled objects, motor vehicle collisions, and falls. The severity of a chest wall defect is directly proportional to its size. Many small wounds will seal themselves. Some large wounds will be completely open, allowing air to enter and escape the pleural cavity. Other wounds function like a ball valve. These wounds allow air to enter when the intrathoracic pressure is negative and block the air's release when the intrathoracic pressure is positive; hence the term "sucking chest wound" (Figure 5-10). These wounds are of particular concern because of their potential to cause a tension pneumothorax.

There are two possible sources of air that can leak into the pleural space: the wound in the chest wall and the

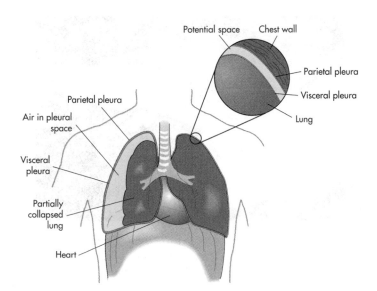

Figure 5-9 Air in the pleural space forces the lung in, decreasing the amount that can be ventilated and therefore decreasing oxygenation of the blood leaving the lung.

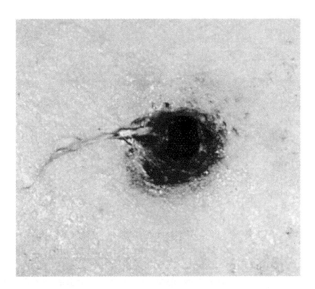

Figure 5-10 A gunshot or stab wound to the chest produces a hole in the chest wall through which air can flow both into and out of the pleural cavity.

lung or bronchus. Even if the injury to the chest wall is sealed, air leakage from injury to the lung can contribute to a pneumothorax (Figure 5-11).

When the chest wall is open, a preferential pathway is created for air to move from the outside environment into the thorax. Rather than passing through the nose, mouth, pharynx, trachea, and bronchi to reach the lungs and thoracic cavity, air simply passes through the chest wound into the thorax. This air remains outside the lung on that side of the chest, generally within the pleura. With reduced or no air coming through the bronchi to expand the lung, and with air accumulating between the pleura but outside the lung, the lung is compressed and cannot expand. The oxygen in the air that enters the thorax in this manner does not enter the lung, cannot become exposed to the alveolar capillaries, and therefore is not diffused into the bloodstream to provide oxygenation to the body's cells.

Assessment

Symptoms of this condition are pain at the injury site and shortness of breath. The signs may include a moist sucking or bubbling sound as air moves in and out of the pleural space through the chest wall defect.

Management

Management is directed first toward closing the hole in the chest, after which pressure-assisted ventilation will provide benefit to the patient. Closing the wound can be done with Vaseline gauze covered with sterile gauze, or any other type of occlusive dressing secured with tape. Blocking airflow completely with a dressing can produce

a tension pneumothorax. If only three sides of the dressing are taped, an effective vent is created that might permit spontaneous decompression of a developing tension pneumothorax (Figure 5-12). Even if a self-venting dressing is applied, any patient who has had an open chest wound sealed by the EMT must be carefully and continually monitored for the onset of a tension pneumothorax until the patient's care can be directly transferred to the hospital emergency department staff.

As for any trauma patient, high-concentration oxygen, ventilatory support, and treatment for hypovolemia must be the EMT's first priority after closure of the chest wound.

TENSION PNEUMOTHORAX
Pathophysiology

A life-threatening situation arises when a one-way valve is created that allows air to enter but not leave the pleural space. As the pressure in the pleural space exceeds the outside atmospheric pressure, the physiologic consequences of a simple pneumothorax are magnified. This injury is called a **tension pneumothorax.** Increasing pressure within the pleural space further collapses the lung on the involved side and forces the mediastinum (heart and blood vessels) to the opposite (contralateral) side (Figure 5-13).

Two extremely serious consequences result: (1) breathing becomes increasingly difficult and (2) the flow of blood into the heart decreases. Breathing is compromised because not only has the lung collapsed on the injured side, but the lung on the other side is compressed by the shift of the mediastinal structures. Normally, the pressure in the great veins leading to the heart is between 5 and 10 millimeters of mercury (mm Hg). As the pressure in the

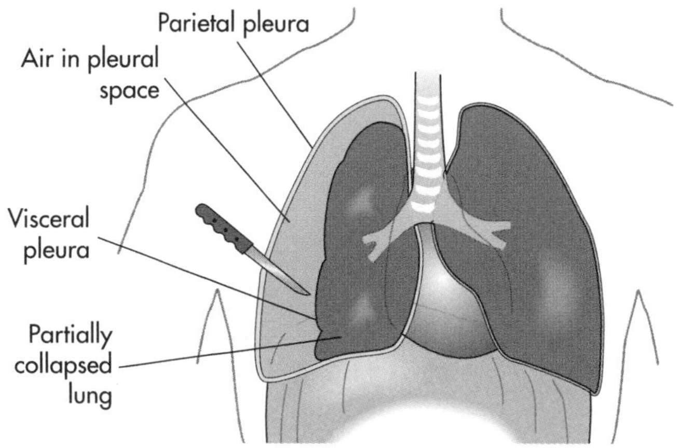

Parietal pleura

Air in pleural space

Visceral pleura

Partially collapsed lung

Figure 5-11 Because of the close proximity of the chest wall to the lung, it would be extremely difficult for the chest wall to be injured by penetrating trauma and the lung not to be injured. Stopping the hole in the chest wall does not necessarily decrease air leakage into the pleural space; leakage can come from the lung just as easily.

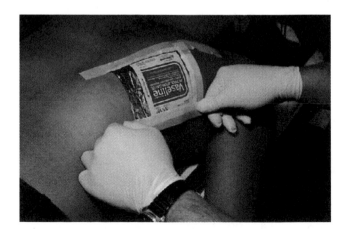

Figure 5-12 Taping a piece of foil or plastic on the chest wall on three sides creates a flutter-valve effect, allowing air to escape from the pleural space but not enter into it.

pleural space increases, the mediastinum shifts (evidenced by tracheal deviation from the midline), resulting in a high venous pressure caused by the increase in intrapleural pressure and kinking of the vena cava, both of which produce decreased blood flow into the heart. The decrease in venous return to the heart results in a decrease in cardiac output. Cardiac output is the amount of blood ejected from the heart at each contraction multiplied by the pulse rate (see Chapter 6: Shock and Fluid Resuscitation). Cardiac output is expressed in liters per minute.

Assessment

The presentation of patients with tension pneumothorax varies according to how much intrathoracic pressure has developed. The signs and symptoms in some patients will be minimal to moderate, whereas in others they will be severe. The signs and symptoms of a tension pneumothorax include extreme anxiety, cyanosis, tachypnea, diminished or absent breath sounds on the injured side, bulging of the intercostal muscles, jugular vein distention (JVD), tachycardia, narrow pulse pressure, hypotension, subcutaneous emphysema, and tracheal deviation.

Although the following signs are frequently discussed, many are not present or are difficult to identify in the field:

- *Tracheal deviation* is usually a *late* sign. In the neck, the trachea is bound to the cervical spine by fascial and other supporting structures; thus, the deviation of the trachea is more of an intrathoracic phenomenon, although if severe, it may be felt. It is not often seen in the prehospital environment. Even when it is present, it can be difficult to diagnose by physical examination.

- *Distended neck veins* are described as a classic sign of tension pneumothorax. However, since the patient with a tension pneumothorax may also have lost a considerable amount of blood, distended neck veins may not be prominent. If the patient has a pneumatic antishock garment applied, the neck veins may be distended by the device and not by a tension pneumothorax (Figure 5-14).

- *Cyanosis* is difficult to see in the poor lighting that frequently exists in the field. Poor lighting, variation in skin color, and dirt and blood associated with trauma often render this sign unreliable.

- The most helpful part of the physical examination is checking for *decreased breath sounds* on the side of the injury. To use this sign, however, one must be able to distinguish between normal and decreased sounds. Such differentiation cannot be done without a great deal of practice. Listening to breath sounds during every patient contact will help.

- *Percussion of the chest* is an excellent method for determining the status of the chest cavity in the relative quiet of the hospital. In the noisy prehospital environment, this sound is much more difficult to detect. Given the difficulty in obtaining this sign and the time and environment necessary with which to perform it, it is not recommended for field diagnosis of tension pneumothorax.

The potential for any patient with a simple pneumo-

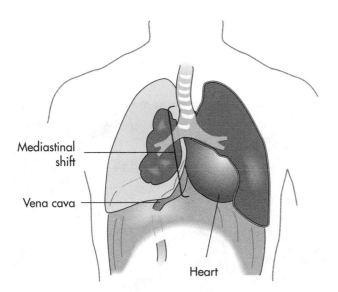

Figure 5-13 Tension pneumothorax. If the amount of air trapped in the pleural space continues to increase, not only is the lung on the affected side collapsed, but the mediastinum is also shifted into the opposite side. The lung on the opposite side then collapses and intrathoracic pressure increases, which decreases capillary blood flow and kinks the vena cava.

Mediastinal shift

Vena cava

Heart

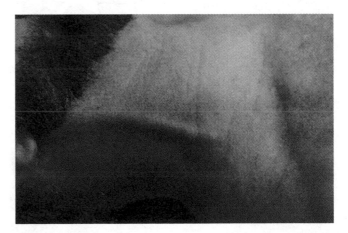

Figure 5-14 Distended neck veins are one of the indications of an increase in thoracic pressure.

The potential for any patient with a simple pneumothorax or hemopneumothorax to develop a tension pneumothorax is very real. The development of a tension pneumothorax is an important concern for any patient who has sustained chest trauma, has been intubated, and requires positive-pressure ventilation. In these cases, it is possible to convert a simple pneumothorax to a tension pneumothorax because air is being pushed into the chest with each ventilation. The patient must be constantly monitored for this possibility, and the EMT must be prepared to rapidly intervene.

Usual signs and symptoms of a developing tension pneumothorax are as follows:

- **early signs:** unilateral decreased or absent breath sounds; continued increased dyspnea and tachypnea despite treatment
- **progressive signs:** increasing tachypnea and dyspnea, tachycardia and subcutaneous emphysema, increasing difficulty ventilating (bagging) an intubated patient
- **late signs:** JVD, tracheal deviation, tympany, signs of acute hypoxia, narrowing pulse pressure, and other signs of increasing decompensating shock

In some cases, the only signs of a developing tension pneumothorax are compromised oxygenation, tachycardia, tachypnea, and unilateral decreased or absent breath sounds.

Management

The management of a patient with a tension pneumothorax involves reducing the pressure in the pleural space.

Penetrating Injury

When there is a wound in the chest wall with signs of a tension pneumothorax, the first step in relieving the increased pressure is to remove the dressing over the wound for a few seconds. If the wound in the chest wall has not sealed under the dressing, air will rush out of the wound. Once the pressure has been released, the wound should be resealed with the occlusive dressing. This short release may need to be repeated periodically if pressure again builds up within the chest. In the rare case that it becomes necessary to keep the defect open to prevent reaccumulation of air in the thoracic cavity, assisted ventilation with an FiO_2 of 0.85 to 1.0 is necessary.

Closed Tension Pneumothorax

If reopening the wound does not immediately solve the condition, or if the pneumothorax developed without a wound in the chest wall, decompression is accomplished by insertion of a large bore needle into the pleural space of the affected side. This procedure can be carried out in the field by an advanced life support (ALS) provider. If ALS personnel are not available, the patient must be transported as rapidly as possible to the appropriate hospital while administering oxygen at a high FiO_2 while en route. A tension pneumothorax or a potential tension pneumothorax is a life-threatening condition. It requires rapid access to an appropriate hospital, as needle insertion or dressing removal is only a temporary solution until more definitive care can be provided.

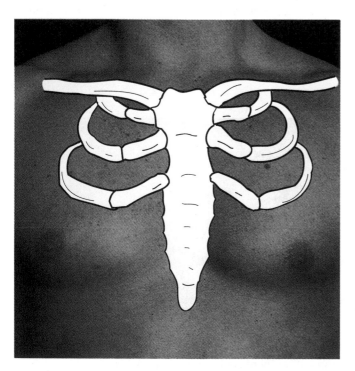

Figure 5-15 Needle decompression of the thoracic cavity is most easily accomplished and produces the least chance for complication if it is done at the midclavicular line through the second intercostal space.

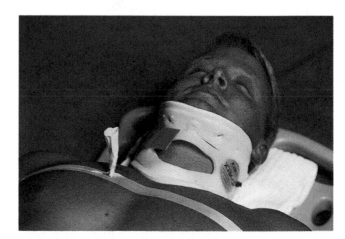

Figure 5-16 Once the needle has been inserted, a one-way valve made with the finger cut from the end of a glove will allow air pressure to flow from within the pleural cavity to an outside wall but not in the opposite direction.

Needle decompression carries minimal risk and can greatly benefit the patient by improving oxygenation and circulation. A 14-gauge or 16-gauge hollow needle is inserted into the affected pleural space at the second intercostal space in the midclavicular line. The landmark for insertion is the angle of Louis on the sternum, which marks the space between the second and third ribs (Figure 5-15). The midclavicular line is at the midpoint of the clavicle. This area lacks anatomic structures that could be injured during needle decompression. The internal mammary artery is just lateral to the sternal border (1 cm), hence the use of the midclavicular line. Since the lung is compressed toward the mediastinum, it will be out of the way if the needle is placed high into the second intercostal space. The nerve, artery, and vein pass just beneath each rib, so the needle should pass just over the third or fourth rib. The midclavicular site is better than the mid-axillary line where chest tubes are inserted in the emergency department. The anterior chest allows better visualization of the needle at the midclavicular line while en route to the hospital. Also, the patient's arm is not strapped down across this area as would be the case if the midaxillary line was chosen. Special situations may require other approaches under the direction of appropriate medical control.

Initially after insertion, air will rush from the needle as the pressure in the chest is relieved. A one-way valve can then be attached to the needle to allow air to escape from the pleural space but not enter it. Such a valve can easily be made by cutting a finger from a sterile glove. Rinse the inside of the glove finger with sterile water or normal saline prior to using it. Rinsing removes the talcum powder and results in a better seal when the valve is closed. Pass the needle and catheter through the length of the glove's finger and puncture the fingertip with it.

If the needle has been inserted in the patient's chest without a one-way valve, the sterile glove finger can be added. Simply cut the finger from the glove, cut a small hole at the fingertip, spread the tip over the catheter hub, and fasten with a rubber band. If available, tubing and a flutter valve can be added to the hub of the needle instead of a glove finger (Figure 5-16).

HEMOTHORAX
Pathophysiology

Blood in the pleural space constitutes a **hemothorax.** In adults, the pleural space on each side of the thorax can hold 2,500 to 3,000 cc of blood, which can come from several sources, such as torn intercostal vessels or the lung itself and its vessels. Hypovolemia (decreased fluid volume) occurs as the blood leaves the cardiovascular space and enters the pleural space. Although a tension hemothorax is an uncommon occurrence, it does happen. A simple hemothorax is much more common, and

the clinically critical component is the associated blood loss (Figure 5-17).

Assessment

The symptoms of a hemothorax are directly related to blood loss and, to a much lesser extent, the amount of lung collapse and the resulting shortness of breath. Depending on the magnitude of respiratory and circulatory compromise, as with any hypovolemic condition, the patient may also be confused or anxious. The signs of a hemothorax include tachypnea, decreased breath sounds with dullness to percussion, and the clinical signs of shock.

Diminished breath sounds with **hyporesonance** (dullness upon percussion) on the same side is found with a hemothorax. This sign is far more difficult to assess in the field than is the hyperresonance of a tension pneumothorax. Often with penetrating trauma, a pneumothorax is associated with a hemothorax and is called a **hemopneumothorax.**

Management

The management of a hemothorax is directed at correcting the ventilatory and circulatory problems. Oxygen should be administered along with ventilatory assistance, using a bag-valve-mask and/or endotracheal tube as necessary. As with other chest injuries, close observation must be maintained. Hypovolemia or shock are the major physiologic defects and should be treated with intravenous electrolyte solutions and rapid transport to a hospital where immediate surgical repair can be achieved.

The use of the pneumatic antishock garment is *not* appropriate in the prehospital management of a hemothorax. The beneficial result of using the garment (increased blood pressure), actually promotes further hemorrhage and can lead to a worsening of the patient's condition. Use of the pneumatic antishock garment with

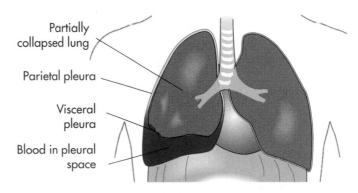

Figure 5-17 Hemothorax. The amount of blood that can accumulate in the thoracic cavity (leading to hypovolemia) is a much more severe condition than the amount of lung compressed by this blood loss.

such patients should only be done under specific instructions from on-line physician medical direction.

MYOCARDIAL CONTUSION
Pathophysiology

The heart occupies a large portion of the center of the chest and is situated between the sternum and the thoracic spine. In severe blunt trauma to the chest, as occurs in frontal motor vehicle collisions, the chest first strikes the dashboard or steering wheel and then the heart is crushed between the sternum and spine (Figure 5-18). Several cardiac injuries may result, but the most common injury is a **myocardial contusion.** The cardiac ventricles can be forcefully compressed and systolic blood pressure can rise to 800 mm Hg, which may cause compression of the myocardial wall. This compression can in turn cause cell wall destruction or frank rupture of the heart itself. The right ventricle is most commonly injured because of its location beneath the sternum.

There are three distinct injury patterns that can occur with myocardial compressive injury: (1) disturbance in the electrical conducting system of the myocardium, (2) contusion (bruise) to the myocardial wall that can be partial or full thickness, and (3) rupture of the myocardial wall. The latter condition may lead to rapid exsanguination (massive loss of blood) or to pericardial tamponade. (See later description of pericardial tamponade.)

Assessment

Myocardial contusion is a frequent injury in patients with chest compression. In the field, a patient with significant chest trauma should be assumed to have a bruised myocardium.

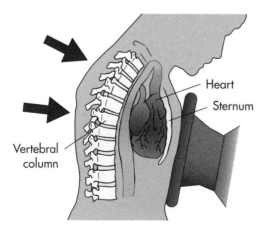

Figure 5-18 The heart can be trapped between the sternum (as the sternum stops against the steering column or dashboard) and the posterior thoracic wall (as the wall continues its forward motion). This can contuse the myocardium.

A partial- or full-thickness contusion may be indicated by reduced cardiac output and arrhythmias; however, there may be no signs at all. When the kinematics and other crash and postcrash evaluations indicate this condition but no clinical indications are present, the hospital personnel must be made aware of the possibility. A frontal collision with vehicle damage that includes a bent steering wheel or a collapsed steering column are indications that must be reported to the emergency department.

There are usually no symptoms of myocardial contusion, but the patient may complain of chest discomfort and pain of fractured ribs or bruised muscles. The patient with arrhythmia may complain of palpitations. Anterior chest tenderness and a bent steering wheel are most common findings and should be tip-offs to the possibility of a myocardial contusion.

Injuries to the electrical system of the heart may be manifest by a variety of arrhythmias, the most common of which is tachycardia out of proportion to other conditions. Premature ventricular contractions (PVCs) are the second most common arrhythmia, followed by atrial fibrillation. Septal injuries may produce conduction defects in the form of a bundle branch block (BBB), most commonly noted on the right (RBBB). Muscle wall damage is identified in the field by ST segment elevation or other electrocardiogram (ECG) changes.

Management

Management of these patients includes oxygen administration and monitoring the patient's pulse. In areas where multiple levels of prehospital response are available and the patient is being treated by EMT-basic personnel, consideration should be given to intersecting with an ALS unit.

Patients who have had a direct trauma to the chest significant enough to suggest a possible myocardial contusion should be placed on an ECG monitor, and any arrhythmia should be treated pharmacologically at the ALS level. Rapid transportation to the appropriate hospital is indicated.

PERICARDIAL TAMPONADE
Pathophysiology

The heart is enclosed within a tough, fibrous, flexible, but inelastic membrane called the pericardium. A potential space—the pericardial space—exists between the heart and the pericardium. As with the pleural space, a few cc's of fluid will normally occupy and lubricate this space. Blood can enter the pericardial space if myocardial blood vessels are torn by blunt or penetrating trauma or if the myocardium is ruptured or penetrated. This condition is called **pericardial tamponade.**

Treatable pericardial tamponade is most frequently associated with stab wounds. Gunshot wounds often create a large enough hole in the pericardium for the blood to exit the pericardial space. Exsanguination into the chest cavity rather than tamponade is the usual result of gunshot wounds. However, with either blunt or penetrating trauma, there may be no means of exit for the blood from the pericardial sac

Because the pericardium is an inelastic sac surrounding the heart, as blood leaks from a wound in the wall of the heart, it fills the sac. As the heart compresses to eject blood during systole, more blood fills the vacant space. Thus, the heart cannot re-expand to refill with blood. Progressively less blood is available to be pumped out with each contraction. Even in patients who are not hypovolemic, the ultimate outcome is inadequate cardiac output (Figure 5-19).

Assessment

The trauma patient with a pericardial tamponade may have no symptoms other than those related to chest injuries and those associated with shock. In an adult, the pericardial space may be able to hold 200 to 300 cc of blood before cardiac tamponade occurs; however, smaller volumes can still significantly reduce cardiac output.

As the amount of blood in the pericardial sac increases, the pulse increases in an attempt to maintain cardiac output. The pulse pressure narrows, and a **paradoxical pulse** may be present. A patient has a paradoxical pulse when the patient's systolic blood pressure drops more than 10 to 15 mm Hg during each inspiration. This blood pressure drop can be clinically determined by noting the radial pulse diminish or even disappear with inspiration. Because the compressed ventricles have reduced expansion during diastole (relaxed phase), only a small amount of blood can enter the heart. Expansion of the pulmonary vascular field during inspiration requires

all or almost all the reduced right heart output. This results in decreased filling of the left heart and reduced left heart output. Back-up of pressure on the right side results in venous pooling and neck vein distention or JVD. The heart sounds may be muffled and distant. Finally, signs of shock appear and progressively worsen. These three findings—elevated venous pressure, shock, and muffled heart sounds—are the classic signs of pericardial tamponade and are known as Beck's Triad. However, all of these signs are not always present with this condition.

Management

These patients require rapid, well-monitored transport to the hospital. It is essential that no delay occurs in the field. As with any type of shock, intravenous electrolyte infusion may improve cardiac output by increasing venous pressure, and it should be established during transport. Although use of the pneumatic antishock garment will increase the right heart filling pressure as well as improve cerebral blood flow, it does not control the cardiac hemorrhage and therefore is contraindicated in such patients.

The management of these patients involves removing the pericardial blood and stopping the source of bleeding. Removing pericardial blood is accomplished by a procedure called needle **pericardiocentesis,** which is almost exclusively a procedure limited to the emergency department. Control of bleeding usually requires surgical repair of the injury.

AORTIC RUPTURE
Pathophysiology

Traumatic **aortic rupture** usually results from a shear injury. With rapid, high G-force speed change in blunt chest injuries, several events take place. The heart and aortic

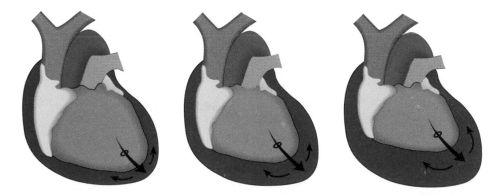

Figure 5-19 Pericardial tamponade. As blood courses from the cardiac lumen into the pericardial space, the expansion of the ventricle is reduced. Therefore the ventricle cannot fill completely. As more blood accumulates in the pericardial space, there is less ventricular space to accumulate blood and cardiac output is reduced.

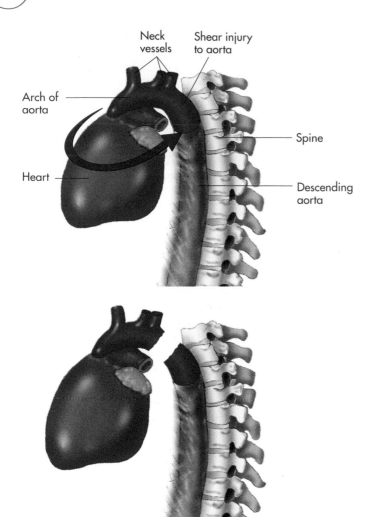

Figure 5-20 The descending aorta is tightly affixed to the thoracic vertebrae. The arch of the aorta and the heart are not attached to the vertebrae. Disruption from shear force usually occurs at the junction of the arch and the descending aorta.

arch suddenly move anteriorly or laterally. The heart and arch of the aorta move away from the descending aorta, which is tightly fixed to the thoracic vertebrae. Severe stress and shear forces occur at the distal portion of the arch where the restrained and unrestrained parts of the aorta meet. If the tensile strength of the aorta is exceeded, these two components can be torn apart (Figure 5-20). The layer of tissue surrounding the aorta may remain intact temporarily and prevent immediate exsanguination.

About 80% to 90% of patients with these injuries sustain aortic rupture and complete exsanguination into the left pleural space within the first hour. The remaining patients will reach the hospital alive. One-third of these initial survivors die within 6 hours, another third die in 24 hours. The final third survive 3 days or longer. Timely surgical repair can prevent most of the deaths of patients reaching the hospital alive.

Assessment

Diagnosis of aortic rupture is extremely difficult. In the hospital, a radiologic study of the aorta—either a computed tomography (CT) scan or an aortogram—is required to make the diagnosis.

Information from the scene concerning the magnitude of the trauma can be very helpful because up to one-third of these patients may have no signs of chest trauma. Patients with unexplained shock and a frontal-impact deceleration injury or lateral-impact acceleration injury must be suspected of having aortic disruption. In some cases, a difference in pulse quality between the arms and the lower torso or between the left and right arms can be detected. Assessment of both radial and femoral pulses is an important diagnostic step.

Management

Management of this condition involves high-concentration oxygen administration (FiO_2 of 0.85–1.0) and ventilatory assistance when indicated. Immediate transport and communication with the hospital are also key factors. Patients suspected of aortic disruption who do not show signs of hypovolemia should not be overhydrated, as the added fluid may accelerate the continued tearing of the remaining aortic wall tissue.

TRACHEAL/BRONCHIAL RUPTURE
Pathophysiology

Any portion of the tracheal/bronchial tree can be injured by penetrating or blunt trauma. These tears allow rapid movement of air into the pleural space, producing a tension pneumothorax that may be refractive to decompression. Rather than a simple one-time rush of air from the needle when inserted, air continually flows from the needle. Assisted ventilation will frequently worsen the condition of a patient with this type of injury. As air is forced into the lungs, it is forced out of the tear in the bronchus or trachea at the same rate.

Assessment

These patients may have severe dyspnea and often cough up bright red blood. Blunt trauma typically ruptures the upper trachea, the larynx, or the major bronchi just beyond the carina. The associated major hemorrhage seen with penetrating trauma is rarely present, but the signs, symptoms, and management are the same as with blunt trauma. With both blunt and penetrating trauma, an associated hemothorax or pneumothorax, or an area of subcutaneous emphysema extend-

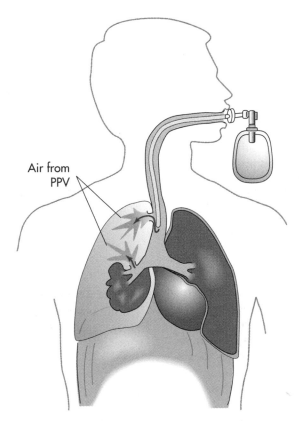

Figure 5-21 Tracheobronchial rupture. Positive-pressure ventilation *(PPV)* can directly force large amounts of air though the trachea or bronchus, rapidly producing a tension pneumothorax.

ing supraclavicularly into the neck and face, may be present.

Management

Assisted ventilation may be extremely difficult (Figure 5-21). If assisted ventilation seems to make the patient worse, allow the patient to breathe on his or her own and ensure an FiO_2 of 0.85 or greater. Otherwise, assisted ventilation with a high FiO_2 (0.85–1.0) should be administered and rapid transportation to the hospital initiated.

TRAUMATIC ASPHYXIATION
Pathophysiology

The term **traumatic asphyxiation** is a misnomer. Although these patients look like victims of strangulation, the condition has nothing whatsoever to do with asphyxia. With severe blunt and crushing injuries to the chest and abdomen, a marked increase in intrathoracic pressure occurs. This forces blood backward out of the right side of the heart and into the veins of the upper chest and neck. This pressure is transmitted to capillaries in the brain, head, and neck, producing microrupture, neurologic ischemia (cerebrovascular accident [CVA]), seizure, and venous distension.

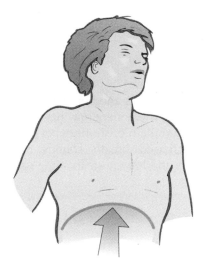

Figure 5-22 Traumatic asphyxiation. The external appearance of traumatic asphyxiation is a bluish discoloration of the face and upper neck.

ASSESSMENT

The patient presents with a bluish discoloration only to the face and upper neck (Figure 5-22). Unless other problems exist, the skin is pink below this area. JVD and swelling or hemorrhage of the conjunctiva may also be present. Most of the discoloration resolves within a few days.

Management

Because of the forces involved, any of the other injuries mentioned earlier may be present. Management includes recognizing the condition, providing airway maintenance, and taking care of the associated injuries.

DIAPHRAGMATIC RUPTURE

Pathophysiology

With high-pressure compression to the abdomen, the intra-abdominal pressure may increase enough to tear the diaphragm and allow abdominal contents to enter the thoracic cavity. Although these defects occur with equal frequency on both sides, those on the left side most often produce changes of clinical significance. The colon, small intestine, and spleen can be forced into the thoracic cavity. The space occupied by these organs restricts lung expansion and reduces ventilation. The reduction in ventilation can be severe enough to be life threatening (Figure 5-23).

Lacerations of the diaphragm can also occur in penetrating trauma because of the slope of the diaphragm, which positions it higher anteriorly than posteriorly. At maximum exhalation, the diaphragm is as high as the fourth intercostal space anteriorly. Any penetrating anterior injury below the nipple line may result in laceration of the diaphragm.

Assessment

Diaphragmatic rupture is another extremely difficult condition to diagnose. The patient may have abdominal complaints or may complain of shortness of breath. Upon examination, decreased breath sounds may be noted, particularly over the left chest. In some cases, it may be

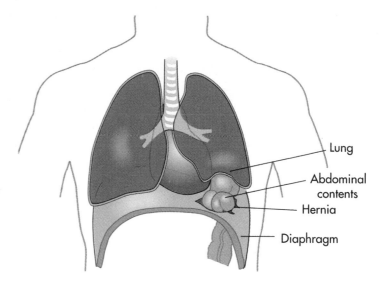

Figure 5-23 Diaphragmatic rupture may cause the result in the bowel or other structures to herniate through the tear, causing partial compression of the lung and respiratory distress.

possible to hear bowel sounds in the left chest. If a considerable quantity of abdominal contents is displaced into the chest, the abdomen may have a hollow or empty appearance.

Management

Assisted positive-pressure ventilation with an FiO_2 of 0.85 to 1.0 will help to provide adequate oxygenation. This condition can be made worse by anything that increases intra-abdominal pressure, such as that associated with pneumatic antishock garment usage. Deterioration of ventilation and oxygenation after inflation of the garment is an indication that such a condition exists. It is one of the few situations where field deflation of this device is indicated.

• Summary •

1. Other than the head, no area of the human body contains such a high degree of vital organs as does the thorax. The thorax also contains the great vessels of the body—the aorta, the vena cava, and the pulmonary arteries and veins.

2. Chest injuries are common in multiple-systems trauma patients and are usually associated with life-threatening injuries. Serious injury to the thorax can easily compromise or disrupt ventilation and circulation.

3. As well as the specific local injuries, trauma to the chest often has the following results:
   - Reduced ventilation of the alveoli can develop due to a lack of adequate chest excursion or loss of thoracic wall continuity, either in its skeletal structure (flail chest) or in its pneumatic integrity (open chest wound) leading to decreased blood oxygenation.
   - Pulmonary shunting and a lack of adequate oxygenation of some of the blood passing through the alveolar-capillary membrane can result from a pulmonary contusion.
   - Loss of pulmonary function can occur even with adequate overall ventilation. Alveolar pulmonary function can be reduced by a pneumothorax, hemothorax, pulmonary contusion, or invasion of abdominal organs through a herniated diaphragm.
   - Circulatory compromise can occur in the thorax through three mechanisms:
     a. Intrathoracic hemorrhage can be moderate (fractured rib) or severe (ruptured aorta).
     b. Loss of cardiac function can result from a pericardial tamponade or from arrhythmia secondary to a myocardial contusion.
     c. Increased intrathoracic pressure associated with a tension pneumothorax can obstruct venous return to the heart and also directly inhibit the heart's ability to function.

4. Bag-valve-mask assisted ventilations, endotracheal intubation, and needle decompression of the chest are among the procedures available in the field. High-concentration oxygen (FiO_2 of 0.85–1.0) should always accompany any of these procedures to maintain oxygen saturation above 90%.

5. The high incidence of other injuries associated with chest trauma necessitates rapid stabilization on a long board (ignoring injuries that are not life threatening until critical problems can be addressed), appropriate use of the pneumatic antishock garment, intravenous fluid administration (usually begun while en route to the hospital), and ECG monitoring for arrhythmia.

6. Many of these patients will require rapid surgical intervention. Although this can frequently be provided in a competent emergency department and does not always require transfer to the operating room, the patient should be transported to a facility where immediate operative intervention and advanced diagnostic techniques such as aortography are available. In smaller communities with only one hospital, this facility should be the initial treatment facility. In larger communities these patients should be transported directly to the trauma center, bypassing hospitals that are not set up to provide definitive management to critical trauma patients.

Scenario Solution

The findings of an apparent gunshot wound to the right chest, subcutaneous emphysema, and decreased breath sounds indicate that the patient has at least a pneumothorax, and given the mechanism, he is also likely to be bleeding into his chest cavity, producing a hemothorax. The patient requires emergent transport to a trauma center. You ask your partner to bring the stretcher and mentally run through the other things you are going to do. Once you have the patient in the ambulance, your partner begins transport to the hospital while you apply supplemental oxygen and obtain venous access. You then check his vital signs and in particular measure his respiratory rate, as you know that a significant change in respiratory rate can indicate that his pulmonary compromise is worsening. You then do a complete examination to be sure you have not missed any other injuries. While you are caring for the patient, your partner has dispatch notify the receiving facility to expect this patient in the next few minutes. On arrival at the hospital, you give your report and turn the patient over to the trauma team.

Review Questions

Answers provided on page 333.

1 In a normal adult, the control of respiration by chemoreceptors in the brain is determined by sensing which of the following chemicals?
A carbon monoxide (CO)
B carbon dioxide (CO_2)
C oxygen (O_2)
D Nitrogen (N)

2 The most important early observation that reveals developing respiratory compromise after trauma is:
A decreased blood pressure
B increased pulse rate
C increased respiratory rate
D decreased respiratory rate

3 The most important concern about a rib fracture is:
A intercostal nerve or vessel injury
B pain with inspiration
C underlying organ injury
D associated thoracic spine injury

4 A patient with a suspected flail chest develops increasing respirations and difficulty breathing. Which of the following interventions would be most likely to help the patient?
A needle decompression
B pericardiocentesis
C administration of an analgesic
D endotracheal intubation

5 Patients with pulmonary contusion should not be given too much intravenous fluid because fluid will:
A increase blood pressure and intra-abdominal bleeding
B increase intracerebral edema
C increase interstitial and intra-alveolar fluid and bleeding
D cause thoracic compartment syndrome

6 A patient with a suspected simple pneumothorax will benefit from which of the following interventions?
A rapid transport
B needle decompression
C administration of an analgesic
D positive-pressure ventilation

7 A patient sustains a stab wound to the right upper chest in the third intercostal space in the anterior axillary line. Your initial examination reveals a pulse of 96, blood pressure of 108/74, and respiratory rate of 22. During transport, you note that the pulse is now 128, blood pressure is 88/62, and respiratory rate is 32. You also note that the patient has developed subcutaneous emphysema from her neck to her mid-abdomen on the right side. The most appropriate intervention is:
A increase intravenous fluid rate
B pericardiocentesis
C endotracheal intubation with positive-pressure ventilation
D needle decompression

8 A patient sustains a stab wound to the left chest in the fifth intercostal space parasternally. He presents with a pulse of 122, blood pressure of 88/78, and respiratory rate of 26. The remainder of the physical examination is unremarkable. The most likely injury is:
A hemothorax
B pericardial tamponade
C tension pneumothorax
D associated abdominal injury and hemorrhage

9 A factory worker is crushed by a truck backing up to a loading dock. Your examination reveals tenderness over his pelvis, diffuse abdominal pain and tenderness, some lower chest wall tenderness, and possibly some rib fractures. The pulse is 116, blood pressure 90/68, and respiratory rate 26. You apply the pneumatic antishock garment (PASG) to stabilize the suspected pelvic fracture. The patient immediately complains of increased respiratory distress. You suspect which of the following additional conditions and perform the associated interventions?

A ruptured aorta, initiate immediate transport
B tension pneumothorax, needle decompression
C ruptured diaphragm, remove the PASG
D bronchial rupture, intubate and initiate positive-pressure ventilation

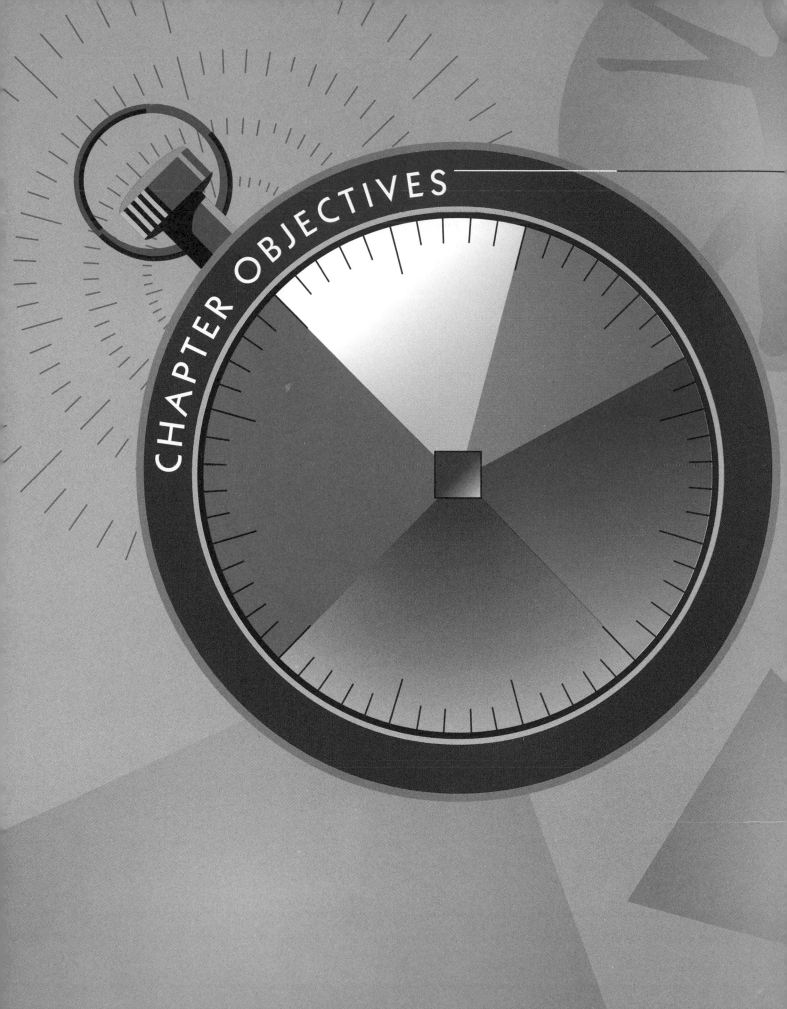
CHAPTER OBJECTIVES

CHAPTER 6

Shock and Fluid Resuscitation

At the completion of this course the student will be able to:

- Define perfusion, hypoperfusion, hypoxia, hypovolemia, normovolemia, hypervolemia, and hypotension.

- Define the pathophysiology of shock, including the three phases of shock and their progression.

- List the signs and symptoms of each phase of shock.

- Explain the proper use of the pneumatic antishock garment.

- List the indications for intravenous fluid replacement.

- Identify the need for rapid transport when confronted with continuing hypoperfusion.

- Demonstrate an understanding for the limits and short-term benefits of crystalloid fluid replacement and pneumatic antishock garment usage.

- Demonstrate an understanding of the need for blood replacement and hemorrhage control as the definitive care for blood loss.

- Explain why severe internal hemorrhage, even if temporarily controlled with a pressure dressing, needs to have direct surgical control in the operating room without delay.

Scenario

You are dispatched to a "motor vehicle collision." Response time will be approximately 15 to 20 minutes to a mountainous rural area. Upon arrival, a bystander informs you that the patient is a 14-year-old male who was riding an all-terrain vehicle. As he was accelerating up a hill, the vehicle slid sideways and rolled over on top of him. He became entangled with the vehicle as it tumbled down the hillside, crushing him as it rolled.

You determine that the patient was not wearing a helmet. Your assessment reveals the following:

- level of consciousness: awake, but disoriented
- airway is open and respirations are rapid and shallow
- pulse is slow and strong
- skin is warm and dry
- capillary refill is normal
- blood pressure reveals hypotension, but with a normal pulse-pressure margin
- contusions and tenderness of the head, neck, chest, and abdomen
- abrasions and lacerations on the hands, arms, and face
- deformed wrist and ankle
- numbness in the lower extremities

What do these findings indicate about this patient's condition? How would you appropriately manage this patient's injuries?

In 1852, the American surgeon, Samuel Gross, defined shock as "a rude unhinging of the machinery of life." Probably no better definition exists today to describe the devastating impact of this process on the patient. More recent definitions tend to be concerned with identifying the mechanism of shock. They are more specific and perhaps give a better picture of the particular pathophysiologic dysfunctions that take place. However, the definition of shock does not lie in low blood pressure, rapid pulse rates, or cool, clammy skin; these are merely systemic manifestations of the entire pathologic process that we call shock. The correct definition of **shock** is lack of tissue oxygenation that leads to anaerobic metabolism.

If the EMT is to understand this abnormal condition and be able to develop a treatment program to prevent or overcome shock, it is important that he or she knows what is happening to the body on a cellular level. The EMT must be able to understand, recognize, and interpret the normal physiologic responses that the body uses to protect itself from the development of shock. Only then can the EMT develop a rational approach for managing the problems of the patient in shock.

Shock can kill a patient early in the field or in the emergency department. Although actual death may be delayed for several hours to several days or even weeks, the most common cause of that death is the failure of early resuscitation. The lack of perfusion of the cells by oxygenated blood produces anaerobic metabolism. Even when some cells are initially spared, death occurs later rather than earlier, because not enough cells are able to carry out the function of that organ indefinitely. This chapter explains this phenomenon and presents methods to prevent such an outcome.

 PHYSIOLOGY

METABOLISM: THE HUMAN MOTOR

Every cell in the body requires oxygen to function. The cells take in oxygen and metabolize it through a complicated physiologic process that produces energy. The metabolism of oxygen requires energy, and cells must have fuel—the sugar glucose—to carry out this process. As in any combustion event, a by-product is also produced. The same process occurs in an engine when gasoline and air are mixed to produce energy, and carbon monoxide (CO) is created as a by-product. In the body, oxygen and glucose are mixed to produce energy and carbon dioxide (CO_2).

Cells in the body do contain an alternate power source. Such an alternate is also available in automobiles; it is possible to drive a car powered only by its battery and electric starting motor if air and gasoline are not available. The automobile could move only as long as the energy stored in the battery lasted. This movement would be much slower and much less efficient than that powered by gasoline and air. However, it would work, in a fashion, although the battery would soon run down and there would be no more energy to move the car, even if air and gasoline again became available.

In animals (humans included) the corollaries are:
gasoline and oxygen present—aerobic metabolism
battery alone—anaerobic metabolism

Aerobic metabolism describes the use of oxygen by cells. This form of metabolism is the body's principal combustion process. It produces energy using oxygen in a complicated process known as the Krebs cycle. **Anaerobic metabolism** occurs without the use of oxygen. It is the back-up power system in the body. The problems with using anaerobic metabolism to power the body are similar to the disadvantages of using a battery to run an automobile: it can only run for a short time, it does not produce as much energy, it produces by-products that are harmful to the body, and it may ultimately be irreversible.

The major by-products of anaerobic metabolism are excessive amounts of acid and potassium. If anaerobic metabolism is not reversed quickly, cells cannot continue to function and they die. If sufficient cells in any one organ die, the entire organ ceases to function. If a large number of cells in an organ die, but not enough cells to kill it, the organ's function will be significantly reduced and the remaining cells in that organ will have to work even harder than usual to keep the organ functioning. These overworked cells may or may not be able to support the function of the entire organ. Even with some cells remaining, the organ may still die. An example is a patient who has suffered a heart attack. Blood flow and oxygen are shut off to one portion of the myocardium (heart muscle), and some cells of the heart die, thus decreasing the cardiac output and the oxygen supply to the rest of the heart. This, in turn, causes a further reduction in oxygenation of the remaining heart cells. If not enough other cells remain, or if they are not strong enough to take over the entire function of the heart to meet the blood flow needs of the body, heart failure can result. Unless major improvement in cardiac output and oxygenation occur, the patient eventually will not survive.

Another example of this deadly process occurs in the kidneys. When the kidneys are injured or are deprived of adequate oxygenated blood, kidney cells begin to die and kidney function decreases. Other cells may be compromised yet continue to function for a while before dying. If enough cells die, the decreased level of function produces an inadequate elimination of toxic byproducts of metabolism. As this systemic deterioration continues, more and more organs die and eventually the organism (the human) dies. Depending on the organ initially involved, the progression from cell death to organism death can be rapid or delayed. It can take as long as 2 or 3 weeks before the damage caused by hypoxia or hypoperfusion in the first minutes posttrauma results in the patient's death. It may not be immediately apparent to recognize the effectiveness of the EMT's actions that reverse or prevent **hypoxia** (insufficient oxygen available to meet cell requirements) and **hypoperfusion** (inadequate blood passing to tissue cells) in the critical prehospital time period. However, these resuscitation measures are unquestionably necessary if the patient is to ultimately survive.

The sensitivity of cells to the lack of oxygen and the usefulness of anaerobic metabolism varies from organ system to organ system. This sensitivity is called **ischemic sensitivity,** and it is greatest in the brain, heart, and lungs. It may take only 4 to 6 minutes of anaerobic metabolism before one or more of these vital organs are injured beyond repair. Skin and muscle tissue have a significantly longer ischemic sensitivity—as long as 4 to 6 hours. The abdominal organs generally fall between these two groups and are able to survive 45 to 90 minutes of anaerobic metabolism (Table 6-1).

Long-term survival of the individual organs and the body as a whole requires delivery of important nutrients (oxygen and glucose) to the tissue cells. Other nutrients are also important, but because the resupply of these materials is not a component of the prehospital EMS system, they are not discussed here. Although these factors are

important, they are beyond the scope of the EMT's practice and resources. The most important supply item is oxygen.

THE FICK PRINCIPLE

The Fick principle is a simple description of the components necessary for oxygenation of the body cells:

1. on-loading of oxygen to red blood cells (RBCs) in the lung
2. delivery of RBCs to tissue cells
3. off-loading of oxygen from RBCs to tissue cells

A part of this entire process is that the patient must have enough red blood cells (RBCs) available to deliver adequate amounts of oxygen to tissue cells throughout the body. (RBC oxygenation has been covered previously in Chapters 2, 3, and 4 of this text.)

The prehospital treatment of shock is directed at the first two critical components of the Fick principle with the goal of preventing or reversing anaerobic metabolism, thus avoiding cellular death and, ultimately, patient death. These two components should be the major emphasis of the prehospital care provider and are implemented in the management of the trauma patient by the following actions:

1. **oxygenation** of the red blood cells by maintaining an adequate airway and ventilation
2. **perfusion** of tissue cells with oxygenated blood by maintaining adequate circulation

The first component (oxygenation of the lungs) is covered in Chapter 3: Airway Management and Ventilation. The second component of the Fick principle involves perfusion, which is the delivery of blood to the tissue cells. A helpful analogy to use in describing perfusion is to think of the RBCs as transport vans, the lungs as oxygen warehouses, the blood vessels as roads and highways, and the body tissue cells as the oxygen's destination. An insufficient number of transport vans, obstructions along the roads and highways, and/or slow transport vans would all contribute to decreased oxygen delivery and the eventual starvation of the tissue cells.

The fluid component of the circulatory system— blood—contains not only RBCs but infection-fighting factors (white blood cells and antibodies), protein for

 Table 6-1 Organ tolerance to ischemia

Organ	Warm ischemia time
Heart, brain, lungs	4–6 min
Kidneys, liver, gastrointestinal tract	45–90 min
Muscle, bone, skin	4–6 hours

cellular rebuilding, nutrition in the form of glucose, and other substances necessary for metabolism and survival. The common term for this fluid movement is *flow* or *blood flow.* The terms blood flow and flow are used throughout this chapter and in the medical care of patients. In most instances, they can be considered synonymous with perfusion, one of the major elements of shock management.

CIRCULATION

The cardiovascular system consists of a pump (the heart), a container (the vascular system, a complex branching pipeline through which the blood travels), and circulating fluid (the blood). Malfunctions or deficiencies in any of these three components will result in decreased or absent delivery of oxygen to the cells, even if the oxygenation of RBCs in the lungs is adequate.

The Pump

The heart consists of two receiving chambers (atria) and two major pumping chambers (ventricles). The function of the atria is to accumulate and store blood so that the ventricles can be filled rapidly, minimizing the delay in the pumping cycle. With each contraction of the right ventricle, blood is pumped through the lungs for oxygenation (Figure 6-1). The blood from the lungs then returns to the left atrium. This oxygenated blood is then pumped by the left ventricle throughout the systemic vascular system (Figure 6-2). As the blood is forced through the "container," a pressure rise occurs in the blood vessels that is greater than the normal resting pressure. The sudden pressure increase in the container takes the form of a pulse wave that pushes blood around the system. The peak of

pressure increase or pulse is the **systolic blood pressure.** It is a representation of the force of the blood produced by ventricular contraction. The resting pressure between ventricular contractions is the **diastolic blood pressure.** The diastolic blood pressure is the pressure force remaining in the system while the heart is refilling (diastole). This is an indirect estimate of vascular resistance (Figure 6-3). Both systolic and diastolic pressures are determined during the initial assessment of patients.

The blood flow out of the heart does not actually create the entire systolic pressure but only the pressure above the diastolic pressure. The term used to describe this difference is called the **pulse pressure,** because it is produced by the pulse (the ventricular contraction) of the heart. The systolic pressure is actually the diastolic pressure (resting pressure) plus the pulse pressure (ventricular contraction force).

Another term used in the discussion of shock management but not directly reported from the field is **mean arterial pressure** (MAP). This is the average pressure in the vascular system. It is estimated by adding one-third of the pulse pressure to the diastolic pressure. As an example, a patient with a pressure of 120/80 would have a MAP rounded to 93:

$$80 + ([120 - 80]/3) = MAP$$
$$80 + (40/3) = MAP$$
$$80 + 13.3 = 93.3$$

The amount of fluid pumped into the system with each contraction of the ventricle is called the **stroke volume.** The amount of blood pumped into the system over a minute is called the **cardiac output.** The formula for cardiac output is a simple one: The volume of each contraction (milliliters) is multiplied by the number of contractions in a given time period.

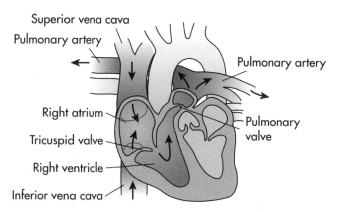

Figure 6-1 With each contraction of the right ventricle, blood is pumped through the lungs. Blood from the lungs enters the left side of the heart, and the left ventricle pumps it into the systemic vascular system.

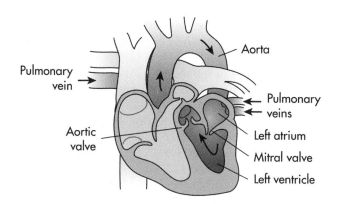

Figure 6-2 Blood returning from the lungs is pumped out of the heart and through the aorta to the rest of the body by left ventricular contraction.

Cardiac output (CO) =

> heart rate (HR) × stroke volume (SV)
> CO = HR × SV

Cardiac output is reported in liters per minute (LPM). Cardiac output is not measured in the prehospital environment. However, the theory of cardiac output and its relation to the stroke volume is important in understanding how to properly manage shock.

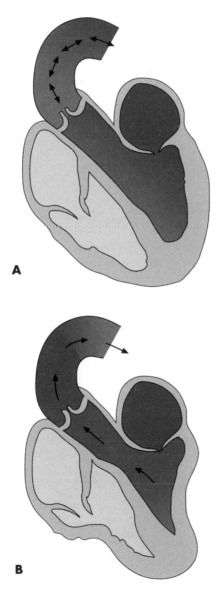

A

B

Figure 6-3 In a relaxed position (diastole), the ventricle fills with blood from the contractions of the atrium. During this time, blood is gradually flowing out of the major vessels as the pressure gradually decreases. During the contraction of the ventricle (systole), a large amount of blood flows into the vascular system, which raises the pressure. Cardiac action and blood flow is demonstrated in A and the pulse wave is seen in B.

For the heart to work effectively, an adequate amount of blood must be present in the intake vessels (vena cava and pulmonary vein), and the systolic blood pressure must be sufficient to cause the fluid to flow into the atria when these chambers expand. Unless pressurized blood is present in the intake vessels, only minimal inflow will occur into the atria. There must be a higher pressure at one end of the vascular system than the other in order for the blood to flow into the atria. The pressure outside the heart in the vena cava is called **preload,** while the pressure against which the left ventricle must pump blood out into the vascular system is called **afterload.**

One major component of the vascular system is the pulmonary pumping system located in the right side of the heart. Consider not one pump, but two; not one system of capillary beds with major inflow and outflow vessels, but two. This doubles the complications, doubles the number of pumping systems that may develop difficulties, and doubles the amount of capillary beds that must be perfused. It also doubles the resistance response within the system. Preload and afterload of both the right heart (pulmonary) and left heart (systemic) pumping systems must be considered (Figure 6-4).

The right ventricle is the pump that receives blood from the systemic circulation and ejects it into the pulmonary circulation. The left ventricle is the pump that receives blood from the pulmonary circulation and ejects it into the systemic circulation. The systemic circulation contains more capillaries and a greater length of blood vessels than the pulmonary circulation. Therefore, the left heart system works at a higher pressure and bears a greater load than the right heart. Anatomically, the muscles of the left ventricle are thicker and stronger than those of the right ventricle.

Although there are two separate systems and two separate pumps, they are connected in the body. They share the same electrical system and respond to the same stim-

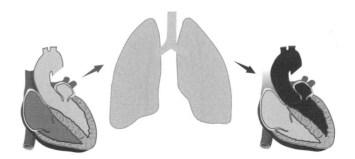

Figure 6-4 Although the heart seems to be one organ, it functions as if it were two. Unoxygenated blood is received into the right heart from the superior and inferior venae cavae and pumped through the pulmonary artery into the lungs. The blood is oxygenated in the lungs, flows back into the heart through the pulmonary vein, and is pumped out of the left ventricle.

uli, either from the internal sympathetic nervous system and hormones or externally by drug administration. However, although they are joined and function as one organ, they must physiologically be viewed as two separate pumping systems. Separate or together, the actions of one affect the performance of the other.

The Container

The blood vessels contain the blood and route it to the various areas and cells of the body. They are the highways of the physiologic process of circulation. Obviously, the single large exit tube from the heart (the aorta) cannot serve every individual cell in the body. The aorta, therefore, splits into multiple arteries of decreasing size that eventually become capillaries (Figure 6-5). A capillary may be only one cell wide; therefore, oxygen and nutrients carried by RBCs and plasma are able to diffuse through the walls of both the capillary and the tissue cell (Figure 6-6). Each tissue cell has a membranous lining called the cell membrane. **Interstitial fluid** is located be-

tween the cell membrane and capillary wall. The amount of interstitial fluid varies tremendously. If little interstitial fluid is present, the cell membrane and the capillary wall are close together and oxygen can easily diffuse between them (Figure 6-7).

The size of the vascular container is controlled by muscles in the walls of the arteries and arterioles, and to

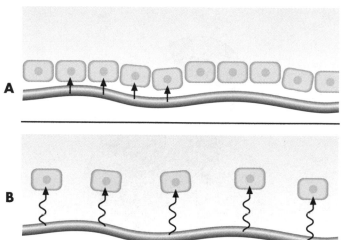

Figure 6-6 If the tissue cells are close to the capillary, oxygen can easily diffuse into them and carbon dioxide can diffuse out (A). If, on the other hand, tissue cells are separated from capillary walls by increased edema (interstitial fluid), it is much more difficult for the oxygen and carbon dioxide to diffuse (B).

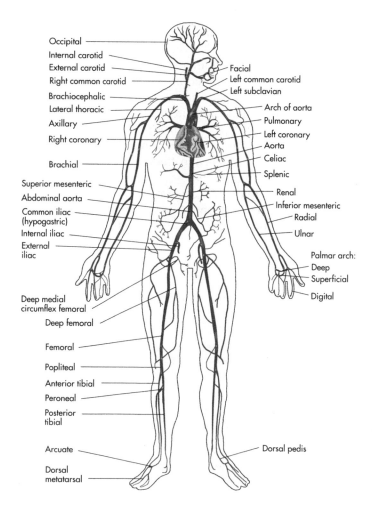

Figure 6-5 Principal arteries of the body. (From Thibodeau, G.A., and Patton, K.T. *Anatomy and Physiology.* 2d ed. St Louis: Mosby–Year Book, Inc., 1993.)

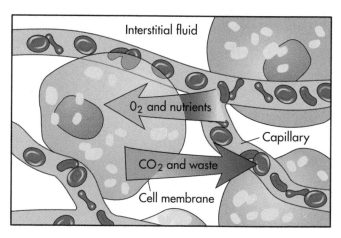

Figure 6-7 Oxygen and nutrients diffuse from the red blood cells through the capillary wall, the interstitial fluid, and the cell membrane into the cell. Acid production is a byproduct of cellular energy production during the Krebs cycle. By way of the buffer system of the body, this acid is converted into carbon dioxide and travels with the red blood cells and in the plasma to be eliminated from the circulatory system by the lungs.

a lesser extent, by muscles in the walls of the venules and veins. These muscles respond to signals from the brain (via the sympathetic nervous system), to the circulating hormones epinephrine and norepinephrine, and to other chemicals present such as nitric oxide (NO). The muscles cause either the dilation or constriction of the blood vessels, thus changing the size of the container component of the cardiovascular system.

The Fluid

The volume of fluid within the vascular system must equal the capacity of the blood vessels if it is to adequately fill the container. Any variance in the size of the vascular system compared with the amount of blood in the system will affect the flow of blood either positively or negatively.

The body's weight is 60% water. A man weighing 70 kilograms contains approximately 40 liters of water. Water is the base of all body fluids. Body water is present in two basic fluids: (1) intracellular and (2) extracellular, which is comprised of both interstitial and intravascular fluids. Each type of fluid has specific and important properties (Figure 6-8). **Intracellular fluid,** the fluid within the cells, accounts for approximately 45% of body weight. **Extracellular fluid,** the fluid outside the cells, can be further classified into two types. The first is interstitial fluid, which surrounds the tissue cells and also includes cerebrospinal fluid (found in the brain) and synovial fluid (found in the joints). It accounts for approximately 15% of body weight. The second is **intravascular fluid.** This fluid carries the formed components of blood as well as oxygen and other vital nutrients within the blood vessels and accounts for approximately 7% of body weight.

In this discussion of how fluids operate in the body, a review of some key concepts may be helpful. Cells require a fluid environment, and that fluid must have cer-

tain properties and a particular chemical balance to support cellular life. A proper volume of fluid under adequate pressure is also essential. A variety of mechanisms constantly adjust chemical balance, fluid volume, and pressure to achieve **homeostasis,** a constant, stable, internal environment. Normally, the total volume of water in the body remains constant; the distribution of fluid also remains relatively constant. In order to maintain these constant conditions, the amount of fluid taken in through the digestive system must equal the amount of fluid lost through the kidneys, lungs, skin, and intestines.

Several mechanisms work to adjust and balance input and output. One way the body maintains this fluid balance is by shifting water from one space in the body to another. When the fluid volume drops, the kidneys reduce their output to allow the vascular volume to build up again. The person feels thirsty and is motivated to drink liquids as an additional mechanism to improve the fluid volume. In the opposite condition, when there is too much fluid in the body, urine output increases.

A person is said to be **normovolemic** if fluid balance is normal. When volume is too high, the person is **hypervolemic;** when volume is too low, he or she is **hypovolemic.**

The body's systems are directed toward maintaining the life of the cells. When death occurs, it is because the body is no longer able to support cellular life. The patient's death is, in reality, the death of the patient's cells. For cellular life to continue, the fluid environment must be maintained and the cells must be adequately perfused—bathed with oxygenated fluid under appropriate conditions. When oxygen and the other nutrients reach the capillaries, they must be able to move through the capillary membrane into the interstitial fluid that bathes the cells. The oxygen and nutrients must then pass into the cell through the cell membrane. At the same time, the capillaries must be able to transfer carbon dioxide (CO_2) and other waste products from the tissue cell into the vascular fluid and eventually transport out of the body. This exchange is accomplished by the processes of diffusion and osmosis.

Diffusion involves the movement of **solutes** (substances dissolved in water) across a membrane. Different membranes have different levels of permeability: that is, different membranes will allow different sizes or types of molecules of the solute to pass through. As noted earlier, the body strives to maintain homeostasis—a state of chemical and metabolic balance. Solutes attempt to move from areas in which they are more numerous to areas in which they are less concentrated as part of the homeostatic drive. When a solute encounters a membrane that will not let its molecules pass through, the solute remains on only one side of the membrane. This lack of passage produces a condition in which there is a greater concentration of that solute on one side of the membrane **(hypertonic state).** On the other hand, water can usually pass through these membranes easily, which will equalize the tonicity on both sides. However,

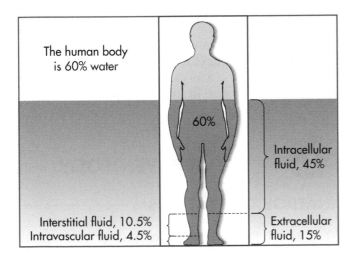

Figure 6-8 Body water represents 60% of body weight. This water is divided into intracellular fluid and extracellular fluid. The extracellular fluid is further divided into interstitial and intravascular fluid.

which will equalize the tonicity on both sides. However, there will be more water on the side of greater pressure, producing a higher pressure (water column) on this side.

Osmosis is the movement of water across a membrane from an area that is hypotonic to an area that is hypertonic. By diluting the solute concentration on the hypertonic side of the membrane, this movement of water brings both sides to equal solute concentrations. If a membrane will not allow water to pass, the concentration of solutes on the side with the increased number of molecules remains hypertonic, and the concentration on the side with fewer or no molecules is hypotonic.

Pressure is required for the fluid to move, not only throughout the circulatory system but into and out of the cells as well. **Osmotic pressure** is produced when differing concentrations of solutes cause water to move from the side of lower concentration to the side of higher concentration (Figure 6-9). Osmosis tends to move fluids from the interstitial space, where solute concentrations are lower, to the intravascular space where concentrations are higher.

Hydrostatic pressure balances osmotic pressure. Hydrostatic pressure can be increased on a body compartment as the result of a constricting band, a compression bandage, a tight cast, increased fluid in a compartment that cannot expand (such as the skull) or in a fascial compartment (e.g., the lower leg), or by an increase in blood pressure that is maintained by the pumping action of the heart.

Nervous System

The **autonomic nervous system** directs and controls the involuntary functions of the body such as respiration, digestion, and cardiovascular function. It is divided into

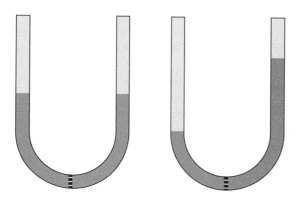

Figure 6-9 A U-tube, in which the two halves are separated by a semipermeable membrane, contains equal amounts of water and solid particles. If a solute that cannot diffuse through the semipermeable membrane is added to one side but not the other, fluid will flow across to dilute the added particles. The pressure difference of the height of fluid in the U-tube is known as osmotic pressure.

two subsystems, the sympathetic and parasympathetic nervous systems. These systems sometimes work against each other to keep vital body systems in balance.

The **sympathetic nervous system** produces the fight-or-flight response, which simultaneously causes the heart to beat faster and stronger, constricts the arteries to raise vascular resistance, and increases the ventilatory rate. The goal of this response is to increase the amount of oxygenated blood circulating throughout the body, especially to critical tissues, so that the individual can respond to an emergency situation.

Without some restrictive control, however, the person's pulse rate and blood pressure could increase too much, overtaxing the heart and killing the individual. The **parasympathetic system** provides that control. The parasympathetic system's vagal response slows the heart rate and reduces the force of contractions, keeping the body within workable limits.

The **medulla** is the primary regulatory center of autonomic control of the cardiovascular system. The medulla receives information from specialized areas in the body that "sense" pressure and chemical balance. **Chemoreceptors** sense changes in chemical balance. **Baroreceptors,** which sense pressure changes, are located mainly around the carotid artery. When these cells sense an increase in the pressure inside the carotid artery, a message is sent to the medulla.

The cardioinhibitory center of the medulla slows or inhibits cardiac activity by sending impulses through the parasympathetic system's vagus nerve. The parasympathetic stimulation causes a decrease in firing of the sinoatrial (SA) node and slows conduction through the atrioventricular (AV) node. The effect is to slow the heart rate. A decreased heart rate will decrease cardiac output, which results in lowered blood pressure.

The cardioaccelerator center of the medulla increases or accelerates cardiac activity. The impulses are sent from the cardioaccelerator center through the sympathetic nervous system. Sympathetic stimulation, through the release of epinephrine, causes an increase in the firing of the SA node and produces increases in conduction velocity, automaticity, irritability, and the force of contraction. The net effect is an increase in cardiac output, which results in an increase in blood pressure.

PATHOPHYSIOLOGY

ANAEROBIC METABOLISM ——————

When there is not enough oxygen to produce energy by aerobic metabolism, the cells produce energy without oxygen (i.e., anaerobically). Anaerobic metabolism is a costly process and results in excess production of acid and potassium.

The body attempts to manage the increased production of acid caused by the switch to anaerobic metabolism by way of its buffer system. A **buffer** is a substance that neutralizes or weakens strong acids or bases. In this case, the hydrogen ion (H^+) of the acid joins with sodium bicarbonate (HCO_3^-) to form carbonic acid (H_2CO_3). This in turn breaks down into water (H_2O) and carbon dioxide (CO_2):

$$H^+ + HCO_3^- \rightarrow H_2CO_3 \rightarrow H_2O + CO_2$$

The resulting increase in carbon dioxide (CO_2) is detected by the brain, which causes the ventilatory rate to increase. Increasing the ventilatory rate has the effect of removing more carbon dioxide from the body. The increased water is removed as the kidneys excrete additional urine. This whole process is the body's normal response to the presence of increased acid. Increased acid is a product of anaerobic metabolism, which is always an element of shock. An increased ventilatory rate, along with an increase in the pulse rate and a reduced level of consciousness, is one of the earliest signs of shock.

The increase in the number of ventilations promotes the increased elimination of carbon dioxide as just discussed. Increasing the concentration of inspired oxygen (FiO_2) increases the amount of oxygen available to be transferred to the RBCs and transported to the tissue cells. These oxygen-depleted tissue cells only survive initially by switching to anaerobic metabolism. When more oxygen is available at the cellular level, the cells can convert back to aerobic metabolism.

The effects of a decreased blood supply, decreased oxygenation, and anaerobic metabolism in an organ can be detected by measuring the performance of that particular organ. In trying to resuscitate a patient, it is important to assess each organ individually whenever possible in order to check its level of function. For example, the kidneys will increase or decrease the output of urine depending on the amount of blood flowing through them. Although urine output is easily measured in the hospital, it is only rarely measured in prehospital situations. It is presented here as an example of what occurs in the body. Another example is that an extremely ischemic heart develops a slow rate (bradycardia), whereas a heart being driven by the brain to increase cardiac output has a rapid rate (tachycardia). However, when the heart becomes oxygen-depleted, it converts to anaerobic metabolism and can no longer perform as directed. Bradycardia and decreased blood pressure results.

EVALUATING BODY SYSTEM FUNCTION

One system that *can* be checked in the field is brain function. Four conditions can produce a reduced level of consciousness and/or a change in behavior as seen in combative or belligerent patients. These conditions are:

- overdose of alcohol or drugs
- brain injury
- metabolic processes such as diabetes or seizure
- hypoxia

Of these four, the easiest to treat—and the one that will kill the patient the most quickly if not treated—is hypoxia. Any patient with a reduced level of consciousness should be treated as if decreased cerebral oxygenation is the cause. A reduced level of consciousness is usually one of the first visible signs of shock.

The brain's function decreases as perfusion and oxygenation drop and ischemia develops. This decreased function evolves through various stages as different areas of the brain become affected. Anxiety and belligerent behavior are usually the first signs, followed by a slowing of the thought processes, and finally a decrease of the body's motor and sensory functions.

All organs react to decreased perfusion and oxygenation by a change, usually a decrease, in their function. The level of cerebral function is an important and measurable prehospital sign of shock. A belligerent, combative, anxious patient or one with a decreased level of consciousness should be presumed to have a hypoxic, hypoperfused brain until another cause can be established. Hypoperfusion and cerebral hypoxia frequently accompany actual brain injury and make the long-term result even worse.

Another system that can be checked in the field is circulation, which is done by assessing capillary refilling time and the color and temperature of the skin. When the body reacts to shock, it closes down the peripheral capillary circulation, and anaerobic metabolism begins in those areas. Slow refilling of a capillary bed indicates poor perfusion of that particular bed and probably the existence of anaerobic metabolism. As the peripheral circulation is closed down, the skin is more poorly perfused. The patient appears ashen, or grey, and the skin temperature drops. Hence, the classic picture of the pale, cool patient in shock.

In some patients, especially the elderly and individuals who have been exposed to a cold environment, a delayed capillary refilling time may also be seen. The EMT should recognize that in such cases, although the extended time period is indicative of poor perfusion, it is not necessarily shock. The EMT must combine this finding with the other results of the assessment before deciding that the patient must be treated for shock.

THE CARDIOVASCULAR SYSTEM IN SHOCK

The container (vascular system) can be artificially divided into three physiologic, not anatomic, parts. The part that serves the heart, brain, and lungs receives the highest priority. The body strives to maintain this part at all costs because its failure would deprive the entire body of circulating oxygenated blood. The blood supply to the abdominal contents and retroperitoneum receives the next highest priority, whereas the component that serves the extremities is the lowest priority. When the circulation of oxygenated blood is reduced for any reason, the system of priorities among these three physiologic components of the vascular system takes effect. Blood is shunted away from the lowest priority area to those areas that are more sensitive to the loss of oxygenated blood and are essential to maintaining life. Blood is not shunted away from the heart, brain, or lungs.

When the blood pressure drops and circulatory flow decreases, the change is detected by the baroreceptors. This information is transmitted by nerves to the brain, which in turn sends signals to the sympathetic nervous system to release norepinephrine, causing constriction of the smooth muscles in the peripheral arterioles and venules. This constriction reduces or completely shuts off the flow of blood to the skin and extremities. If this situation continues, blood flow to the abdominal contents will be reduced or shut off. This reduction of blood flow achieved through constriction of the blood vessels results in increased vascular resistance. If the change affects the entire body, it is known as increased systemic vascular resistance (SVR). This selective reduction in blood flow has two effects on the body, one helpful and one harmful.

The helpful result is that the vasoconstriction is delayed in the blood vessels that provide circulation to the brain, heart, and lungs. The vasoconstriction and resultant reduced circulation occur in areas of the body that are not immediately essential to preserving life and that can tolerate **ischemia** (lack of oxygenated blood) the longest. Liquids flow along the path of least resistance. Blood is a liquid and follows all the laws of physics for liquids. There is less resistance to the flow of blood to the brain, heart, and lungs than to other parts of the body where the blood vessels have been constricted.

The result is improved circulation to the vital organs and decreased circulation to the rest of the body. The increased resistance produced by the peripheral vasoconstriction results in an improved blood pressure. The action of cardiotonic substances such as epinephrine increases cardiac output both in volume and strength, adding to the increase in blood pressure. Although blood pressure is one of the most frequently measured functions of the heart, it is not the most important factor in the management of shock. Delivery of oxygen to the tissues by improving RBC oxygenation in the lungs and perfusion of the cells by these RBCs is the goal of shock management. In this chapter the discussion is concerned mainly with the perfusion portion of management.

There will be decreased or absent blood flow on the distal side of the increased vascular resistance. The decreased circulation through the distal capillary beds and decreased blood flow through distal arteries translate into three of the common signs of shock:

- loss of normal skin color, moistness, and temperature
- absent palpable distal pulse
- delayed capillary refilling time

The decreased blood flow to the skin, abdomen, and extremities also means that these areas receive fewer nutrients and less oxygen than they need. Rather than "starve," these cells convert from aerobic to anaerobic metabolism to survive. Anaerobic metabolism is not as efficient as aerobic metabolism. Less energy is produced for the body to use, and there is an increase in waste by-products (principally acids and potassium). The result is a growing state of metabolic acidosis in the peripheral tissues. This acidosis is entirely related to the tissue cells and has no relationship to the regulation of fluids or electrolytes in the kidney.

If, subsequently, adequate circulation is restored and the peripheral cells receive adequate supplies of nutrients and oxygen, they convert back to aerobic metabolism. At the same time, the toxic by-products of anaerobic metabolism are washed out of the peripheral areas and enter the central systemic circulation. If this accumulation of acids and potassium is large enough, it will now cause systemic metabolic acidosis.

The pathophysiologic process of shock is divided into three stages; **ischemic, stagnant,** and **washout** (Figure 6-10). The ischemic stage is characterized by reduction of capillary blood flow and conversion to anaerobic metabolism with production of toxic by-products. In the stagnant phase, precapillary sphincters open, but postcapillary sphincters remain closed. This results in an increase in hydrostatic pressure within the capillaries. The increased pressure forces fluid out of the capillaries into the interstitial space, resulting in tissue **edema** (swelling). When the postcapillary sphincters open, the washout phase begins. The accumulation of toxic by-products from the first two phases is washed out into the systemic circulation during this third stage. What was once a contained, localized acidosis now becomes a systemic acidosis.

The result is that the heart is forced to function with three handicaps, all of which decrease its efficiency:

1. The resistance to flow in the vessels of the muscles and capillary beds increases the demand on the heart and increases the amount of work required to force blood through these vessels. This increased resistance to flow—systemic vascular resistance—is also known as increased afterload because of the increased cardiac effort needed to push blood throughout the circulatory system against this resistance.

2. The second stressful condition under which the heart must work is decreased oxygenation. The need for oxygen in a harder working (faster beating) heart is greater than the amount needed in an eas-

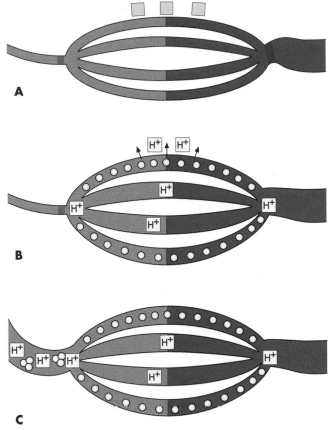

Figure 6-10 The cellular pathophysiologic process of shock is divided into three phases: A, ischemic; B, stagnant; and C, washout.

ier working (slower beating) heart. More work requires more fuel. If the heart must beat faster to overcome the increased afterload, it must have more oxygen. This illustrates the need for the EMT to hyperoxygenate the patient during any period of cardiac stress, thereby helping to prevent further deterioration into shock.

3. The third cardiac difficulty is a lack of available fluid to fill the ventricles during diastole (resting phase). Ejecting blood from the ventricle when the heart is only half full requires more frequent contractions and produces a smaller pulse pressure (and therefore a lower systolic pressure) than when adequate fluid is available. Cardiac work therefore becomes harder but produces less output. One sign of shock is a rising diastolic pressure followed by a decline in both systolic and diastolic pressures.

Edema

If a large amount of fluid is present in the interstitial space (a condition known as edema), the distance between the capillary wall and the cell membrane becomes much greater. Oxygen must diffuse through the capillary wall,

then through the interstitial fluid, and finally through the cell membrane. This increases the amount of fluid separating the capillaries from the tissue cells, and it increases the amount of distance that nutrients and oxygen must travel to reach the cells. The greater the thickness of interstitial fluid, the more difficult the transfer of the oxygen and other nutrients across this space (see Figure 6-6).

If the left heart has some difficulty and fails to pump out all the fluid presented to it while the right heart continues to function normally, there will be an overload of fluid into the pulmonary system. This congestion causes a buildup of pressure in the capillary system between the two pumps. This increased pressure forces fluid from the vascular bed into the tissues and the interstitial space. The pulmonary capillary bed is particularly sensitive to these changes because of limited tissue strength in the lungs. Fluid in the interstitial space increases the distance between the alveoli and capillaries, which makes oxygen exchange into the RBCs more difficult. The increased fluid accumulation, if it persists, will continue to migrate into the alveoli and produce actual fluid in the space normally occupied by air. This produces even more compromise for the patient because now the inspired air cannot enter the alveoli and be absorbed into the RBCs.

Interstitial fluid buildup and alveolar fluid in the lungs because of failure of the left heart is called **congestive heart failure.** Acute fluid buildup in the interstitial space in the posttrauma patient is known as **acute respiratory distress syndrome (ARDS).** Congestive heart failure is cardiac in origin, whereas ARDS is a result of leaky capillary syndrome. Although ARDS is not commonly seen in the field because it occurs 24 to 48 hours after admission, the cause is frequently due to inadequate resuscitation very early in patient care either in the field or in the emergency department. This is one of the causes of patient death that can be prevented or reduced by good prehospital care.

The results of such a condition can be rapidly progressive because a vicious cycle quickly develops. The heart does not receive enough oxygen and therefore works harder and pumps more often to remove the deficit. More oxygen is required to provide fuel for the extra work, but the oxygen is not available. This cycle can produce a rapid downward course—even a fatal course—for the patient unless effective treatment is begun quickly to overcome it. Prehospital treatment is best achieved by increasing the oxygen concentration in the inspired air (FiO_2) to as close to 100% as possible and by taking the necessary steps to improve perfusion (blood flow).

TYPES OF SHOCK

Shock (decreased tissue oxygenation and the resultant anaerobic metabolism) can occur in three ways that are associated with failure of some component of the cardio-vascular system: volume, container, and pump failure.

Volume Failure

When acute blood loss occurs through dehydration or hemorrhage, the volume of fluid and the size of the container become unbalanced. The container retains its normal size, but the fluid volume is decreased. Fluid volume decrease is the most common cause of shock that EMTs will encounter in the prehospital environment.

The heart is stimulated to increase cardiac output by increasing the strength and rate of contractions through the release of epinephrine from the adrenal glands. The sympathetic nervous system releases norepinephrine to trigger constriction of the blood vessels to reduce the size of the container and bring it more into proportion with the amount of remaining fluid. Vasoconstriction results in closing of the peripheral capillaries as discussed earlier and prompts the switch from aerobic to anaerobic metabolism at the cellular level.

These compensatory defense mechanisms work well, up to a point. When defense mechanisms can no longer overcome the volume reduction, the patient's blood pressure drops. A decrease in blood pressure marks the switch from compensated to decompensated shock—a sign of impending death. A patient who is compensating is in shock, not "going into shock." The patient who passes to decompensated shock has only one more stage of decline left—death.

The definitive management for volume failure is to replace the lost fluid. A dehydrated patient needs fluid replacement with water and salt, whereas the trauma patient who has lost blood needs to have the blood replaced and the source of blood loss stopped. Dehydration can be treated with an electrolyte solution that a conscious patient can drink. An unconscious dehydration patient should receive the replacement intravenously. Because blood replacement is usually not available in the prehospital environment, trauma patients who have lost blood should receive an intravenous electrolyte solution and rapid transportation to the hospital where blood is available.

Studies performed during the Korean Conflict and before demonstrated that for lost blood, the replacement ratio with electrolyte solution should be 3 liters of replacement for each liter of blood lost. The studies also showed that replacement with both electrolyte solution and blood was better than blood alone. The use of a limited amount of electrolyte solution before blood replacement is the correct approach. The most commonly used solution for this purpose is lactated Ringer's solution (LR or L/R). Normal saline (NS) is an isotonic crystalloid solution that can also be used for volume replacement.

Other solutions such as hypertonic saline and dextran have been shown to increase blood pressure. This increase in blood pressure will increase the blood flow.

However, if the source of hemorrhage has not been controlled, the increased blood pressure may lead to increased blood loss at the site of the injury and thus increase the mortality.

Short-term assistance with increased vascular resistance, container size reduction, and intra-abdominal hemorrhage control can be provided by the pneumatic antishock garment (PASG). The most important use for the PASG is in intra-abdominal, pelvic, and retroperitoneal hemorrhage control and for patients with a blood pressure below 60 mm Hg. Use of the PASG is fully explained in the "Management" section of this chapter. However, the PASG will increase the blood pressure and may result in increased blood loss at injury sites that are "uncontrolled" by the pressure of the device.

If the preload pressure is low, as when the amount of fluid is insufficient to fill the vascular system (e.g., hemorrhage), there will be a reduced volume of blood into the atria. This results in a reduced volume of blood pumped into the ventricles and less blood for the ventricles to pump out to the body.

Container Failure

Container failure occurs when the vascular container enlarges without a proportional increase in fluid volume. Relatively less fluid will be available for the size of the container. As a result, the amount of fluid available to the heart as preload decreases, and cardiac output decreases as described earlier. It is important to realize that fluid has not been lost from the vascular system. This form of shock is not a case of hypovolemia, where fluid has been lost through hemorrhage, vomiting, or diarrhea. Rather, the problem is with the size of the container. For this reason, this condition is sometimes called relative hypovolemia. However, although some of the presenting signs and symptoms may closely mimic those of hypovolemic shock, the cause of the two conditions is quite different.

In container failure, resistance to flow is decreased because of the relatively larger size of the blood vessels. This reduced resistance decreases the diastolic blood pressure. When combined with the reduced preload and therefore a reduced cardiac output, the net result is a decrease in both the systolic and diastolic blood pressures. Although the pressure is decreased, if normal oxygenation has been maintained, the heart rate does not necessarily increase. In many patients the tissue oxygenation may remain adequate.

Container failure can occur from loss of autonomic nervous system control of the smooth muscles that control the size of the blood vessels. This loss of control can stem from neurogenic causes such as spinal cord trauma (often called spinal shock), psychogenic causes (simple fainting), or loss of vascular support in septic conditions (septic shock; Table 6-2). Management of container fail-

Table 6-2 Signs associated with types of shock

Signs	Psychogenic	Spinal	Septic	Hypovolemic
Skin temperature	Cool, moist	Warm, dry	Cool, clammy	Cool, clammy
Skin color	Pale	Pink	Pale, mottled	Pale, cyanotic
Blood pressure	Drops	Drops	Drops	Drops
Level of consciousness	Altered	Lucid	Altered	Altered
Capillary refill	Slowed	Normal	Slowed	Slowed

ure is directed first toward improving oxygenation of the blood and improving or maintaining blood flow to the brain.

Neurogenic (Spinal) Shock

Spinal shock is the name used to describe the type of neurogenic shock that produces loss of vascular control either below the neck or below the waist. Injury to the spinal cord interrupts the nervous system's communication between the brain and the blood vessels that are served by nerves that branch from the spinal cord below the point of injury. The normal flow of information through the spinal cord is one of the major factors that produces the vascular constriction that causes changes in systemic vascular resistance.

If the flow of information is missing, there is no control of the smooth muscles in the walls of the blood vessels. This results in a loss of control over their internal diameter and thus the area (cross-sectional size) of the lumen of the involved vessels. The result is a lack of control over blood flow and a loss of systemic vascular resistance. Pulse pressure is not affected; therefore the decrease in systolic pressure is caused by a drop in the diastolic pressure.

Hypovolemic shock and spinal shock both produce a decreased systolic blood pressure. However, the other vital signs vary significantly between the two types of shock, and the treatment for each type is also different. (See "Assessment" section of this chapter.)

Hypovolemic shock is characterized by decreased systolic and diastolic pressures and a narrow pulse pressure. These changes are brought about by reduced cardiac output. Spinal shock also displays decreased systolic and diastolic pressures, but the normal pulse pressure margin is maintained. Hypovolemia produces cold, clammy, pale, or cyanotic skin and prolonged capillary refilling time. Spinal shock produces warm and dry skin, especially below the area of injury, and normal or even shortened capillary refilling time. The pulse in hypovolemic shock patients is weak, thready, and rapid; with spinal shock it is strong, and although it can be at a somewhat usual rate for the patient, slow in rate. Hypovolemia produces a decreased level of consciousness, or at least anxiety and often combativeness. The patient with spinal shock is alert, oriented, and lucid.

Psychogenic Shock

Psychogenic shock is mediated through the vagal cranial nerve. Stimulation of the vagus causes the heart to slow down (bradycardia). When the bradycardia is severe enough, insufficient blood flow to the brain results and the patient loses consciousness (faints). There are two main differences between spinal shock and psychogenic shock. First, the patient's vascular tone does not recover readily with spinal shock, although it will recover over several hours or days without treatment. In psychogenic shock patients, the normal blood pressure is quickly restored when the patient is placed in a horizontal position.

Second, the heart rate decreases and becomes thready with psychogenic shock, but it remains slow and strong with spinal shock, although the blood pressure is low. In spinal shock, the skin below the level of injury remains warm and pink because it is well perfused with oxygenated blood, and blood flow to the skin has not been reduced. In psychogenic shock, the skin will be pale, cool, and moist. Initially, psychogenic shock is characterized by hypotension associated with bradycardia. However, by the time the EMT arrives on the scene, the patient is often recovering from the fainting spell and the pulse will be rapid (tachycardia) as the heart rebounds from the vagal stimulation and increases the heart rate to re-establish normal blood flow.

Septic Shock

Septic shock is another condition that exhibits vascular dilation. Septic shock is seen in patients with major infections. Toxins generated by the infection cause damage to the walls of the blood vessels, causing them to lose their ability to constrict. The decrease in circulation produces pooling of blood, which leads to a cyanotic or blotchy skin color and slowed capillary refilling. This condition is usually not seen in the prehospital phase of care.

Pump Failure

Loss of cardiac output usually occurs for one of three reasons:

- decreased contractibility of the cardiac muscle (muscle failure)
- ineffective or unstable contraction rhythms (cardiac dysrhythmia)
- reduced stroke volume

Muscle Failure

Any process that weakens the cardiac muscle will affect its output. The weakness may result from decreased oxygen in the RBCs, a chronic interruption of the heart's own blood supply (as in coronary artery disease), decreased perfusion, or cardiac injury. A vicious cycle may ensue—decreased oxygenation causes decreased contractibility, which results in decreased cardiac output and therefore decreased perfusion. Decreased perfusion results in an even greater decrease in oxygenation and a continuation of the cycle.

A common cause of muscle failure is ischemia caused by lack of adequate oxygenated blood, as described previously by the Fick principle. In trauma, the most common cause is blood loss. Myocardial contusion may also occur, resulting in decreased cardiac output. As with any muscle, the cardiac muscle does not work as well or as efficiently when it becomes bruised or damaged.

Cardiac Arrhythmia

Cardiac arrhythmia can affect the rate and the efficiency of contractions. Because cardiac output is determined by the stroke volume multiplied by the number of contractions per minute, any arrhythmia that interferes with the rate of contractions or with the left ventricle's ability to fill adequately will easily affect cardiac output. Cardiac arrhythmia can also occur secondary to myocardial contusion.

Reduced Stroke Volume

Loss of the heart's ability to expand and receive new blood for pumping also affects cardiac output. Fluid in the pericardial sac (pericardial tamponade) will prevent the heart from refilling completely during the diastolic (relaxation) phase. Incomplete refilling will reduce the amount of available blood during each contraction. As a result, stroke volume is reduced, and thus cardiac output is reduced. A small stroke volume occurs when:

- The heart cannot enlarge to receive fluid (as with pericardial tamponade or tension pneumothorax).
- An insufficient amount of fluid is available to fill the potential size of the ventricle (hypovolemia).
- The heart does not have enough strength to pump efficiently and empty the ventricle (cardiogenic shock).

ASSESSMENT

OVERVIEW

Assessing the patient for shock requires checking each individual organ to identify the presence of shock. Shock was defined earlier as anaerobic metabolism. The question that should be in the EMT's mind when evaluating the performance of each organ system is: "Does anaerobic metabo-

lism exist in this organ?" Specifically identifying anaerobic metabolism is usually extremely difficult; therefore, indirect methods must be used such as cerebral function, cardiac rate, capillary refill time, ventilatory rate, urinary output, and measurement of the body's total acid level. The primary survey (initial assessment) is a gross qualitative estimation of as many organs and organ systems as possible. The goal is to find any abnormalities that might suggest the presence of anaerobic metabolism, or shock.

Simultaneous evaluation is an important part of patient assessment. This initial assessment may not be done at a conscious level, but the EMT's brain nonetheless continues to gather and process information. If all systems are found to be functioning normally, no alarm is set off.

Each patient condition that should be evaluated (status of airway, ventilation, perfusion, skin color and temperature, capillary refill time, and blood pressure) is presented separately in the next section. They are presented in the context of both the primary (initial) survey and the secondary survey (focused physical examination).

PRIMARY (INITIAL) SURVEY AND SECONDARY SURVEY (FOCUSED PHYSICAL EXAMINATION)

The following signs identify the need or lack of need for continued suspicion of life-threatening conditions:

- pale or cyanotic skin color
- presence or absence of radial or carotid pulse
- capillary refill time less than or greater than two seconds.

Any compromise or failure of the airway, breathing, or circulatory systems is managed immediately at this time, before proceeding. The following steps are described in an ordered series. However, when they are carried out in the field, they are all done more or less simultaneously.

Airway

Assessment should include evaluation of patent airway (see Chapter 3: Airway Management and Ventilation).

Ventilation

As noted in the pathophysiology section of this chapter, the anaerobic metabolism associated with decreased cellular oxygenation will produce an increase in carbon dioxide production, the presence of which will lead to increased ventilatory rate driven by the brain. This tachypnea frequently is one of the earliest signs of shock. A rate of 20 to 30 indicates a borderline abnormal rate and the need for supplemental O_2. A rate over 30 indicates the need for assisted ventilation. Both indicate the need to look for the source of anaerobic metabolism.

A patient who tries to remove the oxygen mask, particularly when such action is associated with anxiety and belligerence, is displaying another sign of cerebral ischemia. This patient has "air hunger" and feels the need for more ventilation. The presence of a mask over the nose and mouth creates a psychologic feeling of ventilatory restriction. This action should be a clue to the EMT that the patient is not getting enough oxygen and is hypoxic.

Perfusion

Assessing perfusion begins with a rapid evaluation of the patient's level of consciousness. The EMT must assume that an anxious, belligerent patient has cerebral ischemia and anaerobic metabolism until another cause is identified. Drug and alcohol overdose and cerebral contusion are conditions that cannot be treated rapidly, but cerebral ischemia can. Therefore, all patients in whom cerebral ischemia might be present should be managed as if it is present.

The next important assessment point for perfusion is the pulse. Initial evaluation of the pulse determines whether it is palpable at the artery being examined. In general, a radial pulse will not be palpable if systolic pressure is below 80 mm Hg, a femoral pulse will not be detectable when the pressure is below 70 mm Hg, and a carotid pulse will not be palpable when the pressure is below 60 mm Hg.

If the pulse is palpable, note its character and strength:
- Is it strong or weak (thready)?
- Is it normal, too fast, or too slow?
- Is it regular or irregular?

These conditions can be checked rapidly and the data assimilated to make a quick initial determination of the patient's condition.

In the secondary survey (focused physical examination), the rate will be determined more precisely. The normal pulse range for an adult is 60 to 100 pulsations per minute. Rates below this (except in extremely athletic individuals) are grounds for suspecting either an ischemic heart or a pathologic condition such as complete heart block. A pulse in the range of 100 to 120 identifies a patient who has a probable "shock-like" state, with an initial cardiac response toward tachycardia. A pulse above 120 is a definite sign of shock (unless it is due to pain or fear), and one over 140 is considered critical.

Skin Color

Pink skin indicates a well-oxygenated patient without anaerobic metabolism. Blue (cyanotic) or mottled skin indicates unoxygenated hemoglobin and a lack of adequate oxygenation to the periphery.

Pale, mottled, or cyanotic skin has inadequate blood flow, resulting from one of three causes:

- peripheral vasoconstriction, most often associated with hypovolemia
- decreased supply of RBCs (anemia)
- interruption of blood supply to that portion of the body, such as might be found with a fracture

Pale skin in one area of the body may not represent the remainder of the body. The implications of inconsistent skin color indicate that other findings, such as tachycardia, should be used to resolve these differences and to determine if the pale skin is a localized, regional, or systemic condition.

Skin Temperature

As the body shunts blood from the skin to more important parts of the body, skin temperature decreases. A cool skin temperature (to the EMT's touch) is an indicator of decreased cutaneous perfusion and therefore, shock. A significant amount of core temperature can be lost during the assessment phase; steps should be taken to preserve body temperature.

Capillary Refilling Time

The ability of the cardiovascular system to refill the capillaries after the blood has been "removed" represents an important support system. Analyzing this support system's level of function by compressing the capillaries to remove all the blood and then measuring the refilling time may provide insight for the EMT into the perfusion of the capillary bed being assessed. It is generally true that the body shuts down circulation in the most distal parts of the body first, and restores this circulation last. Evaluating the nail bed of the big toe or thumb provides the earliest possible indication that hypoperfusion is developing. Additionally, it provides the EMT with a strong indication when resuscitation is complete. One of the better signs of completed resuscitation is a warm, dry, pink toe.

Blood Pressure

Blood pressure is one of the least sensitive signs of shock. The blood pressure does not begin to drop until the patient is profoundly hypovolemic (from either true fluid loss or container-enlarged relative hypovolemia). Between 30% to 40% of blood volume must be lost before the systolic blood pressure drops below 90 mm Hg (in patients whose systolic pressure is normally within accepted ranges). For this reason, the capillary refill time, pulse rate and character, and ventilation rate are more sensitive indicators of hypovolemia than is a drop in blood pressure.

When the patient's pressure has begun to drop, an extremely critical situation exists and rapid intervention is required. The severity of the situation and the appropriate type of intervention varies, based on the cause of the condition. For example, low blood pressure associated with spinal shock is not nearly as critical as low blood pressure with hypovolemic shock. The signs used to assess compensated and decompensated hypovolemic shock are presented in Table 6-3.

An important point to remember in the assessment of patients with multiple trauma is that head injuries do not cause hypotension until the cerebellum begins to herniate through the incisura and foramen magnum. Therefore, if a patient with a head injury is found to be hypotensive, the EMT should assume that this condition is due to hypovolemia (usually blood loss) from other injuries and not from the head injury.

MANAGEMENT

OVERVIEW

At the time of publication of the fourth edition of the PHTLS course, the management of the patient in hemorrhagic shock is controversial. There are advocates of three types of treatment:

1. Maintain hypotension in the patient by restricting fluid replacement and avoiding the use of any type of medication or device that will increase the blood pressure until the patient's hemorrhage has been controlled.
2. Overhydrate the patient by replacing the lost whole blood one for one with blood and then the addition of 3:1 blood loss with Ringer's lactate. Resuscitation should be to normal blood pressure.
3. Hydrate the patient with hypertonic solutions. Resuscitation should be to normal blood pressure.

The basis of this controversy is the effect of improved blood pressure on increased bleeding versus the physiologic benefits of good tissue perfusion with oxygenated RBCs.

Table 6-3 Shock assessment in compensated and decompensated hypovolemic shock

	Compensated	Decompensated
Pulse	Increased, tachycardia	Markedly increased, marked tachycardia; can progress to bradycardia
Skin	White, cool, and moist	White, waxy, and cold
Blood pressure	Normal range	Decreased
Level of consciousness	Unaltered	Altered, ranging from disoriented to coma

A review of the physiology as it pertains to fluid resuscitation follows:

- Improved blood pressure increases the blood flow into the organs.
- The positive side of fluid resuscitation is that increased flow improves the oxygenation of the tissue by delivery of RBCs to the tissue.
- The negative side of fluid resuscitation is that as blood pressure is increased to the area of uncontrolled hemorrhage, additional whole blood is lost.
- Initial resuscitation using Ringer's lactate or saline replaces only volume and does not replace the lost RBCs.
- Fluid replacement without RBC replacement lowers the RBC mass and therefore lessens ability of the circulation fluid to carry oxygen.
- The increased bleeding produced by restoration of blood pressure brings about more RBC mass loss.
- Any device, medication, or fluid that increases the blood pressure without increasing the lost red cell mass will produce the same condition. This includes the PASG, vasopressor medications, hypertonic saline/dextran fluids, and crystalloid fluids.

There is, at the time of the publication of this chapter, no data in the literature that demonstrates, to statistical significance, that in any condition, except uncontrolled hemorrhage in the chest, that any of the just mentioned materials (except vasopressor medications) alter outcome. Vasopressor indications decrease the outcome. There are proponents of all arguments, but careful reading of the published literature is inconclusive. It is therefore important that the provider of prehospital care understands the physiology well and makes management decisions based on this knowledge.

There is early information that trauma patients do better with a lower pressure. In *Resuscitation and Anesthesia for Wounded Men*—edited by Henry K. Beecher, published in 1949, and based on World War II data—the following statements are present: "In the treatment of shock preliminary to surgery we can restore blood volume and blood pressure to normal. This is possible but is it necessary? We do not need to guess here . . . It is no . . . The patient will not suffer as long as the systolic pressure is 80 mm Hg and the skin is warm and of good color. Neither will he lose as much blood by renewed bleeding as he will if plasma is used to raise blood pressure higher than necessary during this waiting period."

The management of a patient in shock is directed toward changing the anaerobic metabolism back to aerobic metabolism. Based on the Fick principle, this reversal is produced by delivering more oxygen to the ischemic tissue cells. Improved oxygenation at the cellular level is achieved by oxygenating the RBCs and delivering them to the tissue cells. Without improving the oxygenation and delivery of RBCs, the patient will continue to deteriorate rapidly until reaching the ultimate stabilization—death.

In addition to these first two treatment objectives (oxygenation and delivery), the third objective is to reach definitive care as soon as possible for hemorrhage control and replacement of lost RBCs.

The EMT must ask four questions when deciding what treatment to provide for a patient in shock:

1. What is the cause of the patient's shock?
2. What is the definitive care for the patient's shock?
3. Where can the patient best receive this definitive care?
4. What interim steps can be taken to manage the patient's condition while he or she is being transported to definitive care?

Although the first question may be difficult to answer with a high degree of diagnostic accuracy, having some idea of what is occurring can help the EMT identify the hospital best qualified to meet the patient's needs and to decide what steps to take during transport to improve his or her condition.

AIRWAY

The airway should be evaluated initially in all patients. Patients who are not breathing or have obvious airway compromise, ventilatory rates in excess of 20 breaths per minute, or noisy sounds of respiration should receive immediate management of their airway. Specific techniques are discussed in Chapter 3: Airway Management and Ventilation and Chapter 4, the associated skills chapter.

VENTILATION

When the airway is open, patients in shock or those susceptible to shock (which includes almost all trauma patients) should receive oxygen with an FiO_2 as close to 1.0 (100% oxygen) as possible. This kind of oxygenation can only be achieved with a device that has a reservoir attached and with a high flow rate of oxygen to the device.

It is no longer correct to talk of giving the patient x liters of oxygen or "high flow oxygen." Instead, the EMT should discuss giving the patient an FiO_2 of some defined number. This is achieved by providing a specific flow rate to a specific device. Any device will deliver varying FiO_2s depending on the oxygen flow rate and the design of the device.

A shock patient or a potential shock patient should only be given oxygen with a device that includes a reservoir, so that an FiO_2 as close as possible to 1.0 can be achieved. Nasal prongs cannot deliver anything close to this concentration and therefore should not be used on a patient in shock (see Table 3-1, page 71). If the patient is not breathing, or is not breathing with an adequate depth and rate, ventilatory assistance using a bag-valve-mask unit should be instituted immediately.

CIRCULATION

Difficulties with circulation as identified by decreased capillary refill time, tachycardia, decreased or absent palpable pulses (radial, femoral, or carotid), and pale or cyanotic skin color are treated in several steps.

The first step is to reestablish as much circulation as possible to the brain and to increase the cardiac preload. Placing the patient in the **Trendelenburg position** (head down, with feet elevated) is the initial step for simple fainting. This position is most appropriate for the treatment of psychogenic shock only. It may be the initial step for the management of any type of shock. This position will increase the venous pressure and potentially increase edema in the injured brain. However improved blood flow and oxygenation to the brain is more important initially than is the potential damage done by increased edema.

CONSERVATION OF BODY HEAT

Maintaining the patient's body temperature within a normal range is important. Hypothermia introduces myocardial dysfunction, coagulopathy, hyperkalemia, vasoconstriction, and a host of other problems that negatively affect survival rate. It is very difficult to increase the core temperature once hypothermia has started; therefore, all steps that can be taken in the field to preserve normothermia must be initiated. These steps include the use of warm (104° F [40° C]) intravenous fluids, warm blankets, heated humidified oxygen, and a warm environment for the patient by moving him or her rapidly from the scene into the warm patient compartment of the unit. Any cold, wet clothes should be removed once inside the unit (see Chapter 12: Thermal Trauma).

Although cold does preserve tissue for a short time, the temperature drop must be very rapid and very low for preservation to occur. Such a rapid change is not the correct management for the patient in shock; therefore, body temperature must be preserved to avoid jeopardizing the patient further. Covering a patient with thick plastic sheets (such as heavy-duty garbage bags) or blankets to retain heat and keep the patient dry and placing the patient in a warm environment are important in achieving heat preservation.

Although blankets have been used traditionally, easily available plastic sheets such as 3-mil thick garbage bags are inexpensive, small, easily stored, disposable, and highly efficient devices for heat retention. Fluids, particularly intravenous fluids, given to the shock patient should be warm, not cold. The ideal temperature for such fluids is 104° F (40° C). Most ambulances do not have conventional rapid fluid warmers, but other steps can keep fluids at an adequate temperature. The fluids should not be stored in an air-conditioned compartment, nor should the patient be kept in such a compartment. A convenient storage area for fluids is in a box in the engine compartment. Fluid can also be warmed by wrapping heat packs around the bag. There are commercially available fluid warmer boxes for the patient care compartment, too. The patient compartment should be kept at 85° F (29° C) or more when transporting a severely injured trauma patient.

It is critical that the conditions should be ideal for the patient, not for the EMTs. The patient is the most important person in any emergency. Consider for a moment how you would feel swimming in a pool with a temperature at 72° F (22° C). Very rapidly you would become cold and start to shiver. The patient is in this same situation in a compartment that is air conditioned to 72° F (22° C). The patient has had all or most of his or her clothes removed; the lactated Ringer's that is being run rapidly into his or her veins, heart, and lungs are the same temperature as the compartment. The patient's rate of heat loss into the cold compartment is very high, and the cold fluid is cooling him or her faster. It is easy to cool a patient but very difficult to warm the patient up again.

Hypothermia is the third most serious condition of a trauma patient, ranking close to hypoxia and hypovolemia. It has two causes:

- Anaerobic metabolism results in a reduction of the energy production and the body cannot keep up with heat loss to the outside.
- There is a loss of heat between the body of the patient and the colder environment. This includes the introduction of cold air and fluids into the patient.

Providing warm, humidified oxygen for the patient to breathe and covering the patient with warm blankets or plastic sheets after completing the physical examination are also means for conservation of body heat.

Rapid transportation to a facility that is capable of managing the patient's condition is extremely important. Rapid transport does not mean disregarding or neglecting the treatment modalities that are important in patient care, nor neglecting proper immobilization of trauma patients. It does, however, indicate that such modalities are to be employed rapidly and that time must not be wasted with an inappropriate assessment or with unnecessarily complicated stabilization maneuvers. Many steps, such as warming the patient, starting intravenous therapy, and even performing the focused physical examination, can be accomplished in the ambulance while en route to the hospital.

PNEUMATIC ANTISHOCK GARMENT (PASG)

The PASG, as it has come to be known generically, is a controversial device because its exact role in prehospital care is still not definitively decided. Despite this controversy, it should not be neglected as a prehospital patient treatment tool. Like other medical devices, it should only be used when indicated. Specifically, it is helpful for patients requiring control of blood loss, management of pelvic instability, or long transport times. It may be detrimental to patients with penetrating thoracic trauma or short transport times. It remains contraindicated in patients with pulmonary edema, traumatic diaphragmatic herniation, or known hemorrhage above the diaphragm.

Physiology

Pressure applied by the PASG to the legs and abdomen is transmitted directly through the skin, fat, muscle, and other soft tissue to the blood vessels themselves. The vessels are compressed, and their lumen (internal opening) is reduced in size. The physiologic result is twofold. The vascular container in body areas beneath the device is made smaller, increasing the systemic vascular resistance and thereby raising the systolic and diastolic pressures. The remaining fluid can be distributed and better used in the noncompressed upper half of the body.

Hemorrhage

Compression over a bleeding site is the classic method of hemorrhage control. Effective compression can be achieved with the PASG for body areas such as the abdomen, pelvis, and the legs. The PASG is just a large pneumatic splint. It should be used to control blood loss and stabilize fractures with the same indications as a pneumatic splint.

Increased bleeding in the noncompressed portions of the body is a potential complication of inflating the PASG. The rate of hemorrhage from an open wound is proportional to the blood pressure inside the injured vessel minus the external pressure on the vessel. Less bleeding occurs with a low blood pressure than with a high blood pressure. Open vessels in the upper half of the body may well increase the rate of blood loss when the patient's blood pressure and blood flow are significantly improved, as when the PASG is applied.

Blood Pressure

Reevaluation of several studies indicates that patients with blood pressures below 50 to 60 mm Hg have a better outcome when the PASG is used than when it is not. The increased perfusion of the brain and heart that is provided by the increased vascular resistance in the lower extremities and abdomen is beneficial to such patients.

Immobilization of Fractures

Like any pneumatic splint, the PASG can also be used for fracture immobilization. The two major bones that the PASG immobilizes most effectively are the pelvis and the femur. Because hemorrhage is recognized as a major potential problem with fracture of either of these bones, compression with the PASG provides an extra benefit beyond just immobilizing the fracture. Use of the PASG solely as a splint for isolated lower extremity fractures where shock is not present or expected, however, is not recommended.

Application

The PASG is applied to the patient as quickly as possible and without delay when indications for its use in hemorrhage control or fracture management are present. The PASG is positioned under the patient in one of a number of ways. In many cases, it may be simpler to place the patient on the device (as when moving the patient onto a long board) rather than lifting the patient and inserting the garment beneath the patient.

The PASG is then securely and snugly fastened and inflated. When the Velcro® begins to crackle, between 60 and 80 mm Hg of PASG pressure (not blood pressure) has been achieved.

Deflation

Prehospital deflation of the PASG should not be done except in extreme extenuating circumstances, such as evidence of a diaphragmatic herniation, and even then only with on-line medical direction.

When deflation is necessary, it should be preceded by assessing the patient and confirming that vital signs are within normal limits. Even with vital signs within normal limits, the patient's blood volume might still be depleted: the inflated PASG has reduced the size of the patient's container, and the available blood volume may just fill the artificially reduced container. As the PASG is deflated, the patient's container size will increase. Unless a sufficient amount of fluid is present in reserve, cardiac preload will decrease, systemic vascular resistance will drop, and the patient's blood pressure and level of perfusion will deteriorate rapidly.

INTRAVENOUS FLUID REPLACEMENT

Fluids that are given to the patient fall into four basic groups: (1) water only, (2) water and electrolytes, (3) water and protein or protein substitutes such as colloids, and (4) RBCs. There are other specialty fluids that are used in the hospital, particularly fluids with large amounts of nutrients such as glucose and amino acids, or those that contain blood products such as fresh frozen plasma, platelets, or the various coagulation factors. Perhaps within the next 5 to 10 years, fluids with oxygen-carrying capability such as stroma-free hemoglobin will be available for prehospital use. At the present time, however, no prehospital fluids are capable of carrying oxygen; they

are only volume expanders. Dilution of the remaining blood in the patient by the introduction of volume expanders reduces the percentage of RBCs in the vascular space and therefore the oxygen-carrying capability of the blood. In most trauma patients, a loss of RBCs has already occurred and will remain low until the site of blood loss has been secured.

The definitive care of these patients requires replacement of the RBCs. Even if intravenous access and volume replacement are accomplished in the field, it is extremely important that the patient be delivered as quickly as possible to a facility that can immediately replace the lost RBCs to improve the patient's oxygen-carrying capacity. The facility should have immediate operating room access where hemorrhage can be rapidly controlled.

Water Solutions

Solutions that contain only water and glucose (as opposed to solutions that also contain electrolytes), although isotonic when administered, can be detrimental because the oncotic pressure of the vascular space is reduced by these fluids. For example, 5% dextrose in water (D5W) goes into the body as an isotonic fluid and remains isotonic in its first passage through the vascular system. However, as the glucose is metabolized only water is left behind, reducing the oncotic pressure of the vascular space. Because rapid exchange occurs between the interstitial fluid and the vascular space, interstitial oncotic pressure is likewise reduced. To equalize the oncotic pressure between the extracellular and intracellular fluid, water flows from the extracellular space into the intracellular space. This causes the tissue cells to swell and produces several adverse effects.

Cellular edema, particularly if it occurs in an enclosed space like the skull, puts pressure on the surrounding vessels that reduces the vascular size, especially in the capillary beds. The reduction in vascular size reduces blood flow, therefore reducing the oxygen replenishment capacity. The reduced oxygen replenishment capacity, in turn, increases cerebral ischemia and causes a shift from aerobic to anaerobic metabolism, producing cellular acidosis and more swelling of the cells.

This is a vicious cycle which, although most dramatic in the enclosed skull, also occurs in other organs as well. Some organs are more constrained than others. The kidneys, for example, are each contained in a tight capsule. Swollen cells cannot stretch the capsule; therefore, renal oxygenation may be compromised. The same can occur with the muscles of the extremities that are enclosed in strong fascial compartments.

Crystalloid Solutions

Crystalloid intravenous solutions are isotonic and remain isotonic; therefore, they act as effective volume expanders for a short period of time. Both the water and the electrolytes in the solution can freely cross the semipermeable membranes of the vessel walls (but not the cell membrane), and therefore achieve equilibrium in 2 to 3 hours. The added volume in the vascular space readily translocates to the interstitial space. For a short period, the vascular space is filled by crystalloid intravenous solutions, improving preload and cardiac output. This solution has no oxygen-carrying capacity and contains no protein; therefore, blood must be used eventually to replace the volume that has been lost by the patient.

Rapid infusion of crystalloids such as lactated Ringer's should be used initially for vascular volume replenishment and followed as quickly as possible with blood. A general rule of thumb is that initial crystalloid replacement should not exceed 3 liters before whole blood is instituted. This does not mean that a patient who is severely hypovolemic from acute blood loss should not be given adequate amounts of lactated Ringer's. It does mean that blood should be administered early during the patient's resuscitation. If it is necessary to give the patient more than 3 liters of crystalloid to maintain adequate preload and cardiac output because blood is not available, the detrimental results of such replacement must be accepted.

One hour after administration of a crystalloid solution, only one-third remains in the cardiovascular system. The rest has shifted into the interstitial space. Excessive interstitial fluid shows up as edema. One of the organs most affected is the lungs. The pathologic process of increased pulmonary fluid into the interstitial space is known as pulmonary edema. The solution to this dilemma is rapid transportation to a hospital that has the capability of caring for critical trauma patients.

Colloid and Plasma Substitutes

Administration of human protein to a patient has several drawbacks. Non-A and non-B hepatitis (mostly hepatitis C) are present in 3% of these fluids. The fluids are also expensive and have short shelf lives. "Look-alike" protein molecules that stay in the bloodstream with an increased oncotic pressure are more expensive than lactated Ringer's, require some special techniques in administration, and have some complications such as increased bleeding time and anaphylactic reactions. Recent studies using a combination of hypertonic saline and a colloid (dextran) have proven effective in increasing a patient's blood pressure. However, this increased blood pressure, as explained earlier, may increase hemorrhage and can actually decrease the survival rate. These consequences may or may not have prehospital application; further studies are still needed.

A synthetic colloid solution (Hetrostarch, Hespan) is frequently used as a resuscitation fluid outside the United States.

VASCULAR ACCESS

There are two reasons for obtaining vascular access on any patient in the prehospital phase of care: volume replacement and medication administration. A third, in-hospital reason is to monitor cardiac functions. Whether vascular access is obtained through peripheral or central intravenous lines or through intraosseous infusion, there are several commonalities of use.

The size and location of intravenous line placement are based upon the indication for its use. The rate of fluid administration is directly proportional to the bore of the needle and inversely proportional to its length. When fluid replacement is required, a large bore, short catheter should be used, as it will pass a larger volume than will a smaller, longer tube.

The ideal site for access in a patient requiring fluid replacement is a large vessel in the forearm. The desirable catheter to use is a 14 or 16 gauge and just over 1 inch in length. For administering medications, the chosen vein does not need to be as large, and an 18 or 20 gauge needle will suffice. In a trauma patient, it is best to start a large bore, peripheral intravenous line (preferably two lines). Central intravenous lines are generally not needed in the field or in the emergency department for fluid replacement.

• Summary •

1. Shock has many descriptions, but the most correct is that of cellular anaerobic metabolism.
2. Survival depends on oxygen delivery to the cells. This is accomplished by oxygenation of the red blood cells in the lungs and delivery of the red blood cells to the tissue cells (Fick principle).
3. Getting oxygen into the lungs is a top priority in the management of the shock patient.
4. Besides adequate oxygenation and ventilation, the patient also requires rapid transportation to a facility where hemorrhage can be controlled and blood loss can be replaced.
5. The PASG can assist in controlling hemorrhage by compressing the abdomen and pelvis to control bleeding in those areas while maintaining perfusion through the heart, brain, and lungs. It cannot and should not be used for prolonged periods as the only management technique employed.
6. Fluid replacement is also an important component to prehospital management of shock.

7. Crystalloid solutions function as volume expanders, but they do not have oxygen-carrying capabilities and therefore are not the ideal fluid for replacement. The ideal fluid for replacement of lost blood is blood.

8. The diagnosis of shock is made by recognizing the pathophysiology it produces. Tachycardia, tachypnea, increased capillary refilling time, decreased level of consciousness, and decreased blood pressure are the prehospital findings that indicate hypoperfusion of the various organs and the body's general demand for greater oxygenation.

Scenario Solution

In the scenario at the beginning of the chapter, you encountered a patient with multisystem trauma. Based on the signs and symptoms listed next, you should have concluded that the patient is experiencing spinal shock.

Signs and symptoms include a normal level of consciousness; strong, but slow pulse; warm and dry skin; normal capillary refill; and hypotension.

The management of this patient should include oxygenation, spinal immobilization, rapid transport, and judicious use of intravenous fluids.

Review Questions

Answers provided on page 333.

1 Which of the following statements are correct? (Choose as many as are applicable.)
   A Perfusion is the process of blood passing by tissue cells.
   B Hypoxia is a condition in which cell oxygen requirements are being met.
   C Hypoperfusion is inadequate blood passing by tissue cells.
   D Hypovolemia is a condition occurring when fluid volume is too high.

2 The cellular physiologic process of shock can be divided into all of the following phases, *except:*
   A the ischemic phase
   B the stagnant phase
   C the deceleration phase
   D the washout phase

3 Which of the following is a sign and symptom of shock?
   A warm, dry skin temperature in spinal shock
   B falling blood pressure during compensated shock
   C normal pulse during septic shock
   D pink skin color in hypovolemic shock

4 All of the following statements are true regarding the pneumatic antishock garment (PASG) *except:*
   A Increased vascular resistance in the lower extremities and abdomen is beneficial to patients with systolic blood pressure between 50 to 60 mm Hg.
   B Anterior compartment syndrome is a complication associated with prolonged use of the PASG.
   C The PASG should be inflated until the patient's systolic blood pressure reaches 120 mm Hg.
   D PASG deflation in the field should only be done with on-line physician direction.

5 Which of the following is a reason for intravenous fluid replacement?
   A The PASG is applied, but not inflated.
   B The patient has pulmonary edema.
   C There is a need to replace lost red blood cells with crystalloid solution.
   D There is a need to provide a short-term volume expander.

6 Which of the following statements about the management of shock is true? (Choose as many as are applicable.)
   A Rapid transport is critical when confronted with continuing hypoperfusion.
   B Blood replacement and hemorrhage control are the definitive care for blood loss.
   C Colloid and plasma substitutes have several drawbacks including higher expense, possible contamination with hepatitis, and anaphylaxis.
   D The preferred isotonic solution for the management of a shock patient is 5% dextrose in water (D5W).

7 Which of the following statements is incorrect?
   A Severe internal hemorrhage can be adequately controlled in the prehospital setting without the need for direct surgical control.
   B The IV catheter used for a shock patient should be 18 to 20 gauge.
   C PASG is a short-term treatment modality for shock.
   D A and B

CHAPTER OBJECTIVES

CHAPTER 7

Abdominal Trauma and Trauma in the Pregnant Patient

At the completion of this course the student will be able to:

- Identify the general anatomy of the abdomen.

- Define the physiology and pathophysiology of blunt and penetrating injury to the abdomen.

- Identify the importance of maintaining a high index of suspicion for abdominal trauma.

- List the focused and detailed assessment findings of intra-abdominal bleeding.

- Define the relationship of kinematics to abdominal trauma.

- Explain the importance of abdominal and pelvic hemorrhage control by direct compression using the pneumatic antishock garment along with limitations of its use in certain patients and the later stages of pregnancy.

- Identify the need for rapid intervention and rapid transport when appropriate.

- Identify the anatomic and physiologic changes that occur in pregnancy.

- Identify the proper position for transport of the pregnant trauma patient.

- Understand the physiology of the two lives involved in the management of the pregnant patient.

Scenario

A call is received through the emergency 9-1-1 system for a unit to respond to a single motor vehicle crash. Initial information indicates that the vehicle crashed head-on into a tree at a high rate of speed. There is a single occupant, approximately 20 years of age. Upon arrival at the crash site, the scene is determined to be safe. The vehicle is noted to have significant frontal intrusion and damage to the passenger compartment. The driver is restrained by a lap belt and is trapped by his legs, requiring extrication. The patient is unconscious but responds with localization to painful stimuli. Initial vital signs demonstrate a pulse rate of 85, a respiratory rate of 20, and systolic blood pressure of 120. The decision must be made at this time whether or not the patient should be rapidly extricated.

After extrication, the secondary survey (focused physical examination) reveals a seat belt contusion of the abdomen above the level of the iliac crests. The abdominal examination is otherwise unremarkable. The patient is noted to have facial contusions and swelling, anterior chest contusion, and an obvious fracture of the left femur.

- Does this patient require triage to a trauma center?
- Should the patient be rapidly transported to an appropriate facility?
- Have life-threatening injuries been ruled out in this individual?
- Does this patient have the potential for abdominal injuries?
- If so, how likely is it that abdominal injuries are present, and what type of injuries may exist?

The abdomen is the region of the body in which it is most difficult to correctly diagnose trauma injuries that require surgical repair. When unrecognized, abdominal injury is one of the major causes of death in the trauma patient. It is also the second leading cause of preventable trauma deaths. Because abdominal injury is difficult to correctly diagnose, the correct method of management is to transport patients with even suspected abdominal injuries to the closest appropriate facility.

The extent of abdominal trauma can also be difficult to determine in the prehospital setting. Death may occur from massive blood loss caused by either penetrating or blunt injuries. Late complications and possible death occur from colon, small intestine, stomach, or pancreatic injuries that go undetected. However, blunt trauma often poses a greater threat to life because it is more difficult to diagnose than penetrating trauma. The EMT should not be as concerned with pinpointing the exact extent of abdominal trauma as with treating the clinical findings. It should be noted, however, that the absence of local signs and symptoms does not rule out the possibility of abdominal trauma. A high index of suspicion based on the mechanism of injury should alert the EMT to the potential of abdominal trauma and intra-abdominal hemorrhage.

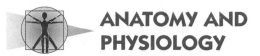

ANATOMY AND PHYSIOLOGY

The abdomen contains the major organs of the digestive, endocrine, and urogenital systems, as well as major vessels of the circulatory system. The abdominal cavity is located below the diaphragm; its boundaries include the anterior abdominal wall, the pelvic bones, the vertebral column, and the muscles of the abdomen and flanks. The cavity is divided into two spaces. The **retroperitoneal space** (potential space behind the "true" abdominal cavity) contains the kidneys, ureters, bladder, reproductive organs, inferior vena cava, abdominal aorta, pancreas, a portion of the duodenum, colon, and rectum (Figure 7-1). The **peritoneal space** (the "true" abdominal cavity) contains the large and small intestines, spleen, liver, stomach, gallbladder, and female reproductive organs (Figure 7-2).

The **cephalad** (toward the head) portion of the abdomen is protected in front by the ribs and in back by the vertebral column (see Figure 1-20). This area contains the liver, spleen, stomach, and diaphragm, any of which may sustain injury as a result of rib fracture or sternal injury. The organs most commonly injured by the same forces that fracture ribs are the liver and spleen. The **caudad** (toward the tail) portion of the abdomen is protected on all sides by the pelvis. This area contains the rectum and much of the intestine (especially when the patient is upright); the urinary bladder and ureters; and in the female, the reproductive organs. Extraperitoneal hemorrhage associated with a fractured pelvis is a major concern in this portion of the abdominal cavity. The abdomen above the pelvis and below the ribs has some soft protection by the abdominal muscles anteriorly and laterally (see Figure 1-20). Posteriorly, the lumbar vertebrae provide protection along with the thick, strong paraspinal and psoas muscles (Figure 7-3; also see inside front and back covers).

Increased intra-abdominal pressure, produced by compression against a car's steering column or similar force, can rupture the abdominal cavity, much like the compression of a paper bag (see Chapter 1: Kinematics of Trauma). Rupture of the left half of the diaphragm is the injury most likely to produce problems in the early care (prehospital phase) of the patient. Translocation of the intra-abdominal contents into the chest can compromise lung expansion (see Figure 1-21).

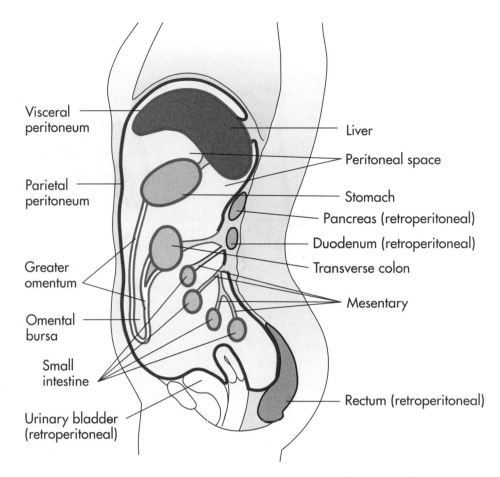

Visceral peritoneum

Liver

Peritoneal space

Parietal peritoneum

Stomach

Pancreas (retroperitoneal)

Duodenum (retroperitoneal)

Transverse colon

Greater omentum

Mesentary

Omental bursa

Small intestine

Urinary bladder (retroperitoneal)

Rectum (retroperitoneal)

Figure 7-1 The abdomen is divided into two spaces: the peritoneal space and the retroperitoneal space. The retroperitoneal space includes the portion of the abdomen behind the peritoneum. The organs are not in contact with the peritoneal cavity. Injury to organs in this area does not necessarily produce peritonitis. (From Thibodeau, G.A., and Patton, K.T. *Structure and Function.* 10th ed. St. Louis: Mosby, 1997.)

Dividing the abdominal organs into hollow, solid, and vascular groups helps provide a basic physiologic understanding of them. When injured, solid and vascular organs bleed, whereas hollow ones spill their contents into the peritoneal cavity or extraperitoneal space. This spilling results in intra-abdominal bleeding, **peritonitis** (inflammation of the peritoneum, or the lining of the abdominal cavity), and **sepsis** (massive infection). Prehospital treatment involves the rapid initiation of shock management and control of hemorrhage with the pneumatic antishock garment (in patients with appropriate indications and per local protocol; see Chapter 6: Shock and Fluid Resuscitation).

For purposes of patient assessment, the surface of the abdomen is divided into four quadrants. These quadrants are formed by drawing two lines, one in the midline from the tip of the xiphoid to the symphysis pubis, and the other perpendicular to this midline at the level of the umbilicus (Figure 7-4).

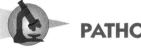

PATHOPHYSIOLOGY

Injuries to the abdomen may be caused by penetrating or blunt trauma. Penetrating trauma, such as a gunshot or stab wound, is more readily visible than blunt trauma. Multiple organ damage can occur in penetrating trauma, although it is less likely with a stab wound than with a gunshot wound. The trajectory of a missile, such as a bullet or the path of a knife blade, can frequently be visualized and can help identify possible injured organs.

Anteriorly, the diaphragm extends cephalad to the fourth intercostal space anteriorly, sixth intercostal space

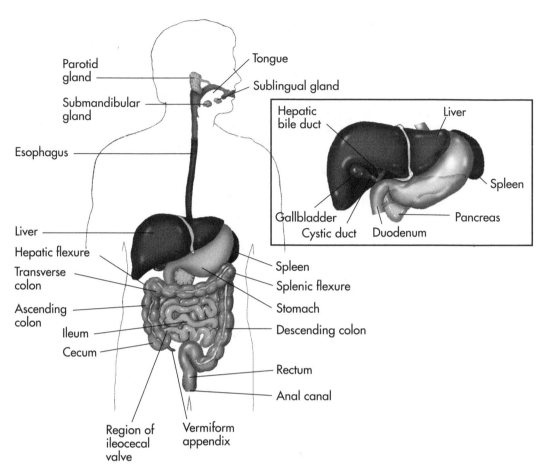

Figure 7-2 The organs inside the peritoneal cavity frequently produce peritonitis when injured. Organs in the peritoneal cavity include solid organs (spleen and liver), hollow organs of the gastrointestinal tract (stomach, small intestine, and colon), and the reproductive organs. (From Thibodeau, G.A., and Patton, K.T. *Anatomy and Physiology.* 2d ed. St. Louis: Mosby–Year Book, Inc., 1993.)

laterally, and eighth intercostal space posteriorly during maximum expiration (see Figure 1-20). Patients with penetrating injury to the thorax or possibly below this line may also have an abdominal injury. Penetrating wounds of the flanks and buttocks may involve organs in the abdominal cavity as well. These penetrating injuries may cause bleeding from a major vessel or solid organ and perforation of a segment of the intestine—the most frequently injured organ in penetrating trauma.

Blunt trauma to the intra-abdominal organs is generally the result of compression or shear injuries. In compression incidents, the organs of the abdomen are crushed between solid objects, such as between the steering wheel and spinal column. Shear incidents create rupture of the solid organs or rupture of blood vessels in the cavity because of the tearing forces exerted against their stabilizing ligaments and vessels. For example, the aorta, liver, and spleen bleed easily, and blood loss can occur at a rapid rate. Pelvic fractures may be associated with bladder or urethral injuries and are usually associated with the loss of large volumes of blood.

Loss of blood into the abdominal cavity, regardless of its source, will contribute to or be the primary cause of the development of shock. The release of acids, enzymes, or bacteria from the gastrointestinal tract into the peritoneal cavity will result in additional organ damage and peritonitis.

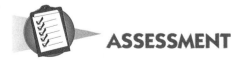

ASSESSMENT

The index of suspicion for injury should be based on the mechanism of injury and on outward signs such as ecchymosis or marks of collision. Intra-abdominal bleeding should be suspected when the patient has external bruising, pain, abdominal tenderness, abdominal rigidity, or distention. Although these signs and symptoms are indicative of intra-abdominal bleeding, patients with sub-

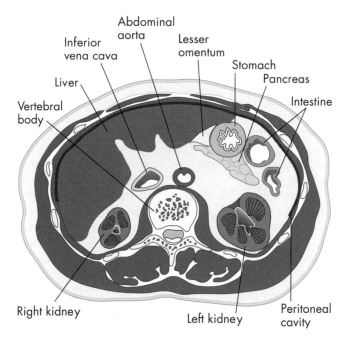

Figure 7-3 This transverse section of the abdominal cavity gives an appreciation of the organs' positions in the anteroposterior direction.

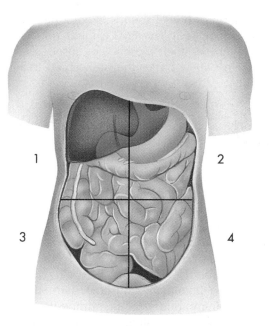

Figure 7-4 As with any part of the body, the better the description of pain, tenderness, and guarding, etc., the more accurate the diagnosis. The most common system of identification divides the abdomen into four quadrants: left and right upper, and left and right lower. (From Thibodeau, G.A. *Anatomy and Physiology.* 3rd ed. St. Louis: Mosby, 1997.)

stantial intra-abdominal hemorrhage often do not display them.

The most reliable indicator of intra-abdominal bleeding is the presence of shock from an unexplained source. Response to physical examination of the abdomen in the conscious patient may or may not be reliable. Pelvic or rib fractures produce pain not necessarily associated with intra-abdominal injury, whereas alcohol, drugs, or spinal fracture may mask such symptoms. Also, fresh blood in the abdomen is not an irritant to the peritoneum and in most cases, will not cause any signs of peritonitis. The adult abdominal cavity can hold up to 1.5 liters of fluid before showing any signs of distention. Therefore, significant amounts of blood may be present in the abdomen, yet the patient's physical examination can be totally normal. In an unconscious patient or a patient who has suffered head injury, it is extremely difficult to determine any appropriate verbal response. Therefore, the EMT must rely on immediate impressions from a variety of other sources of information, including kinematics, bystanders' input, and/or physical evidence. Assessment of abdominal injury may be very difficult. The following are reliable indicators for establishing the index of suspicion for abdominal injury:

- mechanism of injury or damage to the passenger compartment (bent steering wheel)
- outward signs of trauma
- shock with unexplained cause
- level of shock greater than explained by other injuries
- presence of abdominal rigidity, guarding, or distension (a rare finding)

Assessment of the patient with suspected abdominal trauma should include the following:

Observation. The abdomen should be exposed and observed for distension, contusions, abrasions, penetration, evisceration, impaled object(s), and/or obvious bleeding. These signs can all be indicative of underlying injury.

Palpation. Palpating the abdomen can reveal abdominal wall defects or elicit pain in the area palpated. Voluntary or involuntary guarding, rigidity, and/or rebound tenderness may be indicative of bruising, inflammation, or hemorrhage. However, the EMT should avoid deep palpation of an obviously injured abdomen, as palpation can increase existing hemorrhage and worsen other injuries. Pelvic instability is associated with pelvic fractures that are usually accompanied by significant hemorrhage. Pelvic instability is assessed by gently applying pressure to the pelvic girdle.

Auscultation of bowel sounds is *not* a helpful prehospital assessment tool. The EMT should not waste time trying to determine their presence or absence, as this diagnostic sign will not alter the prehospital treatment of the patient.

 ## MANAGEMENT

The management of abdominal trauma is the same regardless of the specific organ injured. The following are the most valuable steps in managing a patient with abdominal injury:

1. Rapidly evaluate the patient and the scene.
2. Initiate basic shock therapy, including oxygen administration (FiO$_2$ >0.85).
3. Apply the pneumatic antishock garment (PASG) to reduce intra-abdominal or retroperitoneal hemorrhage and if indicated, to counter shock [blood pressure 60 millimeters of mercury (mm Hg)]. The major benefit of PASG application to the injured patient is the reduction of intra-abdominal hemorrhage. (See Chapter 6: Shock and Fluid Resuscitation for a complete discussion of the PASG.) In cases in which the use of the abdominal section of the PASG is relatively contraindicated (such as evisceration), if the patient's condition remains critical and unimproved, inflation of the device may be required with appropriate physician approval.
4. Rapidly package and transport the patient to the nearest appropriate trauma facility.
5. Initiate crystalloid intravenous fluid replacement en route to the hospital.

Surgical intervention remains a key need; no time should be wasted in prehospital attempts to determine the exact details of injury. In many instances, identification of specific organ injury will not be revealed until the abdomen is opened.

Transporting a patient with intra-abdominal injuries to a hospital that does not have an operating room and surgical staff immediately available defeats the purpose of rapid transportation. The receiving hospital should be chosen for its ability to provide rapid surgical management.

Special considerations are involved when managing patients who have impaled objects, **eviscerations,** or who are pregnant.

IMPALED OBJECTS

Because removal of an impaled object may cause severe additional trauma and the object's distal end may be controlling bleeding, removal of an impaled object in the prehospital environment is considered relatively contraindicated. An object impaled in the abdomen should neither be moved or removed until its shape and location have been identified by radiograph evaluation, and blood replacement and a surgical team are present and ready. The EMT should support the impaled object and immobilize it, either manually or mechanically, to prevent its further movement in the field and during transport. If bleeding occurs around it, direct pressure should be applied around the object to the wound with the flat of the hand.

The abdomen should not be palpated in these cases, as palpation may produce additional tearing or intrusion by the distal end of the object. Further examination is unnecessary when the presence of objects indicate the need for surgical exploration. The PASG is also contraindicated in such patients.

EVISCERATION

In an abdominal evisceration, a section of intestine or other abdominal organ is displaced through an open wound and protrudes externally outside the abdominal cavity. Protecting the protruding section of intestine or other organ from further damage presents a special problem. *Do **not** attempt to replace the protruding organ back into the abdominal cavity.* Leave the viscera on the surface of the abdomen or protruding as found. Most of the abdominal contents require a moist environment. If intestine or some of the other abdominal organs become dry, cell death will occur. Therefore, eviscerated abdominal contents should be covered with sterile pads that are moistened with sterile saline (normal saline intravenous fluid can be used). These dressings should be periodically remoistened with sterile saline to keep them from drying out.

TRAUMA IN PREGNANCY

Pregnancy causes anatomic and physiologic changes to the body's systems. These changes affect the potential patterns of injuries. The EMT is dealing with two (or more) patients and must be alert to changes that have occurred throughout the pregnancy. The uterus continues to enlarge up through the 38th week of pregnancy. This anatomic change makes the uterus and its contents more susceptible to injury, including rupture, penetration, abruption of the placenta, and premature rupture of membranes.

Heart rate increases throughout pregnancy, rising 15 to 20 beats per minute above normal by the third trimester. This makes the interpretation of tachycardia more difficult. Systolic and diastolic blood pressure will drop 5 to

15 mm Hg during the second trimester but will be normal at term. Some women may have significant hypotension when supine. This condition, supine hypotension syndrome, is caused by compression of the uterus on the inferior vena cava and is usually relieved by placing the woman on her left side (left lateral decubitus position). In pregnant patients with blunt trauma who require spinal immobilization on a backboard, the patient should be quickly placed on the board and the board placed on the stretcher. At this point, the board, with the patient properly secured to it, should be turned to the patient's left side (left lateral recumbant position). If the patient cannot be rotated, the right leg should be elevated and the uterus displaced to the left.

After the tenth week of pregnancy, cardiac output is increased by 1.0 to 1.5 liters per minute. There is a 48% increase in blood volume by term. Because of this significant increase, 30% to 35% of the blood volume can be lost before signs and symptoms of hypovolemia become apparent.

Although a marked protuberance of the abdomen is obvious in late pregnancy, abdominal organs remain essentially unchanged with the exception of the uterus. Intestine that is displaced superiorly is shielded by the uterus in the last two trimesters of pregnancy. The increased size of the uterus, as well as its high blood flow, make it susceptible to both blunt and penetrating injury (Figure 7-5).

The respiratory rate is not altered by pregnancy. During the third trimester, the diaphragm is elevated and may cause mild dyspnea, especially when the patient is supine. Eclampsia, which is a late complication of pregnancy, may mimic a head injury. Careful neurologic assessment and discovery of any pertinent associated past medical history are important.

Peristalsis (the propulsive, muscular movements of the intestines) is slow, so food may remain in the stomach many hours after eating. The pregnant patient may therefore be at greater risk for vomiting and subsequent aspiration. As with the nonpregnant patient, auscultation of the abdomen to assess for abdominal injury is nonproductive. Searching for fetal heart tones at the scene is also nonproductive because their presence or absence is not going to alter the prehospital care. Rapid transport to the trauma center is the correct management.

Blood loss from abdominal injury can be indicated by minimal signs and symptoms up to severe shock. The condition of the fetus depends on the condition of the mother. However, the fetus may be in jeopardy while the mother's condition and vital signs appear stable. The goals of management are essentially the same as for any patient experiencing shock and include increased attention to providing high levels of oxygen to meet the needs of both mother and the fetus.

Vigorous fluid replacement should be started during transport to help combat shock in the mother as well as in the fetus. The PASG may be applied to the leg sections and inflated when indicated. The abdominal section can be inflated if intra-abdominal hemorrhage is suspected. Any evidence of vaginal bleeding or a rigid boardlike abdomen with external bleeding in the last trimester of pregnancy should alert the EMT to possible **abruptio placentae** (separation of the placenta from the uterine wall) or a ruptured uterus. Exsanguination may occur rapidly.

When spinal injury is suspected, the pregnant patient should be immobilized and transported supine. To prevent compression of the vena cava, carefully roll the long board 10° to 15° to the left or elevate the right leg. *Do not delay transport of the pregnant trauma patient.* Every pregnant trauma victim—even those who appear to have only minor injuries—should be transported, because any trauma to the abdomen of a pregnant patient should be evaluated by a physician. *Adequate resuscitation of the mother is the key to survival of the mother and fetus.*

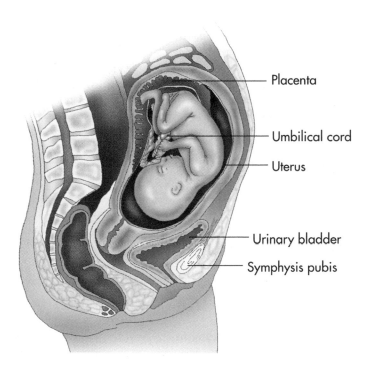

Figure 7-5 In a pregnant patient, as the uterus and fetus enlarge above the symphysis pubis, the fetus becomes more susceptible to both blunt and penetrating trauma. (From Thibodeau, G.A., and Patton, K.T. *Anatomy and Physiology.* 2d ed. St. Louis: Mosby–Year Book, Inc., 1993.)

• Summary •

1. The potential threat to life from intra-abdominal injuries is extremely high. No other area of the body is more susceptible to major hemorrhage without apparent physical evidence of injury. The patient with an abdominal injury can deteriorate rapidly and without warning.

2. The extent of specific abdominal organ injury is seldom identifiable in the prehospital setting. Therefore, rapid evaluation, essential stabilization, and rapid transport are the keys that assure the best chance of survival.

3. Appropriate prehospital care of patients with suspected abdominal trauma requires resuscitation with good airway management and hemorrhage control. This care should be initi-

ated and continued en route to an appropriate facility.

4. The patient should be rapidly packaged and transported without delay. Survival is frequently determined by the length of time from the incident to hemorrhage control in the operating room. Unnecessary time spent in the field doing unnecessary tasks or tasks that can be done just as well en route to the hospital prolongs this critical window of opportunity.

5. It is also essential to transport the abdominal trauma patient to a facility with a trauma team standing by in-house. (See Chapter 2: Patient Assessment and Management for details about choosing the correct facility.)

Scenario Solution

The patient in this scenario has signs of a closed head injury because he has a decreased level of consciousness and only responds to painful stimuli. After the patient's legs are freed, a good argument can be made for proceeding with rapid extrication and packaging of the patient for transport. Although this individual is not tachycardic and has a normal systolic blood pressure, these findings do not rule out the possibility of early, compensated shock in a young, healthy person. The head injury should also convey a sense of urgency and lead to rapid extrication and transport. The patient meets criteria for trauma center transport, including decreased level of consciousness and mechanism of injury.

The secondary survey (focused physical examination) reveals a seat belt contusion above the level of the iliac crests. This

sign indicates an improperly applied seat belt. The potential for intra-abdominal injuries in this situation is very high. Seat belt injuries of this type may include small and large bowel perforations, duodenal and pancreatic damage, and mesenteric tears with hemorrhage. Several of these structures are located in the retroperitoneum, and injuries to these structures may not cause any abdominal physical findings for hours or days. Therefore, the absence of an abnormal abdominal examination does not rule out these injuries. This patient requires rapid surgical evaluation and possible emergent operative intervention if abdominal injuries are found. The patient should be rapidly transported to an appropriate facility with immediately available surgical capabilities.

Review Questions

Answers provided on page 333.

1 The organs most commonly injured in the abdomen by blunt trauma are the:
   A stomach and duodenum
   B small intestines and kidneys
   C colon and pancreas
   D liver and spleen

2 Injuries to hollow organs in the abdomen cause peritonitis secondary to hemorrhage into the peritoneal cavity.
   A true
   B false

3 The loss of 1.5 liters of blood into the abdominal cavity of a normal adult male will most likely produce the following findings on physical examination:
   A distention
   B tenderness
   C involuntary guarding
   D normal examination

4 The use of the abdominal compartment of the PASG is contraindicated in all the following circumstances *except:*
   A pelvic fracture
   B impaled objects in the abdomen
   C evisceration
   D pregnancy

5 By term in pregnancy, the blood volume will increase in the mother by:
A 23%
B 67%
C 48%
D 14%

6 The pregnant patient should be transported appropriately immobilized and the right side of the board elevated 10° to 15° to relieve pressure on the inferior vena cava.
A true
B false

CHAPTER OBJECTIVES

CHAPTER 8

Head Trauma

At the completion of this course the student will be able to:

- Identify the general anatomy of the head.

- Define the physiology and pathophysiology of hypoperfusion, concussion, contusion, laceration, hematoma, and fractures pertinent to the head.

- Define increased intracranial pressure and list the progression of events as pressure rises.

- Define Cushing's triad (response).

- Explain the indications for hyperventilation in the head injury patient.

- Identify the need for cervical spine immobilization with a significant head injury.

- Identify the need for rapid transport of a patient with a decreased level of consciousness from a significant head injury.

Scenario

You and your partner are dispatched to a private residence to aid a man who has fallen. Upon your arrival, you find a 53-year-old man who has fallen down the stairs going to the basement. His wife tells you that he had been drinking most of the evening and that he was quite intoxicated. She states that he has been moaning since he fell, but she has not been able to help him up. As you approach him, you can see that he appears awake and has sustained a scalp laceration that has been bleeding moderately.

- What is your first priority in managing the patient?
- What steps will you take to extricate this patient from the basement?
- What are your initial concerns regarding the likely head injuries?

Head trauma is the leading cause of trauma deaths. Victims of head injuries are commonly young adults who have been involved in motor vehicle collisions. They may also have a history complicated by drug and alcohol intoxication. Because the head injury patient may be unconscious at the scene or unable to provide any past medical history, talking with witnesses and visual evaluation of the scene may provide the only available history. The patient may be combative at the scene or become combative during treatment or transport, adding difficulty to the task of providing patient care. Skilled, rapid care at the scene can often mean the difference between recovery and serious neurologic deficits or death.

Damage to the surrounding environment that may have been caused by the patient's head should indicate a high index of suspicion for a head injury. Common areas of the vehicle that could cause head damage include the windshield, objects within the vehicle, unrestrained occupants, or any other involved fixed objects. Collision of the head with any fixed object can result in multiple skull or brain injuries.

Kinematics also suggests that the damage will depend on the speed at which the head was traveling and its position just prior to contact. Scene assessment, including vehicle damage assessment when necessary, is an important tool. It is essential to report this assessment information to the receiving hospital staff. Some patients who appear stable upon examination may be admitted for further observation based solely on the scene survey or vehicle damage description.

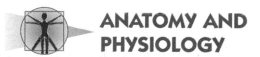

ANATOMY AND PHYSIOLOGY

The incidence of head injuries remains high because there is little support or protection for the head. A knowledge of head and brain anatomy is essential for understanding the causes and results of head injuries.

The scalp is the outermost, thickest layer of body covering. It provides a spongy protection for the skull. The aging process and balding causes the scalp to thin and provide less protection. Because the scalp is highly vascular, uncontrolled bleeding from a laceration may result in significant blood loss. Although scalp injuries may result in copious bleeding, the hemorrhage can be easily controlled with direct pressure.

The skull or cranium (cranial vault) is essentially a closed box encasing the brain tissue (Figure 8-1). The largest opening of the skull is located in the inferior surface of the occipital area (Figure 8-2). This opening is the **foramen magnum,** and part of the brain stem and the spinal cord pass through it.

The cranium provides protection to the brain tissue from most direct injuries originating from the outside. The interior walls of the skull at the base are rough and irregular. These irregularities can cause bruising and lacerations to the brain tissue when the skull and brain move in different directions or at different speeds at the same time. The greater the difference in the direction and/or speed of motion between the skull and brain, the greater the amount of damage possible. The bony tissue of the skull is especially thin in the temporal and ethmoid regions

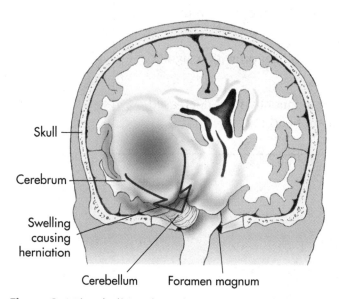

Skull

Cerebrum

Swelling causing herniation

Cerebellum   Foramen magnum

Figure 8-1 The skull is a large bony structure that contains the brain. There is no way the brain can escape the skull if it expands because of edema or if there is hemorrhage in the skull that presses on the brain. (From American College of Emergency Physicians. *Paramedic Field Care: A Complaint Based Approach.* Edited by D. Pons and D. Cason. St. Louis: Mosby, 1997.)

and thus can fracture with less force applied at these sites than elsewhere.

The brain tissue is covered by three different membranes called the **meninges** (Figure 8-3). The outermost layer of the meninges is the **dura mater.** In Latin, this terms means "tough mother." The dura mater is a tough, thick, inelastic, fibrous tissue providing the first line of protection to the brain. The meningeal arteries are located between the internal surface of the bony skull and the dura mater in a potential space called the **epidural space** (Figure 8-4). A potential space means that this area is normally very small but can increase in size with an influx of fluids or blood. An injury causing bleeding in the epidural space can produce an **epidural hematoma.**

The next layer beneath the dura mater is the **arachnoid membrane.** This membrane is spiderweb-like and transparent in appearance. The final layer of the meninges is the **pia mater,** which means "soft (tender) mother." The pia mater both covers and is attached to the brain cortex. It also adheres to the arachnoid membrane in some places. In most places, considerable space exists between the two inner layers of meninges: the **subarachnoid**

space. Rupture of the veins that bridge from the cortex to the sagittal sinus of the brain can result in the formation of a **subdural hematoma.**

The brain is composed of the **cerebrum, cerebellum,** and **brain stem.** Brain tissue occupies approximately 80% of the intracranial space (see Figure 8-1). The cerebrum is divided into two hemispheres, left and right halves. Each hemisphere is further separated into several lobes, each of which is responsible for the control of specific intellectual, sensory, and/or motor functions.

The cerebellum is located in the posterior fossa of the intracranial space, beneath the cerebrum. The cerebellum also surrounds the brain stem and coordinates movement.

The area of the brain responsible for consciousness is called the **reticular activating system** (RAS), which is located in the brain stem. The **medulla,** also part of the brain stem, controls breathing, heart rate, and other automatic functions.

Cerebrospinal fluid (CSF) is produced in the ventricular system of the brain and is found within the subarachnoid space. Cerebrospinal fluid covers the outer surface

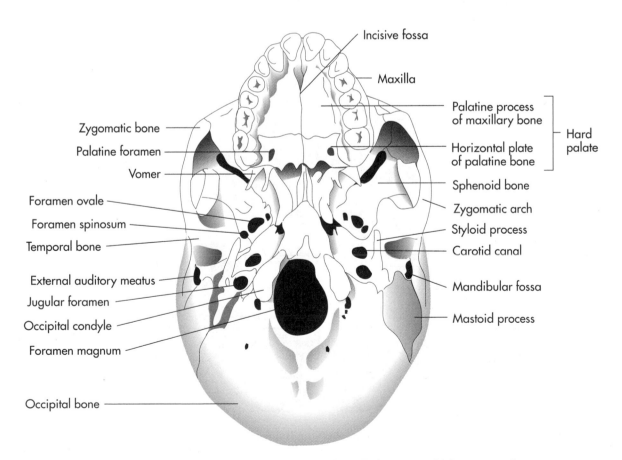

Figure 8-2 Base of skull. Viewed from below, mandible removed.

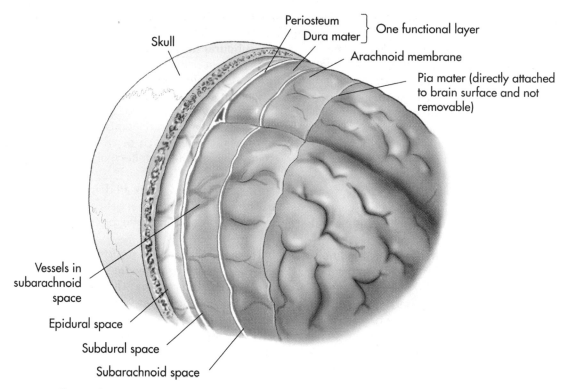

Skull

Periosteum
Dura mater } One functional layer

Arachnoid membrane

Pia mater (directly attached to brain surface and not removable)

Vessels in subarachnoid space

Epidural space

Subdural space

Subarachnoid space

Figure 8-3 Meninges. Meningeal coverings of the brain. (From Seeley, R.R.; Stephens, T.D.; and Tate, P. *Essentials of Anatomy and Physiology*. St. Louis: Mosby–Year Book, Inc., 1991.)

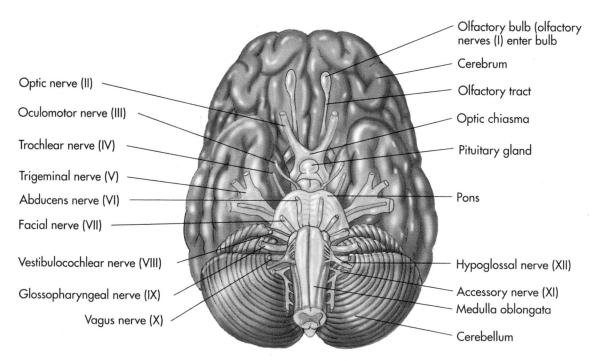

Optic nerve (II)

Oculomotor nerve (III)

Trochlear nerve (IV)

Trigeminal nerve (V)

Abducens nerve (VI)

Facial nerve (VII)

Vestibulocochlear nerve (VIII)

Glossopharyngeal nerve (IX)

Vagus nerve (X)

Olfactory bulb (olfactory nerves (I) enter bulb

Cerebrum

Olfactory tract

Optic chiasma

Pituitary gland

Pons

Hypoglossal nerve (XII)

Accessory nerve (XI)

Medulla oblongata

Cerebellum

Figure 8-4 Inferior surface of the brain showing the origins of the cranial nerves. (From Seeley, R.R.; Stephens, T.D.; and Tate, P. *Essentials of Anatomy and Physiology*. St. Louis: Mosby–Year Book, Inc., 1991.)

of the brain and acts as a liquid shock absorber between the brain and the skull.

The twelve **cranial nerves** originate from within the brain and brain stem and then branch out to their specific target organs (Figure 8-4). During assessment of the patient with a suspected head injury, the function of the third (III) cranial nerve becomes an important tool. The third cranial nerve, the **oculomotor nerve,** is responsible for control of pupillary constriction. A sluggish or a dilated, nonreactive pupil in a patient with an altered level of consciousness generally indicates compression of the third cranial nerve. This compression can be caused by tumors, tissue swelling, or internal bleeding (Figure 8-5).

The **tentorium cerebelli,** a portion of the dura mater, forms a protective covering over the cerebellum. An opening within the tentorium, at the junction of the midbrain and the cerebrum, is called the **tentorial incisura** (see Figure 8-5). The brain stem lies almost directly below the incisura. Any increase in intracranial pressure can force a portion of the temporal lobe of the cerebrum through the tentorial incisura. This process is called **herniation.**

The third cranial nerve passes through the incisura from the brain stem to the pupils. A tentorial herniation will compress the third cranial nerve. Signs of this herniation or pressure can be observed as a fixed and dilated pupil ("blown" pupil) on the same side as the herniation.

Further inferior herniation can result in increased pressure on the tenth (X) cranial nerve (see Figure 8-5). The tenth cranial nerve, the **vagus nerve,** produces a parasympathetic (vagal) response when stimulated. A parasympathetic response will result in a slowing of the heart rate (bradycardia) and some loss in systemic vascular tone.

Blood flow to the brain is remarkably constant despite ever present changes in blood pressure, temperature, and internal activity. Cerebral blood flow begins to decrease when the mean arterial pressure (MAP) drops to 60 millimeters of mercury (mm Hg) or below.

$$MAP = \text{diastolic blood pressure } + \frac{1}{3} \text{ pulse pressure}$$
$$(\text{pulse pressure} = \text{systolic} - \text{diastolic pressure})$$

Arterial $PaCO_2$ concentrations have a profound effect on cerebral blood flow. When $PaCO_2$ levels rise above normal values (35–45 torr), cerebral blood vessels dilate. As with any closed circulatory system, an increase in internal vessel diameter will result in increased blood flow. An increase in blood flow will also cause an increase in bleeding and an increase in intracranial pressure. In addition, the dilated vessels occupy more space inside the confines of the cranial vault. When $PaCO_2$ levels drop

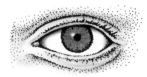
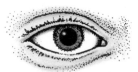

Figure 8-5 Suspect injury to the brain whenever a patient's pupils are unequal in size.

below 30 torr, the vessels will constrict, taking up less space and causing a decrease in blood flow. This decrease in blood flow can result in a temporary lowering of the intracranial pressure. One quick and easy way to decrease $PaCO_2$ levels in the suspected head injury patient is to control ventilation by hyperventilating the patient. Hyperventilation will decrease the level of CO_2 and constrict the cerebral vessels.

The cerebral perfusion pressure (CPP) depends on mean arterial pressure (MAP) and intracranial pressure (ICP).

$$CPP = MAP - ICP$$

The difference between these pressures is normally sufficient to maintain adequate cerebral perfusion. However, if the ICP is increased as a result of cerebral edema or hemorrhage, CPP is decreased and blood flow to the brain will be decreased. The change in CPP is the same with a rising ICP or a falling MAP. If the ICP becomes equal to or exceeds the MAP, blood flow to the brain effectively ceases. Therefore, it is essential to maintain an adequate MAP as well as reducing an elevated ICP in the head injury patient.

PATHOPHYSIOLOGY

Unconsciousness in the head trauma patient results either from an injury to the cerebral cortex or an injury to the brain stem's reticular activating system, which is the area responsible for consciousness. An increase in the intracranial pressure and a decrease in the cerebral blood flow, regardless of the cause, can depress the level of consciousness.

Rising intracranial pressure produces complications because the brain is enclosed in a rigid boxlike structure (the skull). The principal component of blood and edema is water, which is very difficult to compress in comparison to the brain tissue. Whenever fluid volume increases in one area of the brain, the increase will be transmitted throughout the entire intracranial compartment. If cerebral edema increases (brain tissue swells) or a hematoma rapidly enlarges, CSF is pushed out of the intracranial space and the blood volume within the skull is reduced.

This type of fluid shifting within the cranial vault causes poor cerebral blood flow and tissue oxygenation, followed by increasing anaerobic metabolism.

The pressure within the arteries (MAP) of the cranial vault normally exceeds the ICP by a considerable margin. When the ICP increases and approaches the MAP, the vessels will be squeezed from the outside. This increased outside pressure will cause a decrease in the vessels' diameters, resulting in an increased vascular resistance and a decreased blood flow throughout the brain tissue (see Figure 11-4A).

The brain senses the decrease in oxygenation and the increase in anaerobic metabolism and will attempt to correct it. The initial response is to activate the cardiovascular system to increase blood flow by increasing blood pressure. Blood pressure can be increased by increasing the cardiac output through increased heart rate and contractions or by increasing peripheral vascular resistance (systolic blood pressure = cardiac output × peripheral vascular resistance). As the cardiovascular system works to increase blood pressure, the respiratory system will increase its efforts to elevate oxygen content within the blood. The net result of these efforts is an increase in systolic blood pressure and respiratory rate. As the blood pressure and ICP continue to rise, the patient's pulse (heart) rate will then decrease. This threefold phenomenon of (1) rising blood pressure, (2) change in respiratory pattern, and (3) decrease in pulse rate is associated with increasing intracranial pressure and is referred to as **Cushing's triad** or **response.** EMTs should recognize Cushing's triad as a clear but late sign of increasing intracranial pressure.

Increases in intracranial pressure will cause alterations in the patient's level of consciousness. As the ICP rises, cerebral hypoxia and anaerobic metabolism increase, ultimately leading to unconsciousness with deficits in vital functions and finally brain death. Adequate cerebral perfusion (aerobic metabolism) must be maintained to keep the brain tissue viable.

If cerebral edema continues, or the cerebral hematoma continues to enlarge, the brain has nowhere to go except to herniate through the tentorium or the foramen magnum or both. As herniation occurs, one of two types of clinical pictures may be observed:

1. If a hematoma is centrally located, the brain stem is compressed from above. This condition is called **central herniation syndrome.**

2. If the brain stem is compressed from the side, the condition known as **lateral** or **uncal herniation syndrome** occurs.

The main difference between the syndromes is that with lateral or uncal herniation syndrome, cerebral compression and loss of vital functions occur in a random fashion. With central herniation syndrome, the areas of the brain critical for life are compressed in a more orderly or predictable fashion. As the brain stem is compressed

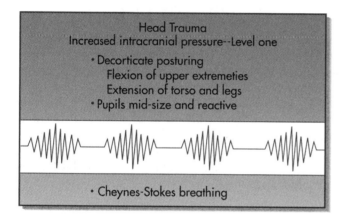

Figure 8-6 The pattern of change in breathing (Cheyne-Stokes respiration) is classic and indicates the changing PaO$_2$ and PaCO$_2$ levels in the patient.

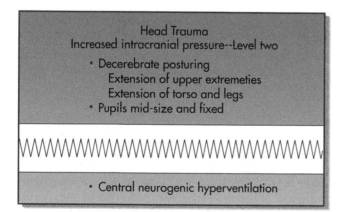

Figure 8-7 A fast, shallow respiratory pattern is associated with brain stem involvement and is called central neurogenic hyperventilation.

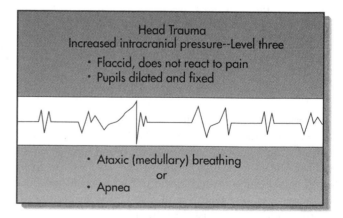

Figure 8-8 Medullary-type breathing has no pattern and is very erratic. Patients frequently become apneic at this stage.

and herniation continues, lower and lower areas of the brain stem are affected. The respiratory, pupillary, and motor patterns change with progressive brain stem compression, and these changes provide clues to the level of brain tissue involvement. As tissue damage continues into lower areas of the brain stem, chances of full recovery or survival decrease.

Three different levels or stages have been identified with increasing intracranial pressure and increasing brain stem involvement. These three levels are associated with characteristic signs and symptoms, such as changes in vital signs, pupil reaction, and response to stimuli.

LEVEL ONE ICP

As the ICP increases and the cerebral cortex and upper brain stem become involved, the blood pressure rises and the pulse rate slows. Pupils at this time may be constricted but still remain reactive. A recognizable, abnormal respiratory pattern appears: the patient may go from slow, shallow breaths to rapid, deep ventilation; then back to slow, shallow respirations followed by a period of apnea; then repeat the pattern. This type of respiratory pattern is called **Cheyne-Stokes respiration** and occurs in response to decreasing PaO_2 levels and increasing $PaCO_2$ levels (Figure 8-6).

The level one ICP patient will initially try to localize and remove painful stimuli. Later, the patient will only withdraw from painful stimuli. As the ICP continues to increase, the patient will show signs of **decorticate posturing** (flexion of the upper extremities with the lower extremities rigid and extended). This stage of cerebral compression is usually reversible with prompt surgical intervention to remove the compressing forces. The need for hyperventilation with high oxygen concentrations and rapid transportation to reduce the ICP is clearly indicated.

LEVEL TWO ICP

As more of the brain stem becomes involved, the patient's blood pressure continues to rise with a decreasing pulse rate. The patient's pupils may become fixed at 3 to 5 mm in size and may not react or will react sluggishly to light. An abnormal respiratory pattern continues. Often, these patients have **central neurogenic hyperventilation**—a very fast, shallow, panting respiratory pattern (Figure 8-7).

When a painful stimulus is applied to a level two ICP patient, the patient may exhibit **decerebrate posturing** (extension of the extremities). Few patients who reach this stage can be expected to recover with normal cerebral function.

LEVEL THREE ICP

As the lower portion of the brain stem is compressed, one or both pupils may become dilated and fixed. A "blown" pupil will usually be on the same side of the brain as the hematoma or swelling that is causing the herniation. The crossover of the nervous system, which creates the well-known effect that the right side of the brain controls the left side of the body and vice versa, occurs at the level of the spinal cord. *Structures innervated by cranial nerves produce signs on the same side of the body as the hematoma or swelling. Structures that are innervated by spinal nerves will show signs on the opposite side of the body as that of the injury.* It is important to note which pupil dilated first, as this information often helps determine which side of the brain has the hematoma. Ventilation may become **ataxic** (erratic breathing with no rhythm) or **medullary** or absent (apneic) at level three (Figure 8-8).

A patient with level three ICP will have no response to painful stimuli and will become flaccid as the medulla becomes involved. The patient's blood pressure will drop, and the pulse will become rapid and irregular.

It is important to recognize the developing signs and symptoms of each level of increased ICP and to react to them rapidly. Any combination of these levels is possible. Although central and uncal herniation syndromes are two distinct and well-recognized syndromes, in the seriously traumatized head injury patient, an overlap of the two syndromes is often seen. Symptoms may not occur with precise definition as the compression involves more of the brain stem.

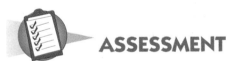

ASSESSMENT

Assessment of the head injury patient includes a number of considerations. As with all trauma patients, ventilation and cardiac functions should be evaluated, while being alert for any special signs indicating head injury.

INITIAL ASSESSMENT
Breathing

The first step is the evaluation of the patient's airway and breathing. Any deficiencies in these areas must be corrected immediately.

Head injuries produce several types of abnormal breathing patterns. An acute rise in intracranial pressure causes a slowing of the patient's breathing rate. As the intracranial pressure continues to rise, the patient's ventilation rate will become more rapid and change in pattern. If not corrected, breathing will deteriorate in both rate and pattern until it finally stops. The respirations of a head injury patient will often be noisy. In the patient with multiple injuries, chest trauma may complicate the EMT's ability to accurately assess breathing. *All head trauma patients must be suspected of having cervical spine involvement* and be managed accordingly. Cervical spine injury may also produce respiratory compromise or arrest and cause difficulties with proper airway management.

Blood Pressure

An elevated blood pressure in a head injury patient without a therapeutic explanation indicates a rise in intracranial pressure. As the intracranial pressure increases, the systolic blood pressure will also rise with a widening of the pulse pressure.

Box 8-1   AVPU

A—patient is Alert
V—patient responds to Verbal stimulus
P—patient responds to Painful stimulus
U—patient is Unresponsive

 Table 8-1 The Glasgow Coma Scale

Eye Opening	Points
Spontaneous eye opening	4
Eye opening on command	3
Eye opening to painful stimulus	2
No eye opening	1
Best Motor Response	
Follows command	6
Localizes painful stimuli	5
Withdrawal to pain	4
Responds with abnormal flexion to painful stimuli (decorticate)	3
Responds with abnormal extension to pain (decerebrate)	2
Gives no motor response	1
Best Verbal Response	
Answers appropriately (oriented)	5
Gives confused answers	4
Inappropriate response	3
Makes unintelligible noises	2
Makes no verbal response	1
Total	

Note: Lowest possible score = 3; highest possible score = 15.

Hypotension resulting directly from head trauma is a rare and terminal event, except in infants who have a large skull and relatively small blood volumes. Infants with significant head injury can become hypotensive from intracranial bleeding. On the other hand, hypotension is frequently found in children and adults who also have head trauma. Look for bleeding or injuries elsewhere to explain the hypotension.

Pulse

Changes in the patient's pulse rate may also be related to increasing intracranial pressure. Elevation of the ICP may produce a slow or bradycardic pulse rate. Bradycardia accompanying hypertension and a change in respiratory pattern suggest a rapidly expanding hematoma and/or herniation (Cushing's triad).

A rapid or tachycardic pulse rate is a grave sign unless it is due to a cause other than head injury, such as hemorrhage elsewhere. Continued elevation of intracranial pressure can result in a tachycardia, which is a late, preterminal event.

Neurologic Examination

The head trauma patient's level of consciousness and a measure of how it is changing over time are the most valuable observations in the head trauma patient. Level of consciousness is measured by use of the acronym **AVPU** (Box 8-1) in the initial assessment and use of the **Glasgow Coma Scale** in the focused assessment. The Glasgow Coma Scale is also used to calculate the trauma score (Table 8-1).

Pupils should be checked using the PEARRL question: **p**upils **e**qual **a**nd **r**ound, **r**eactive to **l**ight? Motor and sensory checks in each extremity are keys to identifying a deficit on only one side of the body (hemiparesis or hemiparalysis), which is an indication of brain damage. In contrast, spinal cord injury usually produces defects on both sides of the body.

Head and Spinal Examination

A physical examination of the head should be done to reveal hidden trauma to the skull or scalp. As stated in the section on neurologic examination, the pupils should be checked. Any fluid escaping from the ears and nose should be examined to see if it contains CSF. This examination can be done rapidly by soaking up a small amount of the drainage onto a clean gauze pad or other light-colored material. If CSF is present, it will appear on the material as a lighter colored ring (a "halo") surrounding the darker center formed by red blood cells that are present.

Any trauma sustained by a patient to the areas above the clavicles suggests cervical spine injury. The patient should be properly immobilized if he or she has any of the following:

- mechanism of injury suggesting violent action to the spine
- any severe blunt head injury
- any trauma resulting in a loss of consciousness or a marked altered level of consciousness
- specific signs of neurologic deficit (motor/sensory)

ONGOING ASSESSMENTS

The initial assessment provides findings that are used as reference points for ongoing assessments. Repeating the elements of the neurologic examination and accurately recording the findings are essential in determining whether a head trauma patient is deteriorating or improving. Several points should be considered:

1. Vital signs can indicate the level of brain stem function and involvement.
2. Drugs, including alcohol, can alter the level of consciousness and cloud significant signs and symptoms in the trauma patient; their presence may mimic signs of head injury.
3. Alterations in the patient's ventilation may also be caused by other injuries, untreated hypovolemia, or metabolic abnormalities.
4. Hypotension as a result of a closed head injury is a rare and terminal sign; other causes of hypotension should be sought and when found, should be treated.
5. Hypertension accompanying tachycardia in the head trauma patient is a preterminal finding.
6. Repeat examinations should be done at regular intervals and the findings recorded accurately. Watch for trends such as vital sign changes or level of consciousness changes that occur on a progressive basis.

SPECIFIC HEAD TRAUMA CONDITIONS

A skull fracture itself does not lead to morbidity and mortality following head injury. Rather, damage to the underlying structures causes problems for the patient, either with or without skull fracture.

CEREBRAL CONCUSSION

A **cerebral concussion** can be thought of as a "shaking up" of the brain. Traumatic, temporary loss of consciousness with associated memory deficit and without underlying brain injury are classic signs and symptoms of a cerebral concussion. Memory deficits include the inability to remember events before the injury (retrograde amnesia) or events after the injury (anterograde amnesia). More commonly, head trauma patients experience concussions with retrograde amnesia. Short-term memory loss generally produces anxiety and may include repetition of questions or seemingly unimportant statements by the patient. A major cause of this type of behavior is frontal lobe brain injury. These patients may also become very combative. Other symptoms and signs consistent with concussion after head trauma include headache, nausea, vomiting, and dizziness.

Concussions are generally associated with only transitory deficits and no identifiable lasting brain injury. Some patients, however, complain of headaches, dizziness, and difficulty concentrating for days or weeks after the traumatic event. This persistence of concussion symptoms is called post-concussion syndrome.

CEREBRAL CONTUSION

When severe acceleration or deceleration forces are applied to the head, the brain is driven into or over the sharp bony outcroppings within the cranial vault. This motion can produce a **cerebral contusion,** or soft tissue damage to the brain. Depending on the location of the contusion, the neurologic deficit may or may not be evident as focal neurologic changes. Focal neurologic findings usually help localize the injury near the site of the blow to the head **(coup)** or to the opposite hemisphere **(contrecoup injury to the brain).** Because the occiput (back) is a frequent site of impact in head injury patients, frontal and temporal lobes are common sites of contrecoup-type contusions. A blow to the occiput area of the skull causes the brain to shift forward within the cranial vault until it strikes the frontal or temporal portion of the skull, causing tissue damage to the frontal or temporal lobe. When a large area of brain tissue is contused, a significant increase in intracranial pressure can occur due to swelling of the contused area.

With contusion of the brain, the period of unconsciousness generally lasts from 5 minutes up to an hour or more. Retrograde or anterograde amnesia may also be associated with cerebral contusions. These signs are caused by impact on the reticular activating system. Persistent vomiting may occur with cerebral contusions as well. Those patients who are unconscious for longer than 5 minutes or who have more than one episode of unconsciousness are usually admitted to the hospital for a period of observation. *Documentation of the patient's level of consciousness, loss of consciousness, neurologic status, and memory deficits at the scene and en route to the hospital are very important parts of the prehospital patient care record.*

CEREBRAL LACERATION

A laceration of the brain (**cerebral laceration**) is much more severe, and because the brain itself has been directly damaged, it has more lasting and permanent complications than a cerebral concussion or contusion. Signs and symptoms differ depending on the part of the brain involved. Cerebral laceration is most often associated with major hemorrhage, mass effect, and unresponsiveness. This injury is severe and life threatening.

SKULL FRACTURE

When the head strikes or is struck by an object, the skull may be deformed at the site of impact, resulting in a **skull fracture.** Eighty percent of all skull fractures are linear and not depressed. These cannot be identified without

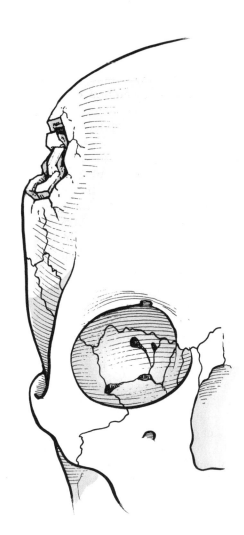

Figure 8-9 A depressed skull fracture may force particles of bone into the brain tissue.

X ray. If the impact force is powerful enough, the area may be depressed and bony fragments may be driven into the brain tissue (Figure 8-9).

Skull fractures may be small and difficult to diagnose even with the use of radiographs. The EMT must suspect skull fractures in head trauma patients when the mechanism of injury suggests it.

Basilar skull fractures are usually the result of the extension of linear fractures onto the floor (base) of the cranial vault. Blood or CSF from the ears or nose should lead the EMT to suspect a basilar skull fracture. Bleeding caused by basilar skull fractures often presents a dramatic appearance within hours of injury. Blood can travel into the periorbital subcutaneous tissue, producing the characteristic **"raccoon eyes"** (distinct ecchymotic area around each eye, limited by the orbital margins). Occipital basilar skull fractures bleed into the subcutaneous tissue behind the ear, producing **Battle's sign** (distinct ecchymotic coloration behind the ear). These two findings are not usually seen immediately after injury. A patient with these types of ecchymotic findings immediately following an injury must be suspected of having old injuries.

High-velocity impacts, such as those associated with gunshot wounds, often perforate the skull. The skull may be without deformity except locally at the entrance site of the missile. The cavitation forces are contained within the hard cranial vault. The lack of expansion of the skull to attenuate this force can produce significant damage to the brain tissue. Occasionally, particularly after gunshot wounds, brain tissue may be found oozing out of the fracture site.

If there are no associated brain injuries, hematomas, subsequent infections, or CSF leaks, skull fractures in and of themselves present no danger to the patient. They may be diagnosed by radiographic exam, or they may be obvious if seen through scalp lacerations.

INTRACRANIAL HEMATOMA

Traumatic intracranial hematomas can produce such devastating neurologic consequences that they must be discussed, not for field diagnosis, but for general consideration in managing the head injury patient. An understanding of the essential facts about hematomas ensures that the EMT reports pertinent clinical information along with the history, and reinforces the need for delivering the patient to a facility capable of providing proper management.

There are three basic types of intracranial hematomas: (1) epidural, (2) subdural, and (3) intracerebral. Although these hematomas are described based upon their specific location, clinical differentiation is often impossible. The signs and symptoms for each of these hematomas have significant overlap, and a definitive diagnosis can often be made only with a computed tomography (CT) scan.

Epidural Hematoma

Epidural hematomas represent about 2% of head injuries that result in hospitalization. They almost always occur from a tear and bleeding from the middle meningeal artery. About 20% of epidural hematoma patients will die (this is true even when the problem is recognized and treated; the mortality rate is even greater when the condition goes unrecognized).

Bleeding occurs when the blood vessels between the dura and the skull are torn. Epidural hematomas are usually produced by low-velocity blows to the head (such as those that occur in fist fights or when hit by a baseball), which result in contrecoup arterial tears and lacerations as the dura is pulled away from the skull by deceleration. Such injuries are often associated with skull fractures (Figure 8-10).

The patient with an epidural hematoma may, after being unconscious, return to consciousness and then—after a period of minutes or hours—lapse back into unconsciousness. Approximately 20% of these patients never regain consciousness again. The intervening period of consciousness is called the **lucid interval.**

An epidural hematoma can create a rapid increase in intracranial pressure. Signs and symptoms include the following:

- loss of consciousness, followed by a lucid interval
- secondary depression of consciousness
- developing hemiparesis on the opposite side of impact
- dilated and fixed pupil common on the side of impact

During the lucid period, the patient may complain of a headache and be sleepy.

Prehospital management involves recognizing that a head injury has occurred and keeping a close watch on the level of consciousness and breathing pattern. This injury requires rapid transportation for surgical intervention. If treated early, prognosis is excellent because underlying brain injury is usually not serious.

Subdural Hematoma

Subdural hematomas differ from epidural hematomas in location, cause, and prognosis. They can be divided into three types: acute, subacute, and chronic. Subdural hematomas usually occur as a result of venous bleeding that takes place between the dura mater and the brain and is frequently associated with damage to the underlying brain tissue. Patients with subdural hematomas may have an early loss of consciousness and focal motor signs immediately following trauma, or they

may not show symptoms until hours, days, or months later.

Acute subdural hematomas display their signs and symptoms within the first 72 hours after onset. They tend to be the result of high-velocity impacts, such as the impacts that occur in motor vehicle collisions. Even when

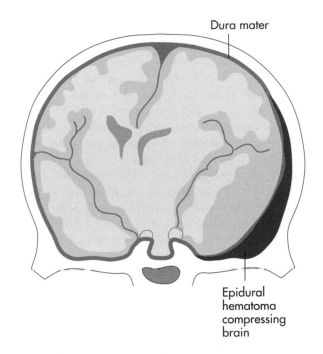

Dura mater

Epidural hematoma compressing brain

A

Dura mater

Subdural hematoma

B

Figure 8-10 A, Epidural hematoma. B, Subdural hematoma.

the problem is recognized early and surgically treated (draining excess fluid from within the cranial vault), the mortality rate remains between 50% to 60%.

Subacute subdural hematomas display signs and symptoms between 3 and 21 days after the insult has occurred. These hematomas also result from high-velocity type injuries but develop more slowly than acute hematomas. This slow development reflects less brain tissue involvement and damage with a better prognosis. The mortality rate for subacute hematomas is approximately 25%.

Chronic subdural hematomas may present weeks or months after a seemingly minor head injury. The smaller vessels that bridge the subdural spaces are torn and bleed more slowly. Because of the slowness in the onset of signs and symptoms, chronic subdural hematomas may go unnoticed. Although slow in onset, these types of hematomas nevertheless cause an increase in intracranial pressure, pressure on the brain tissue, and decreased cerebral perfusion. The mortality rate for chronic subdural hematomas is almost as high as that for acute subdural hematomas, approximately 50%.

The EMT should suspect a possible subdural hematoma postincident, regardless of the time lapse, if the patient exhibits any of the following signs or symptoms at the present time or any time since the injury:

- changes in level of consciousness, including unconsciousness or coma
- confusion or disorientation
- persistent or recurring headache
- blurred vision, double vision, or other affected vision
- nausea or vomiting
- personality changes, including changes in temperament or "out-of-character" behavior
- hemiparesis, hemianesthesia, or hemiparalysis
- slurring or other types of speech impediment

Prehospital management may be called for in a patient who is displaying strange behavior with no rational explanation for his or her actions. While taking the patient's past pertinent history, the EMT may find that the patient suffered a minor head injury in the past. This event may have taken place days, weeks, or even months ago. The patient may not have gone to the emergency department for treatment, or if he or she did, the physical and radiographic examinations may have been normal upon discharge.

Intracerebral Hematoma

Lacerations or tearing of blood vessels within the brain tissue itself can also produce hemorrhage and hematoma formation. This group of hematomas is referred to as **intracerebral hematomas.**

Intracerebral hematomas can occur with penetrating head trauma or when sudden decelerating head injuries drag the brain across the bony outcroppings within the cranial vault area, causing injury to the brain tissue itself.

Seizure activity is one commonly seen sign with this type of head injury. Focal signs and symptoms of intracerebral hematomas depend on the area of the brain involved.

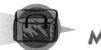 **MANAGEMENT**

Prehospital management of any patient with a suspected head injury should focus on maintaining cerebral perfusion (adequate oxygen and cerebral blood flow). Cerebral perfusion can be accomplished by maintaining the patient's blood pressure and providing oxygen to the hypoperfused cells through the use of hyperoxygenation (high-flow oxygen). The patient's spine must also be protected and the patient rapidly transported to a hospital that is capable of providing definitive treatment.

As with any patient, the airway must have first priority. The head trauma patient may require the insertion of an endotracheal tube to maintain and protect the airway. Because it must be assumed that the patient also has a cervical spine injury, in-line stabilization must be maintained while establishing and maintaining the airway. Intravenous lidocaine (1 mg/kg) has been administered immediately prior to intubation based on animal research showing that lidocaine can blunt the increase in ICP that occurs during the act of intubation.

The head injury patient is also likely to vomit. Suction equipment, including large bore catheters such as the tonsil-tip, should be readily available. The patient must be well secured to a long backboard in case it becomes necessary to quickly turn the patient onto his or her side to prevent aspiration.

Once the head and neck are manually stabilized, the airway controlled, and adequate ventilation established, bleeding can then be controlled and circulation reestablished. Bleeding scalp vessels are easily compressed by gentle, continuous direct pressure. If there is obvious deformity or palpable bony defect or instability, the bleeding can be controlled by compressing the area around the wound while taking care to press against a stable area of the skull. Bleeding from the patient's nose or ears presents still another challenge. While the blood loss needs to be controlled, complete tamponade of the blood flow may result in increased intracranial pressure and cause further brain tissue damage. These areas should be covered with a clean dressing but allowed to "leak" slightly. Hypovolemic shock may occur as a result of gross bleeding since the face and scalp are highly vascular in nature.

If the adult head trauma patient has not experienced excessive bleeding from the face, scalp, or other injuries, shock is rarely due to brain injury unless it is the terminal event. In children, because of their normal lower blood volume, hypotension can be more threatening than in the adult.

The multiply injured patient with head trauma who is in shock should be managed like any other trauma patient in shock. Management should include control of any major hemorrhage, use of the pneumatic antishock garment (PASG) as indicated, and body heat retention. The patient may need fluid resuscitation, which is another reason for rapid transportation to the closest appropriate hospital or for interception with an advanced life support (ALS) unit capable of providing it. The injured brain must be perfused with oxygenated blood under adequate pressure to survive. However, the patient with an isolated head injury needs only maintenance fluids to help minimize cerebral edema. An intravenous line using lactated Ringer's or normal saline (local protocol will dictate which to use) should be initiated with the head trauma patient. If the vital signs are adequate, the intravenous line should be maintained at a maintenance rate of no more than 125 cubic centimeters (cc) per hour and monitored closely to prevent overhydration. If signs of hypovolemic shock appear, the intravenous flow can be adjusted to help maintain pressure.

Surgery to decrease intracranial pressure cannot be performed in the field. The method that can be used to help decrease intracranial pressure and brain stem herniation is hyperventilation. It is well documented that hypoxia and hypercarbia will aggravate or increase brain tissue swelling. The use of 100% oxygen will cause cerebral vasoconstriction and subsequently decrease the intracranial pressure, which will improve cerebral oxygenation. In the deteriorating head injury patient with signs of herniation, a $PaCO_2$ of 30 to 35 mm Hg or lower is desirable. This can be achieved by increasing the patient's oxygen concentration and rate of ventilation from the normal 12 to 16 breaths per minute to a rate of 20 to 24 breaths per minute. It is also essential for the EMT to allow adequate time between each assisted inhalation for exhalation to occur. Failure to allow for adequate exhalation will cause the patient to retain CO_2, thus causing increased intracranial pressure.

A variety of medications such as diuretics (mannitol, Lasix®, etc.) can be used to draw fluid from the interstitial and intracellular spaces in the head injured patient who is showing signs of increased intracranial pressure. Reduction in fluid can decrease cerebral edema and thus decrease the intracranial pressure. These diuretic-type drugs do work well, but like hyperventilation, they are only temporary agents. While causing a decrease in cerebral edema, circulating blood volume, and intracranial pressure, they may also allow for a more rapid expansion of an intracranial hematoma. Because of this potential danger, the use of diuretics and a wide range of other medications should be limited to in-hospital use with the head trauma patient; they should not be administered in the prehospital setting.

Treatment of head injured patients is focused on maintaining cerebral perfusion and oxygenation. Treatment efforts are directed at maintaining the patient's blood pressure, providing supplemental oxygen, and initiating care for increased intracranial pressure when clinical signs are present.

TRANSPORTATION

Not only is it important in prehospital management to transport the suspected head injury patient to the appropriate facility, the EMT must also notify and alert the facility about the patient's type of injury. An example of a radio transmission to alert the receiving facility of a head injury patient might go like this:

Base, this is unit 224, we are transporting to your facility a 26-year-old male patient who was the driver of a motor vehicle involved in a high-speed, sudden deceleration incident. The patient was unrestrained during the incident and was unconscious at the scene upon our arrival. The patient's vital signs are as follows: B/P 124/80 initially, last pressure 138/80; pulse 62 and regular; respirations 38, irregular and shallow; pupils unequal with the right being larger than the left and slow to react to light. The patient's Glasgow Coma Scale is 5 with a score of eyes—1, motor—3, and verbal—1. The patient also responds with flexion on his right side and does not move his left side. The patient is intubated and ventilations are being assisted at a rate of 30 times per minute with a bag-valve device and 100% oxygen. The patient is also secured to a long backboard with head and neck immobilization. We have an ETA to your location of 7 minutes.

This radio traffic should alert the receiving facility that a potential head injury patient is en route, and preparations should be initiated for his arrival and subsequent treatment.

It must be stressed how important it is for the EMT to maintain an accurate record of the suspected head injury patient's vital signs and examinations performed, both at the scene and during transport. Information such as which pupil was "blown" first or any changes in the patient's condition can be key information and helpful in determination of the course of treatment necessary.

The suspected head injury patient should be transported with the head elevated whenever possible to help reduce brain tissue swelling. Elevating the head can be done while still maintaining adequate spinal immobilization by simply elevating the head end of the long backboard. Time is of the essence for the head trauma patient, but so is transporting the patient safely and rapidly to a facility that is capable of providing adequate neurologic care.

• Summary •

1. The brain is encased and thus confined within the rigid skull. Any head injury that causes swelling or bleeding inside the skull results in compression of the brain, which can lead to permanent neurologic damage or death.

2. The assessment of the patient who has sustained head trauma begins with his or her level of consciousness. Any decrease in the level of consciousness should lead the EMT to suspect intracranial injury as the cause and take appropriate steps to intervene.

3. Trauma to the head produces a wide spectrum of injury ranging from mild concussion to life-threatening hemorrhage inside the skull. The significance of visible external injury to the face and scalp as well as skull fractures relate to the potential for injury to the underlying brain.

4. Optimum field management of the head injury patient requires the prompt evaluation of the degree of damage and the areas involved, stabilization of the head and neck, control of the airway, delivery of high concentrations of oxygen for cerebral oxygenation ($FiO_2 = 0.85-1.0$), and hyperventilation at a rate of 20 to 24 breaths per minute to help reduce cerebral swelling and intracranial pressure when clinical signs are present. Treatment for signs and symptoms of shock should be provided as necessary to keep the brain adequately perfused.

5. Transportation should be done rapidly, with the patient in a head elevated position whenever possible, to the closest facility capable of providing adequate neurologic care.

Scenario Solution

You ask your partner to get the scoop stretcher and a cervical collar and to call for more rescuers to help you extricate the patient from the basement. You then turn your attention to the patient. You note he is awake, his airway is clear, and breathing and circulation seem okay. Your first priority is to immobilize his neck and proceed with the assessment.

As you begin your survey, the patient moans and asks you to leave him alone. His speech is slurred, and you can smell alcohol on his breath. He does answer your questions, and he follows commands. The Glasgow Coma Scale (GCS) is 15. His airway is intact, and he has a good strong pulse. You apply the cervical collar and with appropriate help and precautions place him on the scoop stretcher to get him upstairs. Once in the ambulance, you discover that in addition to the scalp laceration, he also has a scalp hematoma over the occiput. His neurologic examination seems unremarkable other than the findings of alcohol intoxication. The head-to-toe examination is also not revealing. You tell you partner that he can drive to the hospital in a non-emergency mode. At this time you consider a possible concussion with alcohol intoxication as well.

While en route to the hospital, you reexamine your patient and note that he now seems more lethargic than he did before. He is much slower to answer your questions and is not making much sense. The GCS is 13. Although it could be the effect of the alcohol becoming more apparent, you prepare yourself and your equipment in case intervention is necessary. As a precaution, you start an IV line and check the patient's glucose, which is normal. The patient suddenly has a seizure. With that you decide to intubate the patient and hyperventilate him. Shortly after leaving the patient at the hospital, you call back to find out what happened and learn that the patient had a brain contusion on the CT scan and is currently being monitored in the ICU.

Review Questions

Answers provided on page 333.

1 A 23-year-old patient is assaulted and struck about the head. He thinks he was unconscious for a few minutes. He has a headache and feels dizzy and nauseated. His physical exam reveals some facial contusions; the neurologic exam is unremarkable with a GCS of 15. Which of the following is the most likely diagnosis?

A cerebral concussion
B cerebral contusion
C epidural hematoma
D subdural hematoma

2 A 45-year-old patient is involved in an automobile accident. She is found unresponsive with a contusion over her forehead. Her pupils are equal and reactive. She moans in response to a painful stimulus, does not open her eyes, and tries to push the examiner's hand away. What is the GCS of this patient?

A 4
B 6
C 8
D 10

3 What is Cushing's triad?
   A increased pulse, decreased blood pressure, distended neck veins
   B decreased pulse, elevated blood pressure, altered respiratory pattern
   C decreased blood sugar, altered mental status, equal pupils
   D odor of alcohol, slurred speech, ataxic gait

4 A 17-year-old patient strikes her head while playing on a trampoline. She is found unconscious with a dilated right pupil. Which of the following is the most likely injury?
   A right-sided skull fracture
   B left-sided cerebral concussion
   C right-sided intracranial hematoma
   D left-sided intracranial hematoma

5 A 55-year-old patient at a bar is beaten about the head and face. He is intoxicated. There was no loss of consciousness, and the GCS is 15. You note a dilated right pupil. The most likely cause is which of the following?
   A right-sided intracranial hematoma
   B left-sided intracranial hematoma
   C right-sided ocular contusion
   D left-sided concussion

6 Hyperventilation is indicated in which of the following scenarios?
   A 17-year-old football player who was knocked out during a play and is found confused and disoriented
   B 34-year-old found in an alley behind a bar with alcohol odor on the breath, scalp hematoma, and slurred speech
   C 56-year-old drinking at home fell down stairs, is lethargic, and cannot move arms or legs
   D 78-year-old found in bathroom with forehead contusion, unconscious with left hemiparesis and right dilated pupil

CHAPTER OBJECTIVES

CHAPTER 9

Spinal Trauma

At the completion of this course the student will be able to:

- Describe the incidence, morbidity, and mortality of spinal injuries in the trauma patient.

- List in order of frequency, four major activities producing spinal trauma in adults.

- List in order of frequency, three major activities producing spinal trauma in pediatric patients.

- List at least four specific mechanisms that can cause spinal injuries.

- Predict spinal injuries based on mechanism of injury.

- Define neurologic spinal shock.

- Describe the pathophysiology of neurologic spinal shock.

- Demonstrate a clear understanding that three indications of spinal trauma must be assessed: (1) mechanism of injury, (2) the presence of other injury due to violent force, (3) specific signs of spinal trauma.

- Discuss the assessment findings associated with spinal injuries.

- Differentiate between spinal injuries based on the assessment and clinical criteria.

- List at least four specific signs or symptoms of spinal trauma.

- Demonstrate a clear understanding that spinal trauma may be asymptomatic, occult, and without neurologic deficits.

- Identify the major goal of spinal trauma management.

Scenario

You respond to a "man down" call. Upon arrival at the scene, you find a male about 30 years old at the bottom of a 15-foot ladder. The scene is safe and there are no overhead hazards. Your initial assessment as you approach the patient reveals an unconscious male who has a large bump on his forehead and pale skin. His airway is open, and his breathing is somewhat shallow. Both radial and carotid pulses are present. There are no obvious signs of external blood loss. His skin is pale, cool, and clammy.

- What should your next action be?
- Is this a priority patient?
- Does this patient require full spinal immobilization?

Spinal trauma, if not recognized and properly managed in the field, can result in irreparable damage and leave the patient paralyzed for life. Some patients suffer immediate spinal cord (cord) damage as a result of an accident. Others suffer an injury to the spinal column that does not initially damage the cord; cord damage may result later with movement of the spine. Because the central nervous system is incapable of regeneration, a severed cord cannot be repaired. The consequences of moving a patient with a missed spinal injury, or allowing the patient to move, can be devastating. Failure to properly immobilize a fractured spine, for example, can produce a much worse outcome than failing to properly immobilize a fractured femur.

Spinal cord injury can have profound effects on human physiology, lifestyle, and financial circumstances. Human physiology is affected because the use of extremities or other areas is severely limited as a result of nerve damage. Lifestyle is affected because spinal cord injury usually results in changes to daily activity levels as well as independence. Financial circumstances are also altered with spinal cord injury. A patient with this injury requires both acute care and long-term care. The lifetime cost of this care is estimated to be approximately $1.25 million for a permanent spinal cord injury.

About 15,000 to 20,000 spinal cord injuries occur annually. Spinal injury can occur at any age; however, it commonly occurs in patients 16 to 35 years old, since this age group is involved in the most violent and high-risk activities. The largest number of spinal trauma patients fall into the group between 16 and 20 years of age. The second largest group is patients between 21 and 25 years of age, and the third largest group is between 26 and 35 years of age. Common causes are motor vehicle crashes (MVCs) (48%), falls (21%), penetrating injuries (15%), sports injuries (14%), and other injuries (2%).

Sudden violent forces acting on the body can move the spine beyond its normal range of motion by either impacting on the head or neck or by driving the torso out from under the head. Four concepts help make the possible effect on the spine clearer when evaluating the potential of injury:

1. The head is like a bowling ball perched on top of the neck, and its mass often moves in different directions from the torso, resulting in strong forces being applied to the neck (cervical spine and/or spinal cord).
2. Objects in motion tend to stay in motion, and objects at rest tend to stay at rest.
3. Sudden or violent movement of the upper legs displaces the pelvis, resulting in forceful movement of the lower spine. Due to the weight and inertia of the head and torso, force in an opposite (contra) direction is applied to the upper spine.
4. Lack of neurologic deficit does not rule out bone or ligament injury to the spine or conditions that have stressed the spinal cord to the limit of its tolerance.

Forty percent of trauma patients with neurologic deficit will have a temporary or permanent spinal cord injury. The remaining group's neurologic deficit will be due to either a local injury or extremity injury not associated with spinal cord injury. Any patient who has sustained an injury indicative of spinal loading or stretching, significant injury above the clavicles, significant blunt trauma to the torso, a head injury resulting in an altered level of consciousness, or a major fall must be presumed to have a potential spine injury. Fifteen percent of patients sustaining trauma above the clavicles will have an actual spine injury. Any such patient must be immobilized in a neutral in-line position (unless contraindicated) before he or she is moved even slightly.

Many spinal cord injuries are due to improper handling. Therefore, due to the potential consequences of a mishandled spinal column or spinal cord injury, the EMT must err on the side of caution when the mechanism of injury suggests a possible spinal cord injury. Findings negative to a spinal cord injury discovered during an examination are not sufficient cause to completely rule out the possibility. A patient who may have suffered spinal trauma should be fully assessed and protected.

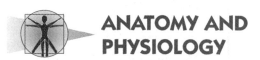

ANATOMY AND PHYSIOLOGY

VERTEBRAL ANATOMY

The **spinal column** is composed of 33 bones called **vertebrae** stacked one on top of the other. Except for the first (C1) and second (C2) vertebrae at the top of the spine and the fused sacral and coccygeal vertebrae at the lower spine, all of the vertebrae are nearly alike in form, structure, and motion (Figure 9-1). The largest part of each vertebra is the anterior part called the **body.** Each vertebral body bears most of the weight of the vertebral column and torso superior to it. Two curved sides called the **neural arches** are formed by the pedicle and posteriorly by the lamina. The posterior part of the vertebra is a tail-like structure called the **spinous process.** In the lower five cervical vertebrae this posterior process points directly posterior, whereas in the thoracic and lumbar vertebra it points slightly downward in a caudad direction.

Most vertebrae also have similarly styled protuberances at each side near their anterior lateral margins, called **transverse processes.** The transverse and spinous processes serve as points for muscle attachment and are therefore fulcrums for movement. The neural arches and the posterior part of each vertebral body form a near-circular shape with an opening in the center. The spinal cord passes through this opening, called the **vertebral foramen** (spinal canal). The cord is protected somewhat from injury by the bony vertebrae surrounding it. Each

vertebral foramen lines up with that of the vertebrae above and the vertebrae below it to form the hollow spinal canal through which the spinal cord passes.

VERTEBRAL COLUMN

As previously mentioned, the individual vertebrae are stacked approximately one on top of the other in an S-like shape (Figure 9-2). This organization allows extensive multidirectional movement while imparting maximum strength. The spinal column is divided into five individual regions for reference. Beginning at the top of the spinal column and descending downward, these regions are the cervical, thoracic, lumbar, sacral, and coccygeal regions. Vertebrae are identified by the first letter of the region in which they are found and their sequence from the top of that region. The first cervical vertebra is called C1, the third thoracic vertebra T3, the fifth lumbar vertebra L5, and so on throughout the entire spinal column.

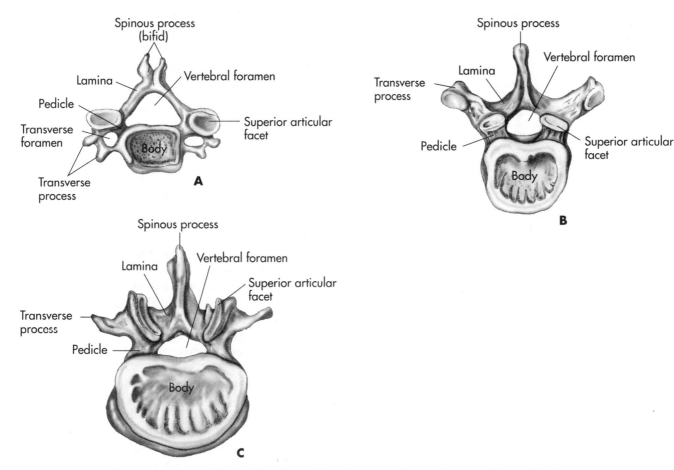

Figure 9-1 Except for the fused sacral and coccygeal vertebrae, each vertebra has the same parts as others. The body (anterior portion of each vertebra) gets larger and stronger as it must support more weight nearing the pelvis. A, Fifth cervical vertebra; B, thoracic vertebra; C, lumbar vertebra. (From Seeley, R.R.; Stephens, T.D.; and Tate, P. *Essentials of Anatomy and Physiology.* St. Louis: Mosby–Year Book, Inc., 1991.)

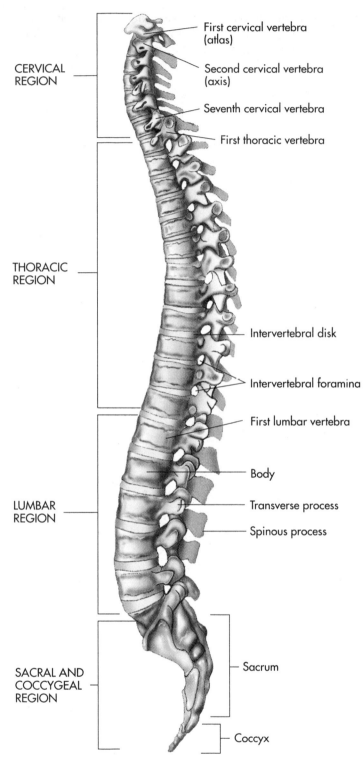

CERVICAL REGION

First cervical vertebra (atlas)

Second cervical vertebra (axis)

Seventh cervical vertebra

First thoracic vertebra

THORACIC REGION

Intervertebral disk

Intervertebral foramina

First lumbar vertebra

Body

LUMBAR REGION

Transverse process

Spinous process

SACRAL AND COCCYGEAL REGION

Sacrum

Coccyx

Figure 9-2 The vertebral column is not a straight rod, but a series of blocks that are stacked in such a manner that allows for several bends or curves. At each of the curves, the spine is more vulnerable to fractures, thus the origin of the term "breaking the S in a fall." (From Seeley, R.R.; Stephens, T.D.; and Tate, P. *Essentials of Anatomy and Physiology.* St. Louis: Mosby–Year Book, Inc., 1991.)

Located at the top end of the spinal column are the seven **cervical vertebrae** that support the head. The cervical region is quite flexible to allow total movement of the head. Next are twelve **thoracic vertebrae.** Each pair of ribs connects posteriorly to one of the thoracic vertebrae. Unlike the cervical spine, the thoracic spine is relatively rigid with very little movement. Below the thoracic vertebrae are the five **lumbar vertebrae** that are the most massive of all the vertebrae. The lumbar area is also quite flexible allowing movement in a number of directions. The five **sacral vertebrae** are fused, forming a single structure known as the **sacrum.** Last, the four **coccygeal vertebrae** are also fused, forming the **coccyx** (tailbone). Approximately 55% of spinal injuries occur in the cervical region, 15% in the thoracic region, 15% at the thoracolumbar junction, and 15% in the lumbosacral area.

Each vertebra supports increasing body weight as the vertebrae progress down the spinal column. Appropriately, the vertebrae from C3 to L5 become progressively larger to accommodate the increased workload (Figure 9-3).

Ligaments and muscles tether the spine from the base of the skull to the pelvis. These ligaments and muscles form a web that sheathes the entire bony part of the spinal column, holding it in normal alignment and allowing movement. If these ligaments and muscles are torn, excessive movement of one vertebra in relation to another occurs. This excessive movement may result in dislocation of the vertebrae, which can compromise the space inside the spinal canal and thus damage the spinal cord.

The anterior and posterior longitudinal ligaments connect the vertebral bodies anteriorly and inside the canal. Ligaments between the spinous processes provide support for flexion-extension movement, while those between the lamina provide support during lateral flexion (side bending).

The head balances on top of the spine, and the spine is supported by the pelvis (Figure 9-4). The skull perches on the ring-shaped first cervical vertebra (C1) referred to as the atlas. The axis, C2, is also basically ring shaped but has a spur called the odontoid process that protrudes like a tooth into the anterior arch of the atlas. The axis allows the head an approximately 180° range of rotation (Figure 9-5).

The human head weighs between 16 and 22 pounds, approximately the same weight as an average bowling ball. The weight and position of the head atop the thin neck, the forces that act upon the head, the small size of the supporting muscles, and the lack of ribs or other bones help make the cervical spine particularly susceptible to injury. At the level of C3, the spinal canal is very narrow and the cord is enlarged. At this point, the spinal cord occupies approximately 95% of the spinal canal (the spinal cord occupies approximately 65% of the spinal canal area at its end in the lumbar region), and there is only 3 mm of clearance between the cord and the canal wall. Even a minor dislocation at this point can produce compression of the spinal cord. The posterior neck muscles are very strong, permitting up to 60% of the range of flexion and 70% of the range of extension of the head without any stretching of the cord. However, when sudden violent acceleration, deceleration, or lateral force is applied to the patient's body, the significant weight of the "bowling ball" on the narrow cervical spine can amplify the effects of sudden movement.

The sacrum is the base of the spinal column, the platform upon which the spinal column rests. Between 70% and 80% of the body's total weight rests on the sacrum. It is important to note that the sacrum is both a part of the spinal column and the pelvic girdle, and it is joined to the rest of the pelvis by immovable joints.

SPINAL CORD ANATOMY

The spinal cord is continuous with the brain and starts from the base of the brain stem, passing through the **foramen magnum** (the hole at the base of the skull) and through each vertebra to the level of the second lumbar

vertebra. Blood is supplied to the spinal cord by the vertebral and spinal arteries. The spinal cord itself consists of gray matter and white matter. The white matter contains the anatomic spinal tracts. Spinal tracts are divided into two types. **Ascending nerve tracts** carry sensory impulses from body parts through the cord to the brain. Ascending nerve tracts can be further divided into tracts that carry the different sensations of pain and temperature; touch and pressure; and sensory impulses of motion, vibration, position, and light touch. **Descending nerve tracts** are responsible for carrying motor impulses from the brain through the cord to the body, and they control all muscle movement and muscle tone.

As the spinal cord continues to descend, pairs of nerves branch off from the cord at each vertebra and extend to the various parts of the body (Figure 9-6). There are 31 pairs of spinal nerves, and they are named according to the level from which they arise. Each nerve has two roots on each side. The **dorsal root** is for sensory impulses and the **ventral root** is for motor impulses. Neurologic stimuli pass between the brain and each part of the body through the cord and particular pairs of these

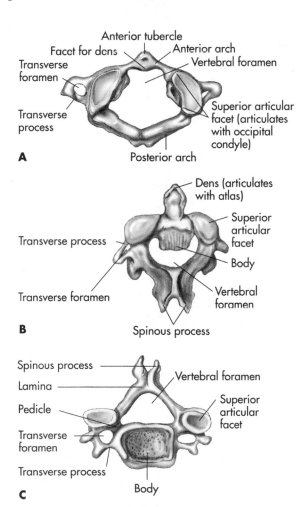

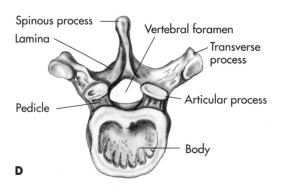

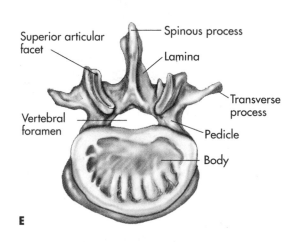

Figure 9-3 Weight bearing increases on the lower vertebral bodies, which are thicker and stronger to carry this load. (From Seeley, R.R.; Stephens, T.D.; and Tate, P. *Essentials of Anatomy and Physiology.* St. Louis: Mosby–Year Book, Inc., 1991.)

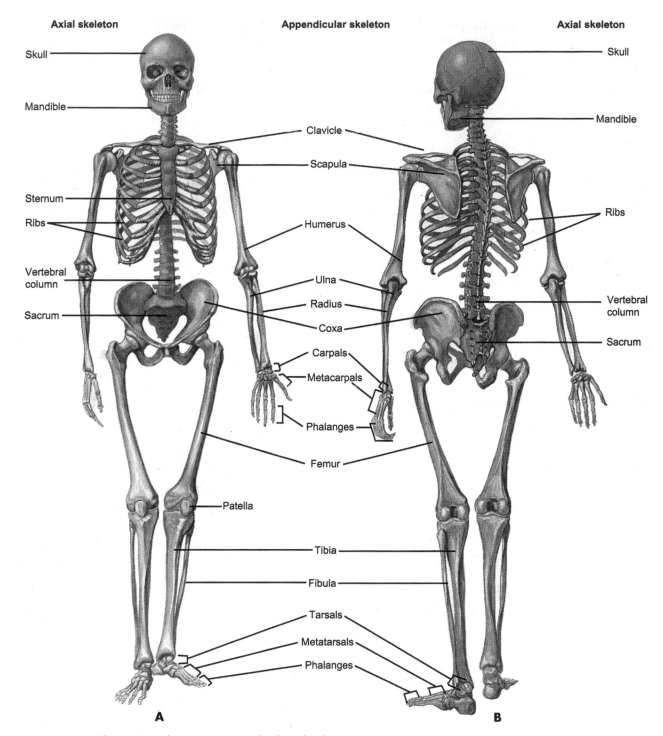

Axial skeleton

Skull

Mandible

Sternum

Ribs

Vertebral column

Sacrum

Appendicular skeleton

Clavicle

Scapula

Humerus

Ulna

Radius

Coxa

Carpals

Metacarpals

Phalanges

Femur

Patella

Tibia

Fibula

Tarsals

Metatarsals

Phalanges

Axial skeleton

Skull

Mandible

Ribs

Vertebral column

Sacrum

A

B

Figure 9-4 The spine is attached to the legs by attachments to the pelvis at the sacroiliac joints. The head is like a bowling ball that balances on top of the spine. (From Seeley, R.R.; Stephens, T.D.; and Tate, P. *Essentials of Anatomy and Physiology.* St. Louis: Mosby–Year Book, Inc., 1991.)

nerves. As they branch from the spinal cord, these nerves pass through a notch in the inferior lateral side of the vertebra, posterior to the vertebral body, called the **intervertebral foramen.** Cartilage-like **intervertebral discs** lie between the body of each vertebra and act as shock absorbers (Figure 9-7).

These nerve branches have multiple control functions and are represented by **dermatomes.** A dermatome is a specific body area through which a nerve impulse travels or controls. Collectively, dermatomes allow the body areas to be mapped out for each spinal nerve (Figure 9-8). Dermatomes can be used to help

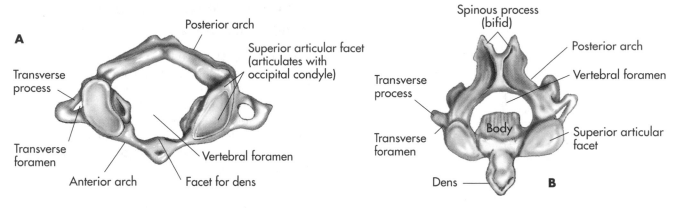

Figure 9-5 The first (A) and second (B) cervical vertebrae are shaped differently than the rest of the vertebrae of the spine. Their function is to both support the skull and to allow rotation and anterior-posterior motion of the head.

determine the level of a spinal cord injury. For example, in adults, the process of inhalation and exhalation requires both chest excursion and proper changes in the shape of the diaphragm. The diaphragm is innervated by the phrenic nerves, which branch from the nerves arising from the cord between the levels of C2 through C5. If the cord at one of these levels or the phrenic nerves are cut or otherwise disrupted, the patient will lose the ability to spontaneously breath. These patients will therefore need positive pressure–assisted or total ventilation.

The spinal cord is surrounded by cerebrospinal fluid (CSF) and is encased in a **dural sheath.** This dural sheath covers the brain and continues down to the second sacral vertebra, where there is a saclike reservoir called the **great cistern.** CSF produced by the brain passes around the cord and is absorbed in this cistern. CSF performs the same function for the cord as for the brain: it is an important cushion against injury during rapid and severe movement.

PATHOPHYSIOLOGY

MECHANISM OF INJURY

The bony spine can normally withstand forces of up to 1,000 foot-pounds of energy. High-speed travel and contact sports can routinely exert forces well in excess of this amount on the spine. Even in a low- to moderate-speed automobile collision, the body of an unrestrained 150-lb person can easily place 3,000 to 4,000 foot-pounds of force against the spine as the head is suddenly stopped by the windshield or roof. Similar force can occur when a motorcyclist is thrown over the front of the cycle or when a high-speed skier collides with a tree.

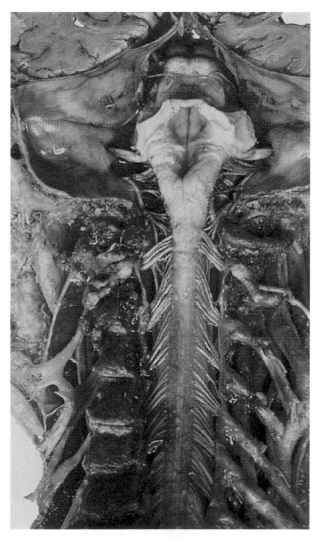

Figure 9-6 The spinal nerves branch from each side of the spinal cord to provide motor and sensory innervation to the torso and extremities. (From Thibodeau, G.A., and Patton, K.T. *Anatomy and Physiology.* 2nd ed. St. Louis: Mosby–Year Book, Inc., 1993.)

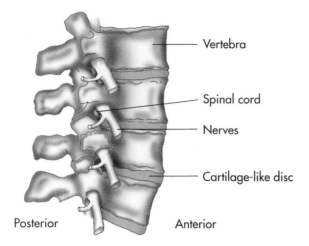

Figure 9-7 The cartilage between each vertebral body is called the intervertebral disc. These discs act as shock absorbers. If damaged, the cartilage may protrude into the spinal canal, compressing the cord or the nerves that come through the intervertebral foramina.

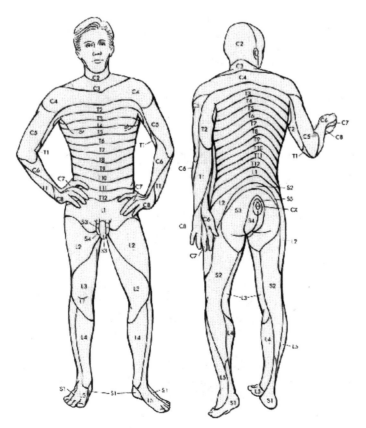

Figure 9-8 A dermatome map shows the relationship between areas of touch sensation on the skin and the spinal nerves that correspond to that area of sensation. Loss of sensation in that area may indicate injury to the spinal nerve.

Using Mechanism of Injury to Assess Spinal Cord Injury

Traditionally, EMTs have been taught that injury is based solely on the mechanism of injury and that spinal immobilization is required for any patient with a motion injury. This generalization has caused a lack of clear clinical guidelines for assessment of spine injuries. Currently, some EMS systems have instituted an *expanded assessment* format to determine the presence of a spinal injury. This expanded assessment still incorporates mechanism of injury as the foundation for determining the presence of a spinal cord injury. However, it also includes assessment of the motor and sensory function, presence of pain or tenderness, and patient reliability as predictors of spinal cord injury.

In most EMS runs a delay in the field to do an in-depth neurologic motor and sensory examination is not a useful expenditure of time. Rather the patient should be immobilized on a backboard and transported to the hospital where the examination can be accomplished by someone much more experienced than the EMT in an environment better suited to the patient. A complete neurologic examination may require an hour or more. The field is not the environment for this to take place. The expanded assessment systems have not received general medical approval. This type of study should take place only with local medical society approval of the experimental protocol and have close supervision by the medical director of the EMS service. The local institutional review board needs to review the protocol to see if an informed consent is required from the patient prior to institution of the study.

Three types of mechanisms of injury are used to assess spinal cord injury:

1. In a positive mechanism of injury, the forces exerted on the patient are highly suggestive of spinal cord injury. The EMT should assume that these patients have a spinal injury, and they should be managed accordingly. An example of a positive mechanism of injury is a high-speed motor vehicle crash.

2. In a negative mechanism of injury, the forces do not suggest the potential for spine injury. An example is a soft tissue injury to the hand from a knife. This would not indicate a need for spinal immobilization.

3. In an uncertain mechanism of injury, it is not clear whether the forces suggest spinal cord injury. Because of a lack of either a positive or negative mechanism of injury, a complete assessment and possible spinal immobilization are indicated. An example is a low-speed motor vehicle crash, e.g., "fender-bender" with no injuries, although in rare situations, even such collisions can produce bony trauma.

The major causes of spine injury in adults in order of frequency are:

1. automobile collisions
2. shallow-water diving accidents

3. motorcycle collisions
4. all other injuries and falls

The major causes of spinal trauma in pediatric patients are different. In order of frequency they are:

1. falls from heights (generally 2–3 times the patient's height)
2. falls from a tricycle or bicycle
3. being struck by a motor vehicle

Specific Mechanisms of Injury that Cause Spinal Trauma

The specific mechanisms of injury that cause spinal trauma are axial loading, excessive flexion (hyperextension), hyperrotation, sudden or excessive lateral bending, distraction, or a combination of any of these motions.

Axial loading can occur in several ways. Most commonly, this compression of the spine occurs when the head strikes an object and the weight of the still-moving body bears against the stopped head, such as when the head of an unrestrained occupant strikes the windshield or when the head strikes an object in a shallow-water diving accident.

Compression and axial loading also occur when the patient sustains a fall from a substantial height and lands in a standing position. This drives the weight of the head and thorax down against the lumbar spine, while the sacral spine remains stationary. Twenty percent of falls from a height greater than 15 feet involve an associated lumbar spine fracture. During such an extreme energy exchange, the spinal column tends to exaggerate its normal curves, and fractures and compressions occur at such areas. The spine is S-shaped; hence, it can be said that the compressive forces tend to break the patient's "S." These forces compress the concave side and open the convex side of the spine. **Excessive flexion, hyperextension,** and **hyperrotation** can cause bone damage and tearing of muscles and ligaments, resulting in impingement on or stretching of the spinal cord.

Lateral bending requires much less movement than flexion or extension before injury occurs. During lateral impact, the torso and the thoracic spine are moved laterally. The head tends to remain in place until pulled along by the cervical attachments. The center of gravity of the head is above and anterior to its seat and attachment to the cervical spine; therefore the head will tend to roll sideways. This movement often results in dislocations and bony fractures.

Distraction—overelongation of the spine—occurs when one part of the spine is stable and the rest is in longitudinal motion. This "pulling apart" of the spine can easily cause stretching and tearing of the cord. Distraction injury is a common mechanism of injury in children's playground accidents and in hangings.

Although any one of these types of violent movements may be the dominant cause of spinal injury in a given patient, one or more of the others will usually also be involved. As a guideline, the presence of spine injury and an unstable spine are frequently assumed with the following situations:

- any mechanism that impacts violently on the head, neck, torso, or pelvis (associated with violent sudden movement of the spine)
- incidents producing sudden acceleration, deceleration, or lateral bending
- falls from a significant height (landing on head or feet), resulting in axial loading and compression
- any fall in which one part of the body was suddenly stopped while the rest continued to fall
- any unrestrained victims in a vehicular rollover, persons ejected from a moving vehicle, or victims of an explosion
- any victim of a shallow-water diving accident

Other situations that are commonly associated with spinal damage include:

- head injuries with any alteration in level of consciousness
- the presence of any significant helmet damage
- significant blunt injury to the torso or above the clavicles
- impacted or other deceleration fractures of the legs or hips
- significant localized injuries to the area of the spinal column

The wearing of proper seat belt restraints has proved to save lives and reduce head, face, and thoracic injuries. However, the use of proper restraints does not rule out the possibility of spine injury. In significant frontal-impact collisions when sudden severe deceleration occurs, the restrained torso stops suddenly, but the unrestrained head attempts to continue its forward movement. Held by the strong posterior neck muscles, the head can only move forward slightly. If the force of deceleration is strong enough, the head then rotates down until the chin strikes the chest wall, frequently rotating across the diagonal strap of the shoulder restraint (Figures 9-9 and 9-10). Such rapid forceful hyperflexion and rotation of the

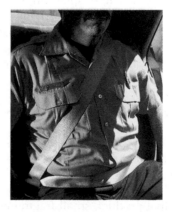

Figure 9-9 The head can rotate forward and to the left (or right) onto the chest wall around the diagonal seat belt strap.

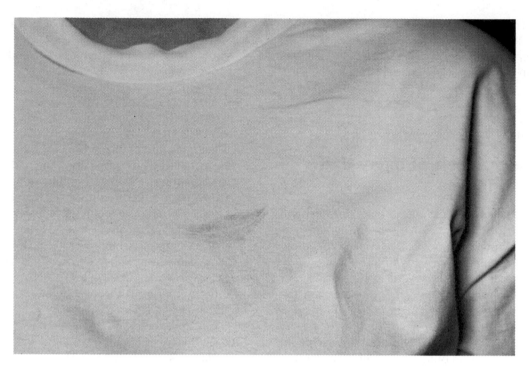

Figure 9-10 The lipstick mark on this patient's left chest indicates that the lips touched the anterior chest during impact. The severe flexion and moderate rotation resulted from head motion around the diagonal shoulder strap. The resultant injury to the patient was a locked facet at C5 and C6. The patient was correctly immobilized due to the EMT's astute recognition of this sign and the proper interpretation of the information.

neck can result in compression fractures of the cervical vertebrae, jumped and locked facets (dislocation of the articular processes), and stretching of the spinal cord. Different mechanisms can also cause spinal trauma in restrained victims of rear or lateral collisions. The amount of damage to the car and the patient's other injuries are the key factors in determining if the patient needs to be immobilized.

The patient's ability to walk should not be a factor in determining whether a patient needs to be treated for spine injury. Almost 20% of patients who required surgical repair of unstable spine injuries were found "walking around" at the scene by arriving EMTs or walked into the emergency department at the hospital. An unstable spine can *only* be ruled out by radiographic examination or a lack of any positive mechanism.

SKELETAL INJURIES

The types of injuries that can occur to the spine are varied. These injuries include:
- compression fractures of a vertebra that can produce total body flattening or wedge compression
- fractures that produce small fragments of bone that may lie in the spinal canal near the cord
- subluxation (a partial dislocation of a vertebra from its normal alignment in the spinal column)

- overstretching or tearing of the ligaments and muscles, producing an unstable relationship between the vertebra

Any of these skeletal injuries may immediately result in the irreversible cutting of the cord, or they may compress or stretch the cord. In many patients, however, damage to the vertebrae results in an unstable spinal column but does not produce an immediate cord injury.

A lack of neurologic deficit does not rule out a bony fracture or an unstable spine. Although the presence of good motor and sensory responses in the extremities indicates that the cord is currently intact, it does not indicate an absence of injured vertebrae or associated bony or soft tissue structures. A significant percentage of patients with an unstable bony spine have no neurologic deficit. A full assessment is still required.

OTHER TYPES OF SPINAL CORD INJURIES

Primary injury occurs at the time of impact or force application and may cause cord compression, direct cord injury (usually from sharp or unstable bony fragments), and/or interruption of the cord's blood supply. **Secondary injury** occurs after the initial insult and can include swelling, ischemia, or movement of bony fragments. **Cord concussion** results from the temporary disruption of

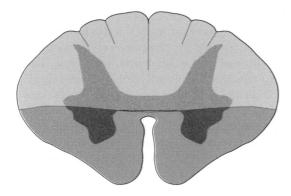

Figure 9-11 Anterior cord syndrome.

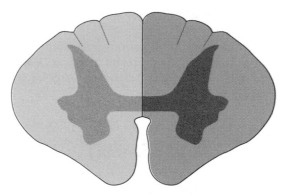

Figure 9-13 Brown-Séquard syndrome.

Area of cord injury

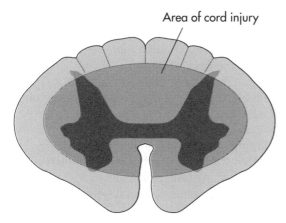

Figure 9-12 Central cord syndrome.

spinal cord functions distal to the injury. **Cord contusion** involves bruising or bleeding into the spinal cord's tissues, which may also result in a temporary loss of cord functions distal to the injury. Cord contusion is usually caused by a penetrating-type injury or movement of bony fragments. The severity of injury resulting from the contusion is related to the amount of bleeding into the tissue. Damage to or disruption of the spinal blood supply can result in local cord tissue ischemia. **Cord compression** is pressure on the spinal cord caused by swelling, which may result in tissue ischemia and in some cases may require decompression to prevent a permanent loss of function. **Cord laceration** occurs when cord tissue is torn or cut. This injury may be reversed if the cord has sustained only slight damage; however, it usually results in permanent disability if all spinal tracts are disrupted.

Spinal cord transection can be categorized as complete or incomplete. In **complete cord transection,** all spinal tracts are interrupted and all cord functions distal to the site are lost. Because of the effects of swelling, actual determination of loss of function may not be accurate until 24 hours after the injury. Most complete cord tran-

sections result in either paraplegia or quadriplegia. In incomplete cord transection, some tracts and motor/sensory functions remain intact. Prognosis for recovery is greater than with complete transections. Types of incomplete cord injuries include the following:

Anterior cord syndrome (Figure 9-11) is a result of bony fragments or pressure on spinal arteries. Symptoms include loss of motor function and pain sensation, temperature, and light touch sensations. However, some light touch, motion, position, and vibration sensations are spared.

Central cord syndrome (Figure 9-12) usually occurs with hyperextension of the cervical area. Symptoms include weakness or paresthesia in upper extremities but normal strength in lower extremities. This syndrome causes varying degrees of bladder dysfunction.

Brown-Séquard syndrome (Figure 9-13) is caused by penetrating injury and involves hemitransection of the cord involving only one side of the cord. Symptoms include complete cord damage and loss of function on the affected side (motor, vibration, motion, and position) with loss of pain and temperature sensation on the side opposite the injury.

Shock secondary to spinal cord injury represents a significant additional finding. **Neurogenic** and/or **spinal shock** is caused by different mechanisms that result from the neurologic deficits produced by injury to the spinal cord. Neurogenic shock from spinal trauma blocks (1) vasoregulatory fibers, (2) motor fibers, and (3) sensory fibers. Injury to the vasoregulatory fibers produces loss of sympathetic tone to the vessels or vasodilation. The skin will be warm and dry, the pulse rate will be slow, but the blood pressure will be low. When the cord is disrupted, the body's sympathetic compensatory mechanism cannot maintain control of the muscles in the walls of the blood vessels below the point of disruption. These arteries, arterioles, and veins dilate, enlarging the size of the vascular container and producing relative hypovolemia and partial loss of systemic vascular resistance. Instead of the tachycardia commonly associated with hypovolemic shock, this type of injury will produce a normal heart rate or a slight bradycardia.

Neurogenic shock results from vasodilation causing hypoperfusion. Spinal shock refers to the appearance of complete spinal cord injury, for which vascular function is later regained.

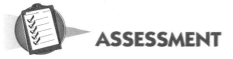

ASSESSMENT

The assessment for spinal injury, as with other conditions, must be done in the context of other injuries and conditions present. Airway, breathing, and circulation problems come first. However, these problems often cannot be assessed or managed without moving the patient. Therefore, a rapid survey of the scene, the situation, and the history of the event should determine if the possibility of a spinal injury exists. If a cervical spine injury *might* exist due to a positive mechanism, it *does exist* until proven otherwise by appropriate radiographic studies. This supposition also holds true for uncertain mechanisms until completion of the critical criteria. Therefore, the patient's spine must be manually protected. The head, unless contraindicated, should be brought into a neutral in-line position. It must be maintained in that position until the manual immobilization is replaced with a spine immobilization device such as a half-spine board, longboard, or vest-type device. *Any necessary movement done by hospital personnel (specifically emergency physicians, trauma surgeons, or orthopedic surgeons) involved in assessing and managing the patient must include continuous manual protection of the spine.*

MECHANISM OF INJURY

Mechanism of injury is used as a determinant for spinal immobilization. Patients with a positive mechanism of injury are always managed as positive for a spinal injury. Positive mechanisms of injury include high-speed MVCs; falls greater than three times the patient's height; injuries near the spine, e.g., stabbings, gunshots, and sports injuries; and any other high-impact injuries. In some situations the mechanism of injury may be such that the EMT feels the mechanism of injury is not indicative of neck injury, e.g., falling on an outstretched hand and producing a Colles' fracture. Uncertain mechanisms of injury are situations in which the forces exerted on the patient are unclear or questionable. In these cases, clinical criteria should be used to determine if spinal immobilization is needed. **Clinical criteria** for suspected spinal cord injury are a set of guidelines used during the assessment process to determine the need for spinal immobilization in uncertain mechanisms of injury.

The patient's other injuries must also be considered when evaluating the mechanism of injury and the forces involved. Any significant blunt trauma to the head, neck, or torso can result in compression or sudden movement of the spine beyond its normal range. For example, any injury to the head that involves enough force to result in unconsciousness (or helmet damage) must be assumed to have produced violent motion of the head, changing the relationship of the various vertebrae. Physical indications of spinal trauma are pain or pain on movement, point tenderness, deformity, and guarding of the spine area. Neurologic signs include bilateral paralysis, partial paralysis, paresis (weakness), numbness, prickling or tingling, and neurogenic spinal shock below the level of the injury. In males, a continuing erection of the penis, called priapism, may be an additional indication of spinal cord injury. Note, however, that the absence of these signs does not rule out bony spine injury.

The signs and symptoms that indicate the need for management of spinal trauma include:

- pain to the neck or back
- pain on movement of the neck or back
- pain on palpation of the posterior neck or midline of the back
- any deformity of the spinal column
- guarding or splinting of the neck or back
- paralysis, paresis, numbness, or tingling in the legs or arms at any time postinsult
- signs and symptoms of neurogenic shock
- priapism (in males)

CLINICAL CRITERIA VERSUS MECHANISM OF INJURY

After the scene survey, the initial assessment of the patient is based solely on the mechanism of injury. Spine stabilization is necessary until assessment is complete. Patients with an obvious positive mechanism of injury are considered positive for spinal injury and should be managed as such. A patient with an obvious negative mechanism of injury, such as an isolated sprained ankle, does not require spine management. However, when a patient has an uncertain mechanism of injury, such as a trip and fall over a hose or a low-speed MVC, further assessment can be made to determine the applicability or need for spine management if time conditions and the education of the EMT permit. In most instances the patient should be immobilized and transported to the hospital, where the physician can provide a better evaluation before the board is removed.

Patient Reliability

A reliable patient is calm, cooperative, and sober. An unreliable patient is any patient exhibiting acute stress reactions (ASR), brain/head injury, intoxication, or altered mental states or one who is suffering from distracting injury or has communication barriers.

Acute stress reactions (ASR) are temporary responses of the autonomic nervous system. Sympathetic ASR is the "flight or fight" response in which bodily functions increase and pain masking occurs. Parasympathetic ASR slows bodily functions and may result in syncope. If signs of sympathetic ASR are present, the patient is considered unreliable.

Brain or head injury may involve temporary loss of consciousness and should necessitate treating the patient as positive for spinal injury. In some instances, belligerence and uncooperative behavior may be the only sign of injury.

Intoxicated patients, those under the influence of drugs or alcohol, are also considered unreliable. These patients should be treated as positive for spinal injury until they are calm, cooperative, and sober.

Patients with abnormal mental status (AMS) include psychiatric patients, Alzheimer's patients, or patients with AMS due to trauma. These patients should be treated as positive for spinal injury and fully immobilized.

Distracting injuries are severely painful or bloody injuries that may prevent the patient from giving reliable responses during the assessment. Examples of distracting injuries include a fractured femur or any other dramatic injury.

Communication problems include language barriers, deafness, very young patients, or patients too distracted by surroundings to communicate effectively. These factors may prevent reliable patient responses during assessment.

Patient reliability should be continually rechecked at all phases of an assessment. If at any time the patient exhibits the just mentioned signs or symptoms, then the patient must be assumed to have a spinal injury, and full immobilization management techniques must be implemented.

MANAGEMENT

The management for a patient with a suspected unstable spine is to immobilize him or her in a supine position on a rigid spine board in a neutral in-line position. The head, neck, torso, and pelvis must *each* be immobilized in a neutral in-line position to prevent any further movement of the unstable spine that could result in damage to the cord. Spinal immobilization follows the common principle of fracture management of immobilizing the joint above and the joint below an injury. Because of the anatomy of the spinal column and the interaction caused by forces affecting any part of the spine, this principle simply needs to be extended. In effect, the "joint above" the spine means that the head must be immobilized, and

the "joint below" means that the pelvis must be immobilized. Moderate anterior flexion or extension of the arms will not cause significant movement of the shoulder girdle.

Any movement or angulation of the pelvis results in movement of the sacrum and of the vertebrae attached to it. For example, lateral movement of both legs together can result in angulation of the pelvis and lateral bending of the spine.

The body is considerably wider at the hips than at the ankles. When a person is rolled to the side and the lower legs are allowed to remain on the ground, they move out of lateral alignment, which may angulate the pelvis and result in moving the lower and midspine. Therefore, in patients with suspected spine injury, the legs need to be maintained in a midline neutral position in line with the rest of the body. Logrolling methods that call for elevating an arm over the head, or methods that do not include keeping the ankles elevated off the ground when the patient is rolled on his or her side, are not recommended because they can cause movement of both the cervical and lower spine.

Fractures of one area of the spine are commonly associated with fractures of other areas of the spine. Therefore, the entire weight-bearing spine (cervical, thoracic, lumbar, and sacral) must be considered as one entity, and the entire spine must be immobilized and sup-ported (splinted) for proper immobilization to be achieved. The supine position is the most stable position to ensure continued support during handling, carrying, and transporting the patient. It also provides the EMT with the best access for further examination and additional resuscitation and management of the patient. When the patient is supine, it is easy to simultaneously access the airway, mouth and nose, eyes, chest, and abdomen.

Patients usually present in one of four general postures: sitting, semiprone, supine, or standing. The patient's spine must be protected and immobilized immediately and continuously from the time he or she is discovered until he or she is mechanically secured to the longboard. Techniques and equipment such as manual immobilization, half-spine boards, immobilization vests, scoop litters, proper logroll methods, or rapid extrication with full manual immobilization are interim techniques that are used to protect the spine while allowing safe movement of the patient from the position in which he or she was found until full supine immobilization on the rigid longboard can be implemented.

Too much focus is often placed on particular immoblization devices without an understanding of the principles of immobilization and how to modify these principles to meet individual patient needs. Specific devices and immobilization methods can only be safely used with an understanding of the anatomic principles that are generic to all methods and equipment. Any inflexible

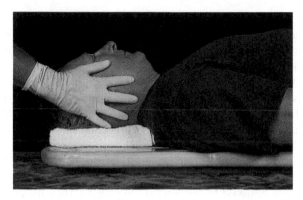

Figure 9-14 In most adults, kyphosis (abnormal forward curvature) of the lumbar spine has moved the origin of the cervical spine forward to a more anterior position in relation to the chest wall and the posterior thoracic wall. Pulling the skull back to the level of the backboard can produce severe hyperextension. Padding is needed between the back of the head and the backboard to prevent such hyperextension.

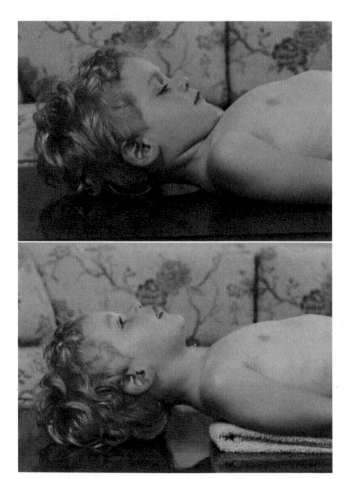

Figure 9-15 The relatively larger size of the child's head, combined with the reduced development of the posterior thoracic muscles, produces hyperflexion of the head when a child is placed on a backboard. Padding beneath the shoulders will prevent this hyperflexion.

detailed method for using a device will not meet the varying problems found in the field. Regardless of the specific equipment or method used, the management of any patient with an unstable spine should follow these general steps:

- Provide manual in-line immobilization.
- Evaluate the patient's airway, breathing, and circulation first. Check motor, sensory, and circulation functions in all four extremities.
- Examine the neck and apply a cervical collar.
- Immobilize the torso to a device so the torso cannot move up, down, left, or right.
- Pad as needed: behind the head for adults and under the thorax for pediatric patients.
- Immobilize the head to the device.
- Once the patient is on the longboard, immobilize the legs and arms to the board.
- Reevaluate the patient's airway, breathing, and circulation and reassess motor, sensory, and circulation functions in all four extremities (if time permits).

As a person grows to adulthood, posture and musculoskeletal changes occur that place the posterior part of the head more anterior than the posterior part of the thorax. In many adults, neutral in-line positioning produces a space between the back of the head and the ground or device (Figure 9-14). When such a space exists, padding must be placed behind the head to maintain neutral alignment. Children are the opposite—the head is large and the posterior musculature is not well developed. If placed on the ground or on a rigid board, a child's head is typically moved to severe flexion (Figure 9-15). When immobilizing children, significant padding under the torso is usually necessary to offset the problem.

Cervical collars alone do not adequately immobilize; they simply aid in supporting the neck and promoting a lack of movement. Generally, cervical collars at best provide only 50% limitation of motion in the three directions of anterior/posterior, lateral flexion, and rotation. *A cervical collar should not be used as an immobilization device.* They can add some comfort and stabilization to the patient placed on a backboard. The backboard should be considered the "gold standard" for cervical spine immobilization. A more detailed discussion of methods and equipment for in-line immobilization is presented in Chapter 10: Spine Management Skills.

• Summary •

1. The vertebral column is composed of 33 separate vertebrae stacked one on top of the other. Their major function is to support the weight of the body and to allow movement.

2. The spinal cord is enclosed within the vertebral column and is vulnerable to abnormal move-

ment and positioning. This large collection of nerves is protected by the bony vertebrae.

3. When support for the vertebral column has been lost due to injury to the vertebrae or to the muscles and ligaments that help hold the spinal column in place, injury to the spinal cord can occur. Because the cord does not regenerate, permanent injury, often involving paralysis, can result.

4. The presence of spinal trauma and the need to immobilize the patient can be indicated either by the mechanism of injury, the presence of other injuries that could only occur with sudden violent forces acting on the body, or by specific signs and symptoms of vertebral or spinal cord injury.

5. Damage to the bones of the spinal column is not always evident. If an initial injury to the cord has not occurred, a neurologic deficit may not be present even though the spinal column is unstable. *The presence of any one of these indications, regardless of the absence of any of the others, should cause the EMT to assume that an unstable spine exists and to manage it accordingly.*

6. Immobilization of spinal fractures, as with other fractures, requires immobilization of the joint above and the joint below the injury. For the spine, the "joints above" are the head and neck, and the "joints below" are the torso and the pelvis.

7. The device used should immobilize the head, chest, and pelvis areas in a neutral in-line position without causing or allowing movement. Interim methods and devices are used to protect the spine until the patient is immobilized in a supine position on a longboard.

Scenario Solution

After responding to a reported "man down" call, you arrive to find a 30-year-old male at the bottom of a 15-foot ladder. Scene size-up reveals a safe area. In your initial assessment you find an unconscious male with a large hematoma on his forehead and pale, cool, clammy skin. His airway is patent with shallow breathing. His radial pulse is present, and there are no obvious signs of external blood loss.

While providing spine stabilization, you place the patient on high percentage oxygen through a non-rebreather mask. Since this is a high-priority patient, you direct your crew to get a cervical collar and longboard while you complete a focused assessment for a trauma victim.

During the focused assessment, you examine the patient from head to toe, looking and feeling for any abnormalities, and you apply the cervical collar. There are no abnormalities other than the hematoma on the forehead, and you also note a bruise in the left upper quadrant of the abdomen.

You logroll the patient onto the longboard and initiate transport to the hospital. Because you have a short transport time, you elect not to call an advanced life support (ALS) intercept. You assess vital signs en route. You find a blood pressure of 180/110, pulse 62, and respirations of 34/shallow. The patient remains unconscious, and you reassess every 5 minutes.

Review Questions

Answers provided on page 333.

1 The decision to immobilize a suspected trauma patient's spine should be based on:
   A mechanism of injury
   B the presence of other sudden, violent, force-produced injuries
   C specific signs and symptoms of vertebral or spinal cord injury
   D All of the above

2 Immobilization of the spine should follow the same standard as any other splinting technique: immobilize the joint above (head) and the joint below (pelvis).
   A True
   B False

3 The first step in providing spinal immobilization for any suspected trauma patient should be:
   A measurement and application of a rigid cervical collar
   B neurovascular checks
   C manual stabilization of the head and neck
   D check of dermatomes

4 The most common (frequent) cause of spinal trauma in the pediatric patient would be:
   A falls from a tricycle or bicycle
   B falls from heights (generally 2 to 3 times the patient's height)
   C being struck by a motor vehicle
   D diving injuries

5 When immobilizing the spine of a suspected adult trauma patient, padding should be placed under the patient's:
   A legs
   B thorax
   C pelvis
   D head

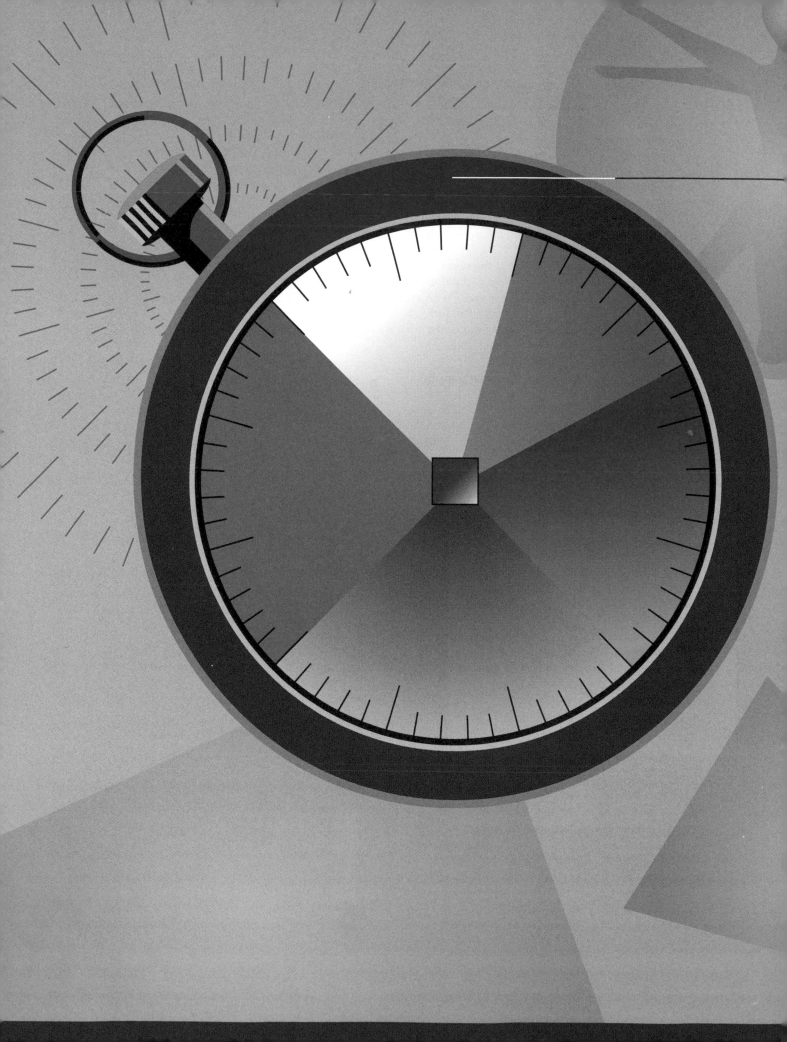

CHAPTER 10

Spine Management Skills

A wide variety of devices and methods exist for immobilizing the sitting, lying, or standing patient. The use of any specific device or method should follow an understanding of a generic sequence. Use of a general method focuses the EMT on the patient and his or her needs regardless of the device used, and it avoids the need to remember countless different methods for each of the wide range of equipment that is presently available.

GENERAL METHOD

Once safety, the scene, and the situation have been assessed, and the EMT has determined that the possibility of an unstable spine exists due to the mechanism of injury, the following steps should be taken:

1. Move the head into a proper neutral in-line position (unless contraindicated). Continue manual support and in-line immobilization without interruption.
2. Evaluate using A B C D E method and provide any immediately required intervention.
3. Check motor ability, sensory response, and circulation in all four extremities (MSC × 4).
4. Examine the neck and measure and apply a properly fitting, effective cervical collar.
5. Position the device (i.e., shortboard, vest-type) on the patient or the patient on the device (i.e., long backboard) and immobilize the torso to the device so that it cannot move up or down, left or right.
6. Evaluate and pad behind the head or chest as needed.
7. Immobilize the head to the device, being sure to maintain the neutral in-line position.
8. Once on the longboard, immobilize the legs so that they cannot move anteriorly or laterally.
9. Fasten the arms to the board.
10. Recheck using A B C D E method and reassess motor ability, sensory response, and circulation in all four extremities.

To ensure a full understanding of these steps, and the potential problems associated with them, the following pages discuss the general method in greater detail.

MANUAL IN-LINE IMMOBILIZATION OF THE HEAD

Once it has been determined from the mechanism of injury that an unstable spine must be suspected and managed, the first step is to provide manual in-line immobilization immediately. The head is grasped and carefully moved to a neutral in-line position unless contraindicated. A proper neutral in-line position is maintained without any significant traction. Only enough pull should be exerted on a sitting or standing patient to cause axial unweighting (taking the weight of the head off the axis and the rest of the cervical spine). The head should be constantly maintained in the manually immobilized neutral in-line position until the completion of mechanical immobilization of the torso and head. In this way the patient's head and neck are immediately immobilized, and they remain so until after examination at the hospital. Moving the head into a neutral in-line position represents less risk than if the patient were carried and transported with the head left in an angulated position. In addition, both immobilizing and transporting the patient are much simpler with the patient in the neutral position.

In a few cases, moving the patient's head into a neutral in-line position will be *contraindicated*. If careful movement of the head and neck into a neutral in-line position results in any of the following, the EMT must *stop* the movement:

- neck muscle spasm
- increased pain
- the commencement or increase of a neurologic deficit such as numbness, tingling, or loss of motor ability
- compromise of the airway or ventilation

Neutral in-line movement should not even be attempted if the patient's injuries are so severe that the head presents with such misalignment that it no longer appears to extend from the midline of the shoulders.

In these situations the patient's head will have to be immobilized in the position in which it is initially found. Fortunately such cases are extremely rare.

CERVICAL COLLARS

Cervical collars do not immobilize. Although they assist in reducing some of the range of movement of the head, they do not limit motion enough to provide immobilization. The best collar will still allow 25% to 30% of motion by flexion and extension and the range of other motion by 50% or less. Cervical collars are an important adjunct to immobilization but *must always be used in conjunction with manual immobilization or mechanical immobilization* provided by a suitable spine immobilization device.

The unique *primary purpose* of a cervical collar is to protect the cervical spine from compression. Prehospital methods of immobilization (using a vest, halfboard, or longboard device) still allow some slight movement, since these devices only fasten externally to the patient, and the skin and muscle tissue move slightly on the skeletal frame even when the patient is extremely well immobilized. Most rescue situations involve movement when carrying and loading the patient. This type of movement also occurs when the ambulance accelerates and decelerates in normal driving conditions.

An effective cervical collar sits on the chest, posterior thoracic spine and clavicle, and trapezius muscles, where the tissue movement is at a minimum. This still allows movement at C6, C7, and T1 but does prevent compression of these vertebrae. The head is immobilized under the angle of the mandible and at the occiput of the skull. The rigid collar allows the unavoidable loading between the head and the torso to be transferred from the cervical spine to the collar, eliminating or minimizing the cervical compression that could otherwise result.

Secondarily, even though it does not immobilize, the cervical collar aids in limiting head movement. Also, the rigid anterior portion of the collar provides a safe pathway for the lower head strap across the neck.

The collar must be the correct size for the patient. A collar that is too short will not be effective and will allow significant flexion. Too large a collar causes hyperextension or full motion if the chin is inside of it. The collar must be applied properly. Too loose a collar will be ineffective in helping to limit head movement and can accidentally cover the anterior chin, mouth, and nose, obstructing the patient's airway. A collar that is too tight can compromise the veins of the neck (Box 10-1).

A collar should only be applied to a patient *after* the head has been brought into a neutral in-line position. Use of any of the collars presently available for prehospital use, if the patient is not in a neutral in-line position, is difficult and should not be considered. *A collar that does not allow the mandible to move down and the mouth to open without motion of the spine will produce aspiration of gastric contents into the lungs if the patient vomits. Such a cervical collar should not be used.* Alternative methods to immobilize the patient when a collar cannot be used may include using such items as blankets, towels, tape, etc. The EMT may need to be very creative when presented with these types of patients. Whatever method is used, always follow the basic concepts of immobilization.

IMMOBILIZATION OF DEVICE TO THE TORSO

Regardless of the specific device used, the device must be immobilized to the torso so that it cannot move up, down, left, or right. The rigid device is strapped to the torso *and* the torso to the device. The device is secured to the torso so that the head and neck will be supported and immobilized when affixed to it. The torso and pelvis are immobilized to the device so that the thoracic, lumbar, and sacral sections of the spine are supported and cannot move. ***The device should be immobilized to the torso before it is immobilized to the head.*** In this way, any movement of the device that may occur when fastening the torso straps is prevented from angulating the cervical spine.

Many different specific methods for immobilizing the device to the torso exist. Protection against moving in any direction—up, down, left, or right—should be achieved at both the upper torso (at the shoulders or chest) and at the lower torso (at the pelvis) to avoid compression and lateral movement of the vertebrae of the torso. Immobilization of the upper torso can be achieved with several specific methods. It is important that the EMT understand the basic anatomic principles common to each method. Cephalad movement of the upper torso is readily prohibited by a strap on each side, fastened to the board inferior to the upper margin of each shoulder, which then passes over the shoulder and is fastened at a lower point. Caudad movement of the torso can be readily prohibited by straps that pass snugly around the pelvis.

In one method, two straps (one going from each side of the board over the shoulder, then across the upper chest and through the opposite armpit to fasten to the board on the armpit side) produce an **X**, which stops any upward, downward, left, or right movement of the upper torso (Figure 10-1A).

> ### Box 10-1 Cervical Collars
>
> - Do not immobilize by themselves
> - Must be properly sized for each patient
> - Must not inhibit the patient's ability to open his or her mouth or the EMT's ability to open the patient's mouth if vomiting occurs
> - Should not obstruct or hinder ventilation in any way

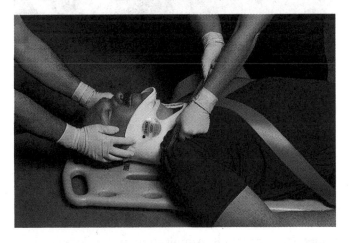

A

Figure 10-1 A, Close-up of upper thorax with X straps applied by EMTs. *Continued*

The same immobilization can be achieved by fastening one strap to the board and passing it through one armpit, then across the upper chest and through the opposite armpit to fasten to the second side of the board. Then a strap or cravat is added to each side and passes over the shoulder to fasten to the armpit strap (like a pair of suspenders) (Figure 10-1B).

Immobilizing the upper torso of a patient with a fractured clavicle can be achieved by placing backpack-type loops around each shoulder through the armpit and fastening the ends of each loop in the same handhole. In this method the straps remain near the lateral edges of the upper torso and do not cross the clavicles. With any of these methods the straps are over the upper third of the chest and can be fastened tightly without producing the ventilatory embarrassment that is commonly produced by tight straps placed lower on the thorax.

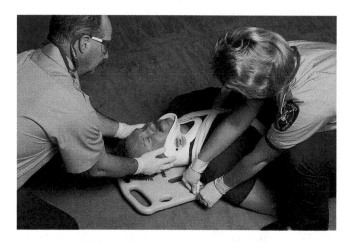

B

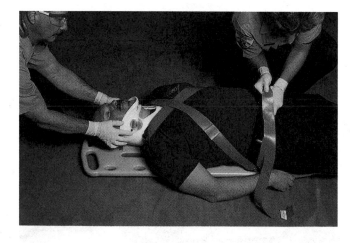

C

Figure 10-1, cont'd B, Armpit strap: a strap or cravat over each shoulder is fastened to armpit strap by EMT. C, Patient with X strap at upper torso with single lower strap over iliac crests.

Immobilization of the lower torso can be achieved by a single strap fastened tightly over the pelvis at the iliac crests (Figure 10-1C). If the longboard will have to be up-ended or carried on stairs or over any distance, a pair of groin loops will provide stronger immobilization than the single strap across the iliac crests.

Lateral movement or anterior movement away from the rigid device at the midtorso can be prevented by an additional strap around the midtorso. Any strap that surrounds the torso between the very upper thorax and the iliac crests should be snug, but not so tight as to inhibit chest excursion or cause a significant increase in intra-abdominal pressure.

MAINTENANCE OF NEUTRAL IN-LINE POSITION OF THE HEAD

In many patients, when the head is placed in a neutral in-line position, the outer measurement of the occipital region at the back of the head is between 1/2 inch and 3-1/2 inches anterior of the posterior thoracic wall (Figure 10-2A). Therefore, in *most* adults a space occurs between the back of the head and the device when the head is in a neutral in-line position, and suitable padding *must* be added prior to securing the head to the device (Figure 10-2B). To be effective, this padding must be made of a material that does not readily compress. Firm semirigid pads designed for this purpose or folded towels can be used. The amount of padding needed must be individualized for each patient. A few individuals require none. If too little padding is provided, or if the padding is of an unsuitable spongy material, the head will be hyperextended when the head straps are applied. If too much padding is inserted, the head will be moved into a flexed position. Both hyperextension and flexion of the head can increase spinal cord damage and are contraindicated.

The same anatomic relationship between the head and back is true when most people are supine—whether on the ground or on a backboard. When most adults are supine, the head falls back into a hyperextended position. Upon arrival, one EMT should move the head into a neutral in-line position and manually maintain it in that position, which in many adults will require holding the head up off the ground. Once the patient is placed on the longboard, and prior to fastening the head to the board, the proper padding, as previously described, should be inserted between the back of the head and the board to maintain the neutral position.

In small children (generally those having a body size of a 7-year-old or younger) the size of the head is much larger relative to the rest of the body than it is in adults, and the muscles of the back are less developed. When a small child's head is in a neutral in-line position, the back of the head usually extends between 1 inch and

2 inches beyond the posterior plane of his or her back. Therefore, if a small child is placed directly on a rigid surface, the head will be moved into a position of flexion (Figure 10-3A).

Placing small children on a standard longboard results in unwanted flexion. The longboard needs to be modified either by creating a recess in the board or by inserting padding under the torso to maintain the head in a neutral position (Figure 10-3B). The padding placed under the torso should be of the appropriate thickness so that the head lies on the board in a neutral position; too much will result in extension, too little in flexion. The padding under the torso must also be firm and evenly shaped, and extend the full width and length of the torso from the buttocks to the top of the shoulders. Using irregularly shaped or insufficient padding, or placing it under

only part of the torso, can result in movement and misalignment of the spine.

IMMOBILIZATION
Head

Once the rigid device has been immobilized to the torso and appropriate padding has been inserted behind the head as needed, the head should be secured to the device (only after the torso has been secured). Due to the rounded shape of the head, it cannot be stabilized on a flat surface with only straps or tape. Use of these alone will still allow the head to rotate and move laterally. Also, because of the angle of the forehead and the slippery nature of moist skin and hair, a simple strap over the forehead is unreliable and can easily slide off. Although the

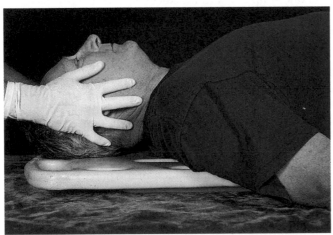

A

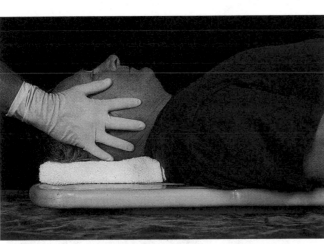

B

Figure 10-2 A, Head immobilization without padding. B, Adult on longboard with padding behind head.

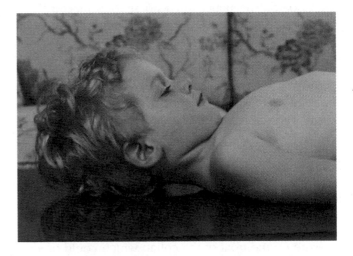

A

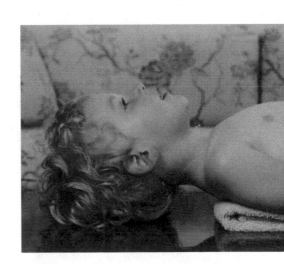

B

Figure 10-3 A and B, Child on backboard without and with padding.

human head weighs about the same as a bowling ball, it has a significantly different shape. The head is ovoid, being longer than it is wide and having almost completely flat lateral sides. It may be helpful to think of a bowling ball that has had about 2 inches cut off its left and right sides. Adequate external immobilization of the head, regardless of method or device, can only be readily achieved by placing pads or rolled blankets on these flat sides and securing them with straps or tape. In the case of vest-type devices, this is accomplished with hinged side flaps that are part of the vest.

The side pieces, whether they are preshaped foam blocks or "homemade" rolled blankets, are placed on the flat lateral planes of the head. The side pieces should extend to an area at least as wide as the opening of the patient's ears or beyond. Two straps or pieces of tape surrounding these head pieces draw the sides together. When packaged between the blocks or blankets, the head now has a flat posterior surface that can be realistically fixed to a flat board. The upper forehead strap is placed tightly across the front of the lower forehead (across the supraorbital ridge) and helps prevent anterior movement of the head. This strap should be pulled tightly enough to indent the blocks or blankets and rest firmly on the forehead.

The use of chin cups or straps encircling the chin prevents opening of the mouth to vomit; these devices should not be used. The device holding the head—regardless of type—also requires a lower strap to help keep the side pieces firmly pressed against the lower sides of the head and to further anchor the device and prevent anterior movement of the lower head and neck. The lower strap passes around the side pieces and across the anterior rigid portion of the cervical collar. Care must be taken to ensure that this strap does not place too much pressure on the front of the collar, which could produce an airway or venous return problem at the neck. Using

sandbags secured to the spine board on the sides of the head and neck represents a dangerous practice. Regardless of how well secured, these heavy objects can shift and move. Should the patient and board have to be rotated to the side, the combined weight of the sandbags can produce localized lateral pressure against the cervical spine. Raising or lowering the head of the board when moving and loading the patient, or any sudden acceleration or deceleration of the ambulance, can also produce shifting of the bags and movement of the head and neck.

Legs

Significant outward rotation of the legs may result in anterior movement of the pelvis and movement of the lower spine. To eliminate this possibility the feet should be tied together.

Immobilize the legs to the board with two or more straps: one strap proximal to the knees at about midthigh and one strap distal to the knees (Figure 10-4A).

The average adult measures between 14 and 20 inches from one side to the other at the hips, and only 6 to 9 inches from one side to the other at the ankles. When the feet are placed together, a V-like shape is formed from the hips to the ankles. Because the ankles are considerably narrower than the board, a strap placed across the lower legs can prevent anterior movement but will not prevent the legs from moving laterally from one edge of the board to the other. If the board is angled or rotated, the legs will fall to the lower edge of the board. This can angulate the pelvis. Angulation of the pelvis can produce movement of the spinal column.

One way to effectively hold the lower legs in place is to encircle them several times with the strap before attaching it to the board. The legs can also be kept in the middle of the board by placing blanket rolls between

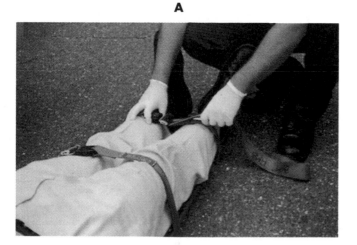
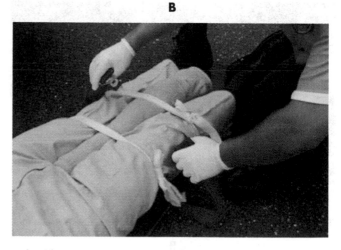

Figure 10-4 A, Immobilize the legs to the board with two or more straps. One strap should be proximal to the knees at about midthigh and one strap distal to the knees. B, Patient's legs immobilized to each other with blanket between each leg and edge of board, then fastened to the board.

each leg and the edges of the board before strapping (Figure 10-4B).

Arms

For safety, the patient's arms should be secured to the board or across the torso prior to moving the patient. One way to achieve this is with the arms placed at the sides on the board with the palms in, secured by a strap across the forearms and torso. This strap should be made snug but not so tight as to compromise the circulation in the hands.

The arms should not be included in either the strap at the iliac crests or in the groin loops. If they are tight enough to provide adequate immobilization of the lower torso, they can compromise the circulation in the hands. If they are loose, they will not provide adequate immobilization of the torso or arms. Use of an additional strap exclusively to hold the arms also makes it possible to open the strap for taking a blood pressure measurement or starting an intravenous line once in the ambulance without in any way compromising the immobilization. If the arm strap is also a torso strap, loosening it to free just an arm has the side effect of loosening the torso immobilization as well.

MOST COMMON MISTAKES

The three most commonly noted immobilization errors follow:

1. **Inadequate immobilization**—either the device can move significantly up or down on the torso or the head can still move excessively.
2. **Immobilization with the head hyperextended.** The most common cause is a lack of appropriate padding behind the head.
3. **Readjusting the torso straps after the head has been secured,** causing movement of the device on the torso, which results in movement of the head and cervical spine.

CRITERIA FOR EVALUATING IMMOBILIZATION SKILLS

Immobilization skills need to be practiced in hands-on sessions using mock patients prior to the EMT's use with real patients. When practicing, or when evaluating new methods or equipment, the following generic criteria will serve as good tools for measuring how effectively the "patient" has been immobilized:

- Was manual in-line immobilization initiated immediately, and was it maintained until it was replaced mechanically?
- Was an effective, properly sized cervical collar applied appropriately?
- Was the torso secured before the head?

- Can the device move up or down the torso?
- Can it move left or right at the upper torso?
- Can it move left or right at the lower torso?
- Can any part of the torso move anteriorly off the rigid device?
- Does any tie crossing the chest inhibit chest excursion, resulting in ventilatory compromise?
- Is the head effectively immobilized so that it cannot move in any direction, including rotation?
- Was padding behind the head used if necessary?
- Is the head in a neutral in-line position?
- Does anything inhibit or prevent the mouth from being opened?
- Are the legs immobilized so that they cannot move anteriorly, rotate, or move from side to side, even if the board and patient are rotated to the side?
- Are the pelvis and legs in a neutral in-line position?
- Are the arms appropriately secured to the board or torso?
- Have any ties or straps compromised distal circulation in any limb?
- Was the patient bumped, jostled, or in any way moved in a manner that could compromise an unstable spine while the device was being applied?
- Was the procedure completed within an appropriate time frame?

There are many methods and variations to meet these objectives. The EMT should select the specific method and equipment to be used based on the situation, the patient's condition, and available resources.

• Summary •

This chapter presents a variety of spine immobilization skills and techniques, whenever possible in a generic manner. The skills presented have been identified from national experience as those needing particular attention or remediation by EMTs, or those that present new and effective approaches to old problems. This is not meant to be an exhaustive or complete portrayal of every possible spine immobilization skill.

For every technique shown:

1. Local medical protocols and guidance should be sought for the variations presented herein.
2. The EMT should practice the skills and techniques presented, under a variety of situations and conditions, to prepare for actual experiences.
3. The general principles and concepts presented here can be applied to many different kinds and models of equipment. The EMT who understands these general principles can make any piece of equipment work properly in virtually any situation.

INDIVIDUAL IMMOBILIZATION SKILLS

Most methods of immobilization require three operators to perform them properly and to ensure the maintenance of manual immobilization throughout. When only two EMTs are available, one should maintain manual immobilization at the head while the second applies the device. When first responders or others are enlisted to help, care must be taken to assign them tasks that do not require previous training (such as positioning the longboard) or are the least sensitive (such as moving the legs), and to furnish them with precise directions.

The skills demonstrations in the following pages describe only the skills—they are not scenarios. In real life the EMTs would have evaluated the scene and situation and ensured their safety and that of the patient. They would have also completed any higher priority care that the patient required prior to performing the demonstrated skill. Assessment of motor ability, sensory response, and circulation should be done in all four extremities (MSC × 4) before and after each procedure. The EMT should reassess the patient using the A B C D E method when the immobilization is completed.

MANUAL IN-LINE IMMOBILIZATION
BEHIND

1 From behind the patient, place the hands over the patient's ears without moving the head (Figure 10-5A). Place the thumbs against the posterior aspect of the skull. Place the little fingers just under the angle of the mandible. Spread the remaining fingers on the flat lateral planes of the head and increase the strength of the grasp. If the head is not in a neutral in-line position, slowly move the head until it is. Bring the arms in and rest them against the seat, headrest, or your torso for support.

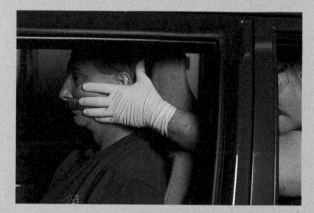

Figure 10-5A

SIDE

1 Stand at the side of the patient (Figure 10-5B). Pass your arm over the patient's shoulder and cup the back of his or her head with your hand. Be careful not to move the head. Place the thumb and first finger of your other hand, with one on each side of the face, on the cheeks in the notch where the upper teeth join the maxilla. Tighten the anterior and posterior pressure of the hands. If the head is not in a neutral in-line position, move the head until it is. Brace your elbows on your torso for support.

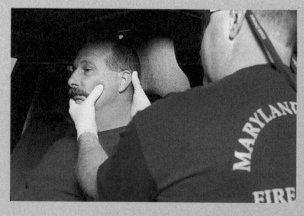

Figure 10-5B

FRONT

Manual immobilization can be provided from the front using the same principles but with different finger placement.

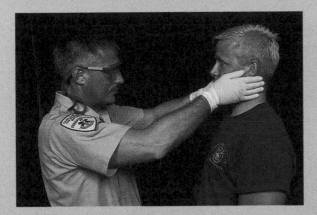

Figure 10-6

Stand directly in front of the patient. Place the hands on the sides of the head as shown (Figure 10-6). Front method of manual immobilization by EMT: Place the little fingers at the posterior aspect of the skull. Place one thumb in the notch between the upper teeth and the maxilla on each cheek. Spread the remaining fingers on the flat lateral planes of the head and increase the strength of the grasp. If the head is not in a neutral in-line position, slowly move the head until it is. Bring your arms in and brace your elbows against your torso for support.

1

Note: This method can also be used when kneeling alongside the thorax of a supine patient and facing toward his or her head.

SUPINE PATIENT

Note: Except that the fingers point in a caudad direction (toward the tail) instead of in a cephalad direction, hand placement for a supine patient when immobilizing from a position kneeling above the head is the same as when immobilizing a sitting patient from the front.

The little fingers are placed at the posterior aspect of the skull. A thumb is placed in the notch between the upper teeth and the maxilla at each cheek. The other fingers are spread across the flat lateral planes of the head (in this case facing the patient's feet) (Figure 10-7).

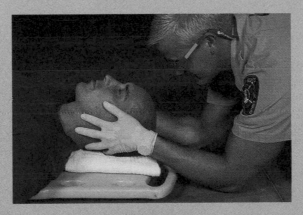

Figure 10-7

SELECTING A METHOD FOR PLACING THE SUPINE PATIENT ON A LONGBOARD WHILE MAINTAINING PROPER IMMOBILIZATION

Several methods are available to maintain immobilization of the spine while moving a supine patient onto a longboard. Recent studies have clearly demonstrated that previously taught logroll techniques in which an arm is elevated over the head or in which the arms are moved anteriorly result in undue movement of the spine. Only logroll techniques in which the arms are maintained in extension and pressed palm-in against the patient's sides, with the patient being rolled onto his or her own arm on one side, minimize the referred movement of the spine. Therefore, only such logroll methods should be used.

To minimize the potential for accidentally translocating part of the patient's spinal column when performing a logroll, the patient as a unit should be rolled to one side only as far as is necessary to insert the board under the patient. When a flat board without runners is used, the required degree of rotation is minimal. When using boards with runners or molded boards with raised edges, more rotation will be required.

A variety of alternative methods are available for placing a supine patient onto a longboard without logrolling. Several techniques involve placing the longboard on the ground beyond the patient's head. While maintaining manual immobilization, the patient is slid longitudinally into position on the board. Use of a scoop stretcher (sometimes called a split litter) is also an effective alternative. When a scoop stretcher is used, each side is separately inserted under the patient from the side while manual immobilization of the head and neck is maintained. The sides are then refastened, the patient is securely immobilized to the stretcher with straps, cravats, and/or tape, and the stretcher and immobilized patient can be lifted a few inches off the ground while a longboard is inserted underneath.

The EMT will have to select the best method for placing a supine patient onto a longboard based on the situation, the patient's injuries, and the resources at the scene.

LOGROLL: SUPINE PATIENT

Logrolling methods that elevate an arm over the head or allow lateral movement of the lower legs can easily result in angulation of the pelvis and movement of the spine and should not be used. The following method uses the patient's arms to splint the patient's body, maintains neutral alignment of the pelvis and legs, and eliminates or minimizes any unwanted movement.

1 While neutral in-line immobilization is maintained by the EMT at the patient's head (EMT #1), a cervical collar is applied and a longboard is placed alongside the patient as shown (Figure 10-8A). A, Patient is immobilized in the supine position and prepared to logroll after cervical collar is applied.

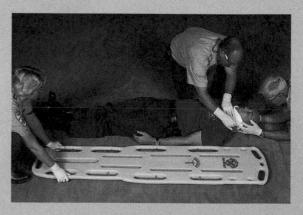

Figure 10-8A

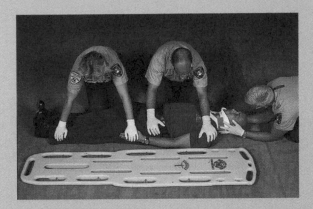

Figure 10-8B

EMT #2 kneels at the patient's midthorax and **2** EMT #3 kneels next to him or her at the patient's knees. The arms are straightened, and placed palm-in next to the torso while the legs are brought together into neutral alignment by EMT #3. Then EMT #2 extends the patient's arms, locking the elbows, and grasps the far side of the patient at the shoulder and wrist (Figure 10-8B). B, EMT #1 supports the head while EMTs #2 and #3 grasp the patient. EMT #3 grasps the hip just distal of the wrist and tightly grasps both pants cuffs at the ankles. (If the patient is wearing shorts or a skirt or if the pants have been cut off, a cravat around the ankles will provide a similar hold on the lower legs.)

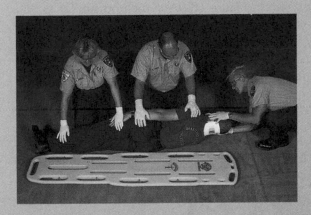

Figure 10-8C

With arms locked firmly at sides, the patient **3** is rolled slowly onto his or her side until rotated just enough to allow proper insertion of the longboard under his or her back (Figure 10-8C). C, Patient is partially rotated. The EMT at the head watches the thorax turn and maintains neutral in-line support of the head, rotating it exactly with the torso and being careful to avoid any flexion or hyperextension. EMT #3, at the legs, assists the rotation of the torso with his or her hand at the patient's hip. EMT #3 rotates the legs, moving in line with the torso at all times. As well as rotary alignment, the EMT at the legs must also maintain lateral and anterior/posterior alignment. To maintain lateral alignment the ankles must be kept elevated.

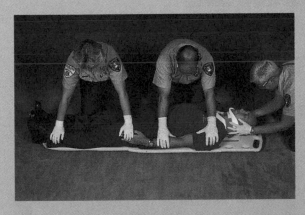

Figure 10-8D

A helper slides the board into position under **4** the patient's back and next to the side remaining on the ground (Figure 10-8D). D, Patient is partially rolled onto the longboard. Whether the board is placed flat on the ground, is held at an angle, or is placed flat against the patient's back is solely a matter of individual preference.

5 The patient is then rolled back onto the board in the same manner (Figure 10-8E). E, Patient has been completely logrolled onto the longboard. If the board was angled or upright, the patient and board are then lowered to the ground together. Keeping the patient in neutral alignment, adjust the patient's position so that he or she is centered on the board and a proper space exists between the top of the patient's head and the head end of the board.

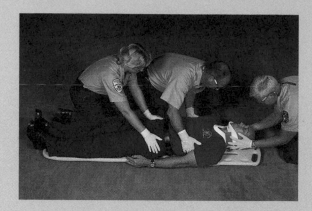

Figure 10-8E

LOGROLL: SEMIPRONE PATIENT

When the patient presents in a semiprone position, as shown in Figure 10-9A, a method similar to that for a supine patient is used. EMT #1 supports the head of the semiprone patient while EMT #2 positions the longboard. The method incorporates the same initial alignment of the patient's limbs, the same positioning of EMTs and hand placement, and the same responsibilities for maintaining alignment.

The EMT at the head positions his or her arms in anticipation of the full rotation that will occur. *With the semiprone logroll method, a cervical collar can only be safely applied once the patient is in an inline position and supine on the longboard, not before.*

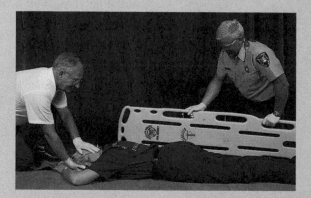

Figure 10-9A

1 The patient is rolled away from the direction in which his or her face initially points (Figure 10-9B). B, Patient is turned in the opposite direction from which his or her head was facing, while EMT #1 maintains neutral head support. EMTs #2 and #3 grasp the torso and lower extremities. This determines which side the EMTs place themselves. The head is rotated *less* than the torso, so that by the time the patient is on his or her side (perpendicular to the ground), the head and torso have come into proper alignment. EMT #3 must keep the pelvis and legs in alignment with the torso throughout the entire procedure.

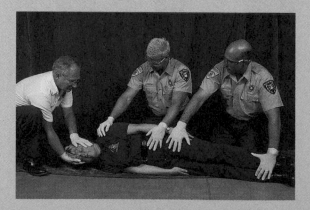

Figure 10-9B

Note: Two options exist in placing the long-board. Either (1) it can initially be placed on the ground 4 to 5 inches from the patient's side with the EMTs kneeling on it *or* (2) once the patient has been rolled onto his or her side, it can be inserted (on its side) longitudinally between the patient's back and the two EMTs at the patient's side. In either case the two EMTs supporting the body, while continuing to hold the patient steady, shuffle backward one at a time to provide space to continue rotating the patient.

Rotation of the patient is continued in the **2** same direction as before, and the patient or patient and board are rolled until on the ground and supine (Figure 10-9C). C, Patient is completely turned as a unit and maintained in a neutral position on the longboard. Neutral alignment is maintained throughout. A cervical collar is then applied and the patient's position on the board is adjusted as needed.

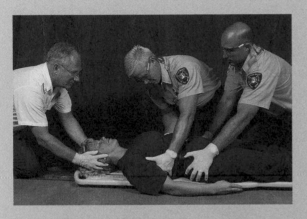

Figure 10-9C

LONGBOARD IMMOBILIZATION
ADULT

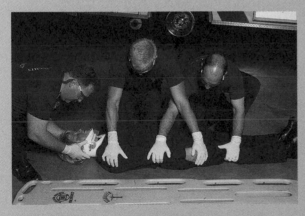

Move the head to a neutral in-line position **1** (unless contraindicated) and provide manual in-line immobilization. Using an acceptable method, position the patient on the longboard (Figure 10-10A).

Figure 10-10A

Immobilize the upper torso to the board so that **2** it cannot move up, down, or laterally. Then immobilize the lower torso (pelvis) to the board so that it cannot move up, down, or laterally, using either a strap over the iliac crests or groin loops. Readjust the torso straps as needed. Pad under the head as needed. Place pads or rolled blankets on each side of the head (Figure 10-10B).

Note: Immobilize the head to the board. Fasten a strap tightly over the pads and the lower forehead. Place a second strap over the pads and the rigid cervical collar and fasten it snugly to the board.

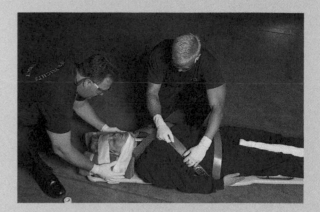

Figure 10-10B

3 Secure the legs to the board with straps proximal and distal to the knees. The distal strap must be tied so as to prevent lateral movement (Figure 10-11). EMTs immobilize the legs of a patient who has an X strap supporting the chest. Blanket rolls may be added at the lower legs for this purpose. Place the patient's extended arms palm-in along his or her sides and secure them (Figure 10-11). Patient is now completely immobilized on longboard.

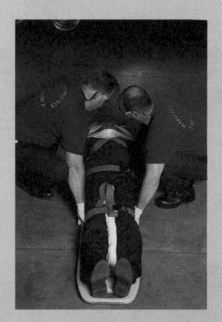

Figure 10-11

PEDIATRIC

Two major adjustments in the previous method are necessary when immobilizing a small child to a longboard.

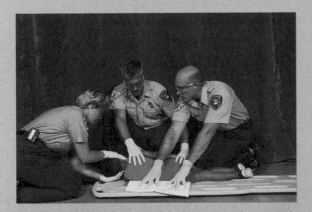

Figure 10-12

Due to the relatively large size of the child's head, padding is needed under the torso to elevate it and maintain the spine in neutral alignment. Figure 10-12 shows EMTs immobilizing a pediatric patient. The padding must extend from the lumbar area to the top of the shoulders, and to the right and left edges of the board. A folded blanket usually works well.

Note: Small children are usually narrower than an adult-size board. Blanket rolls can be placed between the child's sides and the sides of the board to prevent lateral movement. Pediatric-size devices take these differences into account and are preferable if available.

SPLIT LITTER/SCOOP STRETCHER (LONGBOARD ADAPTATION)

Always use the split litter in conjunction with a rigid longboard.

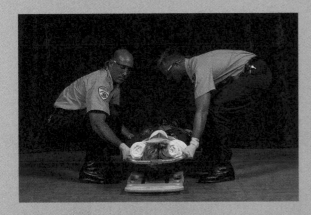

Figure 10-13A

The split litter is adjusted to the correct length, separated, inserted, and fastened according to its design. The patient is immobilized to it in the same way as to a longboard. Lift the split litter from the sides about 4 to 6 inches off the ground while a longboard is slid lengthwise under it (Figure 10-13A). **1**

Note: The split litter should *not* be picked up from the head and foot ends or used to carry the patient before it has been placed on a longboard, since it can sag without center support.

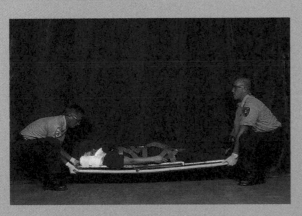

Figure 10-13B

Secure the split litter to the longboard. Since the patient is already fully immobilized, no additional immobilization should be necessary (Figure 10-13B). The longboard, split litter, and patient are then secured to the ambulance cot. **2**

STANDING LONGBOARD APPLICATION

There are two general methods for immobilizing a standing patient. One, for stable patients, involves strapping the torso, neck, and head prior to lowering the patient. The other method is intended for unstable patients who are unable to remain upright long enough to complete the immobilization using straps and ties. If the patient's condition or conditions at the scene do not allow time to mechanically immobilize the patient with straps while he or she is standing, the manual method should be used.

UNSTABLE PATIENTS (MANUAL METHOD)

1 Apply manual in-line immobilization from behind the patient and apply the cervical collar (Figure 10-14A).

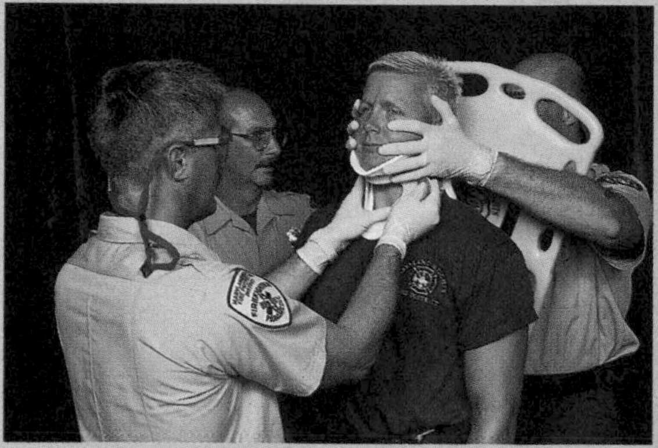

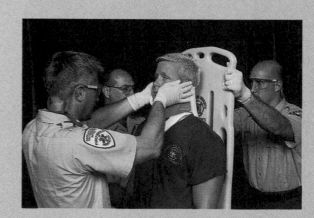

Figure 10-14A

OR

Apply manual in-line immobilization while facing the patient and apply the cervical collar (Figure 10-14B).

Figure 10-14B

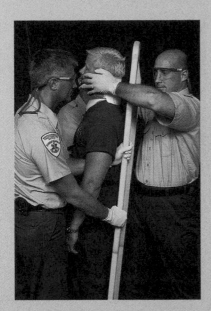

Figure 10-14C

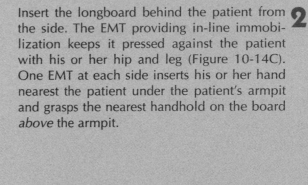

Insert the longboard behind the patient from the side. The EMT providing in-line immobilization keeps it pressed against the patient with his or her hip and leg (Figure 10-14C). One EMT at each side inserts his or her hand nearest the patient under the patient's armpit and grasps the nearest handhold on the board *above* the armpit.

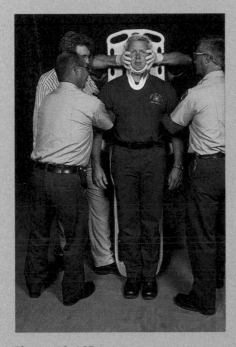

Figure 10-14D

Another rescuer or spectator places his or her foot or hands at the bottom of the board so that it cannot move. Next, each EMT grasps a handhold near the top of the board with a free hand. The EMTs lower the board partway to the ground, stopping about halfway down (Figure 10-14D).

4 The EMT holding the head must rotate his or her hands as shown without losing immobilization (Figure 10-14E). The EMTs at the sides may have to reposition their arms so that they will clear those of the EMT at the head when the board is fully lowered.

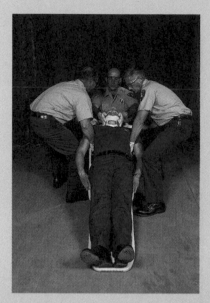

Figure 10-14E

5 Lower the board to the ground (Figure 10-14F). The EMT at the head must go from a standing to a kneeling position to avoid moving the head out of line, then immobilize the patient to the board.

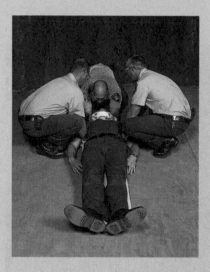

Figure 10-14F

STABLE PATIENTS

The rapid method for immobilizing a standing patient shown in the preceding method provides protection to the spine. However, if the patient is stable, mechanical immobilization of the torso, neck, and head prior to lowering provides more positive immobilization and is safer, affording less chance of movement. If time is not a key factor, it is the method of choice and should be used. The stability of the patient and scene should be the determining factors and not individual preference.

Note: Once manual in-line immobilization has been obtained from behind the patient, a cervical collar is applied and the longboard is inserted behind the patient from the side. Using any of the accepted methods for longboard immobilization, immobilize the upper and lower torso to the board. Rapidly reevaluate and adjust the torso straps. Pad behind the head as needed. Secure the head to the board. (Do not tie or immobilize the legs of a standing patient.) Once the torso, neck, and head have been immobilized to the board, the EMT at the head can release his or her hold on the patient's head. Have the patient hold his or her hands in front of him or her. With one EMT at each side of the board and one person holding the bottom of the board, lower the board to the ground. Do this in two distinct steps, stopping halfway down to adjust your hands. Once on the ground, complete the immobilization and tend to the patient's overall condition and injuries.

SITTING IMMOBILIZATION (VEST-TYPE EXTRICATION DEVICE)

Several brands of vest-type devices are available. Each model is slightly different in design, but any one can serve as a general example. The KED® is used in this demonstration. The EMT will have to modify the details (but not the general sequence) when using a different model or brand.

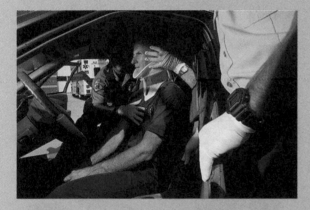

Figure 10-15A

Once manual in-line immobilization has been **1** initiated and a cervical collar applied, position the patient so he or she is sitting upright and an adequate space exists between his or her back and the seat. Insert the device between the patient and the vehicle seat (Figure 10-15A).

Note: Release and prepare the straps. Unfasten the two long straps (groin straps). Open the side flaps and place them around the patient's torso, under the arms.

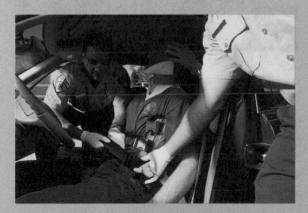

Figure 10-15B

Correctly position and fasten the torso straps. **2** Hold the vest so that its top is level with the top of the patient's head. (In other vests, it is usually with the flaps snugly in the armpits.) The middle strap is secured first, followed by the lower strap (Figure 10-15B). **B,** Once the vest is snugly fit under the armpits, the middle strap is secured first, followed by the lower strap. Connect the buckle, pull the strap tight, and adjust the buckle. Next, fasten the upper torso strap. The upper torso straps only support the midtorso from moving forward or laterally, but they do not prevent the vest from moving up or down; therefore they only need to be snug. Fastening them too tightly may result in inhibiting respiration.

3 Position and fasten each groin loop (Figure 10-15C). C, The groin straps are adjusted. Insert one of the long groin loop straps above the knee and, with a back-and-forth motion, work it under the thigh and buttock until it is in a straight line in the intergluteal fold from back to front. Position it in the crotch on one side of the genitalia. Bring the strap up the inner thigh, over the pelvis, and fasten it to the buckle on the same side of the vest so that the strap has formed a loop over one side of the pelvis. Repeat this procedure with the other strap. Fastening and adjusting only one side at a time prevents unwanted movement of the patient.

Note: Evaluate and readjust all torso straps as needed. Pad behind the head as needed. The square orange pads can be combined to fit a variety of dimensions. Position the head flaps. This will involve some careful changing of hand positions by the EMT supporting the head as another EMT places the flaps against the patient's head.

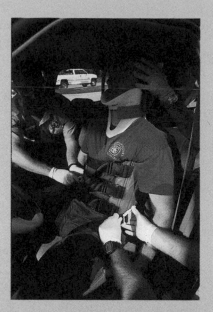

Figure 10-15C

4 Fasten the forehead strap (Figure 10-15D). D, Patient's forehead strap is applied. Place the nonskid surface over the supraorbital ridge as shown. Bring the ends straight back around the outside of the side flaps and affix them to the Velcro® so that the strap is very tight. Fasten the lower head strap. Place the center (open part) of the black neck strap over the rigid cervical collar. Fasten the ends to the Velcro® on the head flaps snugly, but not too tightly.

Warning: Avoid fastening these straps too high on the flaps, which can inhibit motion of the mandible and the patient's ability to open his or her mouth.

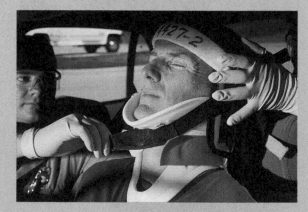

Figure 10-15D

Once the neck strap is secured, the sitting immobilization is completed and the torso, neck, and head are immobilized. The EMT behind the patient can now release manual immobilization and simply support the patient by holding the top of the vest.

With any vest or halfboard device, based on preference, the head straps can be replaced by using any type of self-adhering firm wrap, or with 2 to 3 inches of adhesive tape. Elastic or gauze bandages do not generally provide adequate secure fixation and immobilization and are therefore not recommended.

A NOTE ABOUT RIGID HALFBOARD DEVICES

Immobilization with a vest, halfboard, or shortboard follows the same basic steps and sequence. Once the device is inserted behind the manually immobilized patient who has had a cervical collar applied, the following steps are taken.

1. The device is immobilized to the upper torso.
2. The midtorso is fastened.
3. The device is then immobilized to the pelvis using a strap over the iliac crests or groin loops.
4. The torso straps are readjusted.
5. Padding is provided as needed behind the head.
6. The head is held between head pillows or blanket rolls.
7. Lastly, the head is immobilized by tape or straps.

Because these are the same steps that were described for vest-type devices, no separate detailed halfboard section has been included in this text.

Some halfboards only have a narrow head piece. Fastening the head with only straps does not adequately arrest rotation. Such a "sculptured board" should either be used with tape holding the head, or preferably by placing it upside down (sculptured part at the coccyx and the broader base at the upper torso and head) in conjunction with a commercial head immobilizer or blanket rolls and straps or tape.

Using a commercial head immobilizer system with a halfboard, or a halfboard system such as the Kansas Board®, which includes an effective head immobilizing system and prefastened torso straps, is easier and faster to use and therefore should be considered.

TRANSITION FROM VEST OR HALFBOARD TO FULL LONGBOARD

Once the application of a vest or halfboard has been completed, the patient is ready to be safely moved onto a longboard.

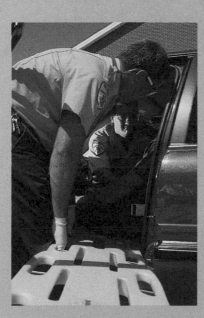

Figure 10-16A

If possible, the ambulance cot with a longboard on it should be brought to the opening of the car door. The board should be placed under or at least next to the patient's buttock, so that one end is securely supported on the car seat and the other end is on the ambulance cot (Figure 10-16A). A, The longboard is placed under the patient in a vest-type device. If a cot is not available, the longboard can be held by others while the patient and device are lifted out of the seat as a unit and placed on the longboard.

1

2 Rotate the patient and device in place and elevate the legs, lowering the patient and the device onto the longboard (Figure 16B). B, Patient is then turned onto the longboard. Slide the patient and device along the board until he or she is properly positioned. Lower the legs onto the board. If the groin straps have been placed over the pelvis correctly, they will only need to be loosened in obese or extremely muscular patients. Position the longboard on the ambulance cot.

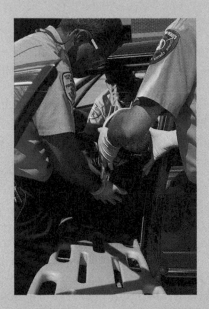

Figure 10-16B

3 Securely fasten the device to the longboard so that it cannot move in any direction. Remember, the torso, neck, and head are already immobilized. Immobilize the legs to the board. Secure the longboard and patient to the ambulance cot (Figure 10-16C).

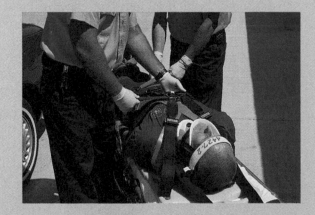

Figure 10-16C

RAPID EXTRICATION (SITTING PATIENT)

With sitting patients who are cardiodynamically unstable and who are suspected to have an unstable spine, the EMT will have to make an appropriate choice from two alternative methods: mechanical immobilization using a device as shown in previous methods, or use of the rapid extrication method, which provides only manual immobilization while the patient is turned and lowered directly to the longboard.

Immobilization to an interim device prior to moving provides more stable immobilization than when using only a manual method. However, it requires an additional 4 to 8 minutes to complete. The vest or halfboard methods should be used in the following situations:

- When the scene and patient's condition are stable and time is not an overriding primary concern.
- When a special rescue situation involving substantial lifting or technical rescue hoisting exists, and significant movement or carrying of the patient is involved before it is practical to complete the supine immobilization to a longboard or Stokes litter.

The rapid extrication method should be used only in the following situations:

- When the scene is unsafe and clear danger to the EMT and patient exists, necessitating rapid removal to a safe location.

- When the patient's condition is so unstable that he or she needs immediate intervention that can only be provided in a supine position and/or out of the vehicle, or when his or her condition requires immediate transport to the hospital without delay.
- When the patient blocks the EMT's access to other more seriously injured patients in the vehicle.

Rapid extrication should be selected only when time is a factor and not on the basis of personal preference.

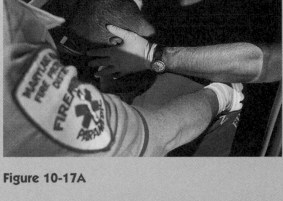

Figure 10-17A

EMT #1 gets behind the patient and brings the head into a neutral in-line position and provides manual immobilization (Figure 10-17A). **1**

OR

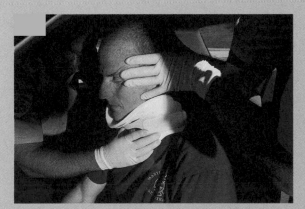

Figure 10-17B

When he or she cannot be behind the patient, this will have to be done from the side (Figure 10-17B). B, EMT #1 supports the patient's head from the side of the car while EMT #2 prepares to affix the cervical collar. EMTs #1 and #2 bring the patient to an upright sitting position.

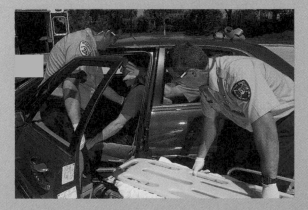

Figure 10-17C

A rapid assessment is performed and a cervical collar is applied. C, EMT #2 performs a rapid survey. While the patient is being assessed, the longboard is placed near the door (Figure 10-17C). D, EMT #3 brings a longboard and cot to the car and supports the patient's torso. If the open door presents an obstacle to two EMTs working outside the car in the doorway, the door can be manually forced back, springing the hinges as far as possible. **2**

3 While EMT #1 maintains manual immobilization of the head and EMT #2 supports the midthorax, EMT #3 works from the passenger's seat to free the patient's legs from the pedals and prepares to move them (Figure 10-17D). At EMT #2's command, EMT #2 and EMT #3 begin to rotate the patient until his or her back faces the open doorway and his or her feet are brought up onto the passenger's seat. This usually takes three or four short moves. EMT #1 follows the rotation, maintaining the neutral in-line positioning of the patient's head throughout. The rotation is coordinated with good voice commands by EMT #2, and it is done in short moves that quickly follow each other.

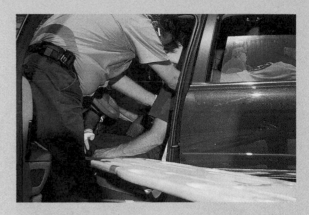

Figure 10-17D

Note: In many vehicles, EMT #1 will not be able to extend his or her arms far enough to complete the rotation from his or her original position. Either EMT #3 from the passenger's seat, or another EMT from outside the driver's door, will have to provide manual stabilization of the head when EMT #1 runs out of room. If EMT #3 does this, EMT #1 can get out of the car, reposition him or herself in the driver's doorway, and retake the manual immobilization.

4 The rotation is completed when the patient's back is squarely facing the open doorway and his or her feet are on the passenger's seat (Figure 10-17E). The longboard is now inserted on the car seat at the patient's buttock, and EMT #2 and the EMT holding the patient's head lower him or her onto the longboard (Figure 10-17F). F, At the command of EMT #2, the patient is rotated onto the longboard.

Note: In the previous steps, exact roles and positioning of each of the three EMTs has been indicated. This only represents one example, as very few field extrication situations are ideal. As long as the manual immobilization of the head is maintained without interruption and the spine is maintained in-line without unwanted movement, any positioning of the

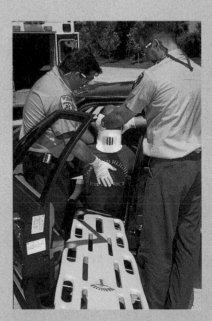

Figure 10-17E

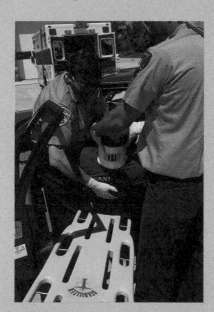

Figure 10-17F

EMTs that works can be used. However, care should be taken to avoid numerous position changes and hand position takeovers, as they invite a lapse in immobilization.

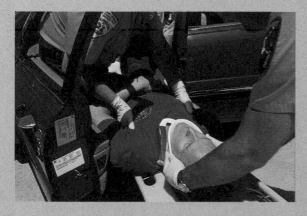

Figure 10-17G

Once the patient's torso is down on the board, **5** EMT #2 places his or her hands in the patient's armpits and EMT #3 positions him- or herself to move the patient's legs and hips, and all EMTs prepare to slide the patient up the longboard (Figure 10-17G).

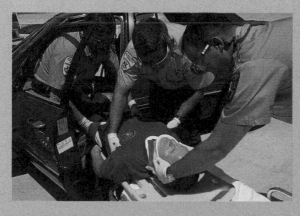

Figure 10-17H

With the EMT at the head setting the pace, the **6** patient is slid in 6 to 12 inch increments up the board until his or her hips are fully on the board (Figure 10-17H). The EMT at the legs will have to move across the inside of the car on the seat. Do not attempt to move the patient all the way in one step. Moving in increments, teamwork, and good communication are all necessary in order to move the patient as a unit without compressing or distracting the spine.

Note: When the patient's hips are on the board, EMT #3 (at the feet) can exit the car and come to the driver's door to assist in further moving of the patient onto the longboard. Frequently EMT #2 takes over responsibility for the hips and legs at this point, and EMT #3 takes over control of the upper torso. If additional EMTs are available, time can be saved by having one of them assume this position. With the EMT at the head now giving the orders, the patient is again slid in 6- to 12-inch increments up the board until he or she is fully positioned on it. Once the patient is properly positioned on the longboard, and with the EMT at the head giving the commands, the patient and the board are lifted and moved away from the car.

What is important now is that the EMTs act in accordance with whatever caused them to use the rapid extrication method in the first place. If the scene is dangerously unsafe, the EMTs (while maintaining the manual in-line immobilization) should immediately carry the board and the patient away from the danger without spending time tying or strapping the patient to the board. If rapid removal was done due to the seriousness of the patient's condition, then the EMTs should immediately begin resuscitation and treatment without carrying the patient away. If the ambulance cannot be positioned near the patient, a decision must be made whether the patient's condition will allow him or her to be moved to the vehicle or if treatment must be started immediately with portable equipment before the patient is moved to the ambulance.

Note: The rapid extrication technique can effectively provide manual in-line immobilization of the head, neck, and torso throughout the patient's removal from the vehicle. Three points are key factors:

1 At all times one EMT must immobilize the head, another must rotate and immobilize the torso, and a third must move and control the legs.

2 In-line immobilization of the head and torso will be nearly impossible to maintain if the EMTs attempt to move the patient in one continuous motion. It is important to limit each movement, stopping to reposition and prepare for the next step. Undue haste will actually cause delay and may result in movement of the spine.

It has already been noted that many acceptable variations exist, and each is "right" as long as it follows the general principles for this maneuver. It is also important to note that each victim (body size) and each vehicle (design and body size) require some variation from others. A "luxury" size four-door car is relatively easy to work in, while a four-wheel drive pickup truck presents a different environment. The EMTs must practice this technique with different crews and in different vehicles to be best prepared to deal with a real situation.

RAPID EXTRICATION (SUPINE PATIENT)

When a patient is found lying on the seat or floor of a car or on the ceiling of an overturned car, a modified version of the rapid extrication technique can be used to provide manual immobilization while moving and sliding him or her directly onto the longboard.

HELMET REMOVAL

Patients wearing full-face helmets must have the helmet removed early in the assessment process to provide immediate access to the airway and face, to ensure that hidden bleeding is not occurring into the posterior helmet, and to allow the head to be moved (from the flexed position caused by large helmets) into neutral alignment. Explain to the victim what is going to happen. If the patient indicates that he or she was told that the helmet should not be removed, explain that untrained spectators should not remove a helmet, but that properly trained personnel (you) can remove it by protecting the victim's spine. Two EMTs are required for this maneuver.

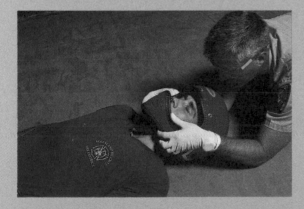

Figure 10-18A

The first EMT kneels above the patient's head. With palms pressed on the sides of the helmet and fingertips curled over its lower margin, he or she immobilizes the helmeted head in as close to a neutral in-line position as the helmet allows (Figure 10-18A). A, EMT #1 performs manual immobilization of the head and neck. To ensure that immobilization is not lost if the helmet is loose, the curled fingers should use the mandible as support for the head, not the helmet.

2 The second EMT kneels alongside the patient's torso and opens (or removes) the face shield, checks the airway and breathing, and undoes (or cuts, if necessary) the chin strap (Figure 10-18B). Then the second EMT places one hand so that the mandible is grasped between the thumb at the angle of the mandible on one side and the first two fingers at the angle at the other side. He or she places the other hand under the neck on the occiput of the skull and takes over the in-line immobilization of the head.

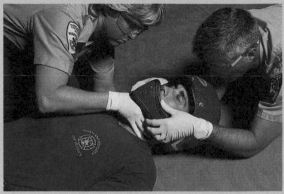

Figure 10-18B

3 The first EMT now releases his or her hold on the mandible. EMT #1 pulls the sides of the helmet slightly apart, away from the sides of the head (Figure 10-18C). The helmet is rotated so that the lower end of the facepiece rotates toward him or her and is elevated, clearing the patient's nose. EMT #1 then carefully pulls the helmet in a straight line off the patient's head.

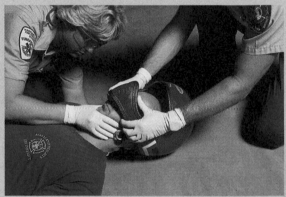

Figure 10-18C

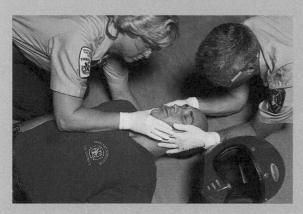

Figure 10-18D

The first EMT is now ready to remove the helmet completely. The helmet is rotated about 30° following the curve of the head. This causes the posterior lower margin of the helmet to point caudally rather than anteriorly. Now the helmet can safely be removed in a straight line toward the EMT's abdomen. Once the helmet has been fully removed, the first EMT again takes hold of the head and provides manual in-line immobilization from that position. The assessment is continued and a cervical collar is applied (Figure 10-18D). D, EMT #1 maintains head immobilization while EMT #2 prepares to apply the cervical collar.

Note: Two key elements are involved in removing a helmet.
- While one EMT provides immobilization, the other moves. Both EMTs *never* move their hands at the same time.
- The helmet must be rotated in different directions: to first clear the nose, and then to clear the back of the head.

CHAPTER OBJECTIVES

CHAPTER 11

Musculoskeletal Trauma

At the completion of this course the student will be able to:

- List the four groups used to classify patients with extremity injuries and relate this to priority of care.

- Describe the primary and secondary surveys as related to extremity trauma.

- List the five major pathophysiologic problems that require management in extremity injuries.

- Indicate an understanding of the relationship between hemorrhage and open and closed fractures.

- List the four primary signs and symptoms of extremity trauma; list other signs and symptoms that can indicate less obvious extremity injury.

- Explain the management of extremity trauma, especially in the presence of life-threatening injuries.

- Indicate an understanding of splints and splinting methods.

- Describe the special considerations involved in femur fracture management.

- Describe the management of amputations.

Scenario

You are called to the scene where a 22-year-old woman was playing in a football game. The patient states that she was going out for a pass when she was hit by the cornerback while jumping to catch the ball. The patient, Lisa, states that she has no pain except for in her right leg. Upon assessment, no other trauma is noted except for a swelling approximately 5 to 6 inches in diameter to her right midfemur region. Her vitals are as follows: pulse 120, respiratory rate of 22, BP 106/78. While packaging the patient for transport, she asks, "What are you doing? What is taking so long?" She then begins thrashing about. While trying to calm Lisa, she becomes more agitated and tries to hit your partner.

- What would you do at this point?
- What other interventions might you perform at this time?
- What is your number one concern at this time? And why?
- Outline the steps you would take in order of priority.

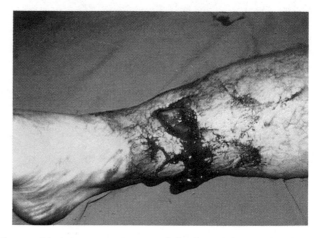

Figure 11-1 An open injury of the lower leg with protruding bone ends. (From Vallaton, J., and Dubas, F. *Color Atlas of Mountain Medicine,* London: Wolfe Medical Publications, Ltd., 1991.)

Extremity injury, though quite common in most trauma patients, will rarely pose an immediate life-threatening condition. Extremity trauma can be life threatening when it produces severe blood loss (hemorrhage), either externally or from internal bleeding into an extremity.

The first priority in the management of patients with extremity injuries is the same as for patients with injuries to other areas of the body: care for life-threatening conditions first. When caring for the multisystem trauma patient, the EMT has two primary considerations with regard to extremity injuries. First, the EMT must not overlook a life-threatening condition in the extremities or a life-threatening condition caused by an extremity injury. Second, the presence of horrible looking but noncritical extremity injuries must not distract the EMT from caring for life-threatening injuries to other areas of the body (Figure 11-1).

If a life-threatening or potentially life-threatening condition is revealed anywhere in the body during the primary assessment, the EMT should not continue with an itemized secondary assessment. Any deficiencies found during the primary assessment *must* be corrected before moving to the secondary assessment. This may mean delaying secondary assessment until en route or even until arrival at the emergency department.

Each multisystem or critical trauma patient should be secured to a longboard in a supine position, with as much normal anatomic positioning as possible, to allow for resuscitation. This positioning is called **anatomic splinting.** Securing the patient to the longboard can effectively support and splint every bone and joint. This can be done in an efficient manner and will not detract from focusing on

critical conditions. It *is not* the responsibility of the EMT to differentiate between the types of musculoskeletal injuries. It *is* the responsibility of the EMT to identify and treat life-threatening injuries and, if time permits, to identify and stabilize extremity injuries—either grossly with anatomic splinting on a spine board, or if time and condition of the patient allows, with specific splinting devices.

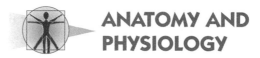

ANATOMY AND PHYSIOLOGY

Of the 206 bones in the human body, those of the upper extremity (beginning at the clavicle and ending at the distal phalanx of each finger) and those of the lower extremity (beginning with the pelvis and ending at the distal phalanx of each toe) are the main consideration of this chapter (see Figure 9-4, p. 190). All of these bones have muscles attached to them that allow each bone to perform its designated function for the body (Figure 11-2). It is not the purpose of this chapter to review these muscles and bones in detail; that is part of the EMT-Basic and the EMT-Paramedic training program. However, to function properly as an EMT in caring for the trauma patient, it is important to be aware of each of these bones and muscles. Loss of integrity at the proximal aspect of an extremity can cause functional damage to the distal aspect of the extremity. Therefore, the EMT should understand the location of the major bones and muscles. The exact names of some are important, whereas with others a knowledge of their existence and what they do may be all that is necessary to properly care for the patient. Figures 9-4 and 11-2 will aid in a review of the bones and muscles. The types of joints should also be reviewed and are listed in Table 11-1.

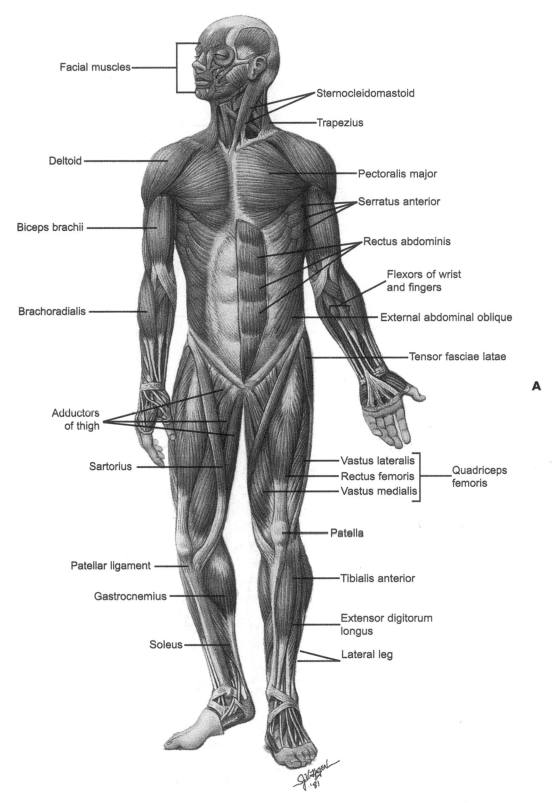

Figure 11-2 The muscular system. A, Anterior view. (From Seeley, R.R.; Stephens, T.D.; and Tate, P. *Essentials of Anatomy and Physiology.* St. Louis: Mosby–Year Book, Inc., 1991.)

Continued

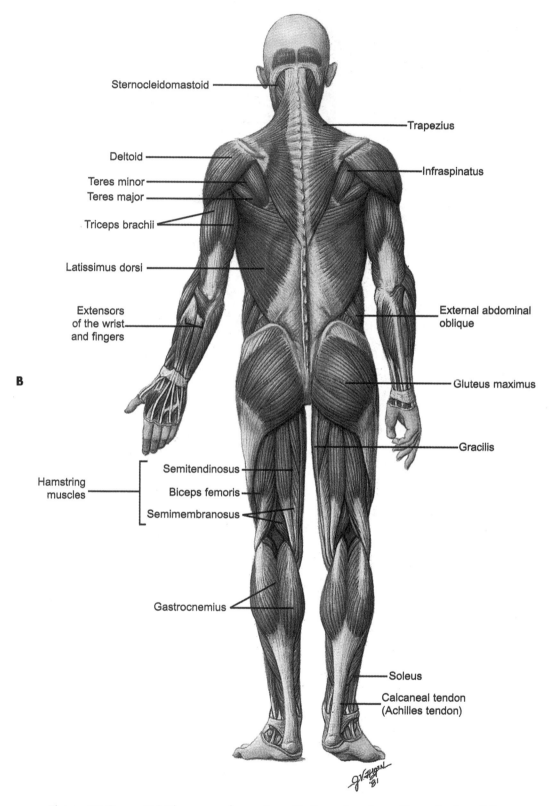

B

Figure 11-2, cont'd The muscular system. B, Posterior view. (From Seeley, R.R.; Stephens, T.D.; and Tate, P. *Essentials of Anatomy and Physiology.* St. Louis: Mosby–Year Book, Inc., 1991.)

Table 11-1 Types of joints

Joint	Example
ball-and-socket	shoulder, acetabulum
hinge	elbow, knee
gliding	vertebrae, radioulnar
saddle	carpal-metacarpal
minimal motion	sacroiliac
pivot	atlas-axis

PATHOPHYSIOLOGY

MECHANISM OF INJURY

Determining mechanism of injury is one of the single most important aspects of the EMT's job (see Chapter 1: Kinematics of Trauma). The EMT should be able to reconstruct in slow motion and visually picture the series of events that caused the injuries to the patient's body. If the patient fell 20 feet off of a ladder, this should help the EMT know what parts of the body to assess for injuries, such as calcanus, hip, lumbar spine, or C-spine fractures. If a driver of a vehicle that struck a pole head on did not have his or her seat restraint applied properly, or not at all, the EMT would look for injuries to the head, neck, back, and so on. Did the patient take an up-and-over path or a down-and-under path in the car at the time of impact? It is the responsibility of the EMT to be the eyes and ears of the physician. Information may be obtained from bystanders, the patient's family, or anyone that might have witnessed the incident. It is particularly important to determine the mechanism of injury because it raises suspicion of injuries that may not be immediately apparent. This information should be reported to the receiving hospital and documented on the run report.

INJURIES TO THE BONES

Injuries to the extremities have four major problems that require management by the EMT. These are hemorrhage, instability (fractures and dislocations), soft-tissue injury (strains and sprains), and loss of tissue (amputation).

Hemorrhage

Hemorrhage is the escape of blood from the vessels of the vascular system. The torn vessels can be large or small. The ability of the body to respond to and control these tears is a function of the size of the vessel, the presence of clotting factors, and the ability of the vessel to go into spasm. Initially, the rate of blood loss is directly propor-

tional to the size of the opening in the vessel and the pressure inside the vessel. This was described by Bernoulli, the Swiss mathematician, with the following equation. (The specifics of the equation are "nice-to-know information"; the principle itself is very important.)

$$Q = \frac{AP + 2V}{E}$$

where Q = rate of leakage, A = area of laceration, P = transmural pressure (intraluminal pressure minus extraluminal pressure), E = density of fluid media, and V = velocity of fluid flow (inside the vessel).

The blood flow or rate of leakage out of the laceration in the vessel is proportional to the difference in the intraluminal pressure and the extraluminal pressure, and the size of the hole in the vessel wall. The first step in the management of hemorrhage should be to increase the extramural pressure (pressure on skin or over laceration) by increasing external pressure on the area overlying the injury. Increasing external pressure actually serves two purposes: (1) It reduces the differential pressure (intraluminal pressure minus the extraluminal pressure), and (2) it compresses the sides of the torn vessel, reducing the area of the opening, both of which reduce blood flow out of the vessel. Although the body has other mechanisms of hemorrhage control such as clotting factors and vessel spasm, the EMT has the most control over the mechanical measures (compression).

Instability of the Bone or Joint

Tears of the supporting structures of a joint, fracture of a bone, or major muscle/tendon injury can diminish the capability of the extremity to support itself. Any of these circumstances may require some type of external support for the extremity. The two divisions of instability to the bone or joint are fractures and dislocations.

Fractures

If a bone is fractured, the bone should be immobilized so that it reduces the potential of continued injury and pain to the patient. Movement of the sharp ends of bone inside the soft tissue of muscle and in the vicinity of vessels and nerves can produce significant additional injuries.

The two general types of fractures that the EMT should recognize are open fractures and closed fractures.

Closed fractures are fractures in which the bone(s) has(ve) been broken, but there is no loss of skin integrity (Figure 11-3). Closed fractures can range in seriousness from a hairline fracture (a crack along the shaft of the bone) to a comminuted fracture (splintering or crushing of a bone).

Closed fractures may produce additional sources for major internal hemorrhage into the tissue compartments. An example is the closed femur fracture. Closed fractures can result in blood loss of approximately 500 cc per

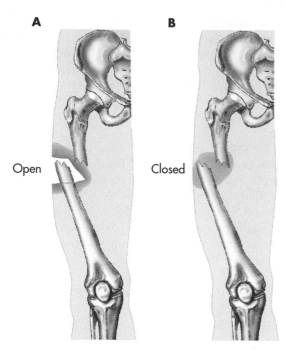

A **B**

Open   Closed

Figure 11-3 Open vs. closed fracture. (From Thibodeau G.A. *The Human Body in Health and Disease.* 2nd ed. St. Louis: Mosby, 1997.)

fracture. A femur may be broken in several places or the fracture may be comminuted. Each site has potential for large amounts of blood loss by laceration of the vessels or the very vascular muscles near the fracture site. A total blood loss of 1,000 cc to 2,000 cc per thigh can occur. Due to the natural tamponade effect of the surrounding tissue, muscles, and skin, smaller quantities of hemorrhage are more common.

Another example of a fracture that may result in a large volume blood loss is a pelvic fracture. As a blood manufacturing center of the body the pelvis has a large blood supply, and there are multiple vascular plexes that lie adjacent to the pelvis especially on the inner surface. An unstable pelvis associated with a rapidly distending abdomen is an indication of large blood loss, and rapid transportation to the hospital is required. As with other fractures, compression and fracture stabilization are important to control hemorrhage. The pneumatic antishock garment (PASG) is very helpful in doing this job. This is one of the conditions where there is no controversy that the PASG works and works well (see Chapter 6: Shock and Fluid Resuscitation).

Open fractures are those in which the integrity of the skin has been interrupted. They are usually caused by the bone ends perforating the skin from the inside or by crushing or laceration of the skin by an object at the time of the injury. A laceration caused by the bone ends is common. This laceration may or may not cause a gross hemorrhage. The EMT should not try to replace the bones;

however, the bones occasionally return to almost near normal position due to realignment by the EMT or by the muscle spasms that usually occur with fractures. Complications of open fractures include external hemorrhage, further damage to the muscles and nerves, and contamination.

Dislocations

Joints are held together by ligaments between the bones and are held to muscles by tendons. Joint movement is accomplished by muscles contracting (shortening). This reduction of the muscle length pulls on the tendons that are attached to a bone and then moves the extremity. A **dislocation** is a separation of two bones at the joint, whereas a fracture is a separation of two pieces of bone. A dislocation produces an area of instability that must be secured. Dislocations can produce a great deal of pain, difficult to distinguish from a fracture. Individuals with prior dislocations have a more lax supporting structure and can have frequent dislocations. These patients usually know what the problem is and can help in assessment and stabilization. This is another situation where the patient has important information about his or her own condition; you should listen to what the patients have to say.

Soft Tissue Injury

Injuries to the muscles and ligaments are more common than injuries to the bones. Injuries to these soft tissues occur when a joint or muscle is either torn or stretched beyond its normal limits. Strains and sprains are two types of these injuries. Although it is not necessary for the EMT to differentiate between these two injuries, it is necessary to understand the pathophysiology of each.

Strains

A **strain** is a soft tissue injury or muscle spasm that occurs around a joint anywhere in the musculature. This injury involves only the muscles surrounding the joint, not the ligaments or tendons. Strains are characterized by pain with movement, with little or no swelling.

Sprains

A **sprain** is an injury in which ligaments are stretched, or even partially torn. Sprains are characterized by extreme pain, swelling, and possible hematoma. Externally, they may look like a fracture. Sprains are caused by a sudden twisting of the joint beyond its normal range of motion. The only definitive differentiation between a sprain and a fracture is through use of an X ray.

Loss of Tissue

When tissue has been totally separated from the extremity, the tissue is completely without nutrition and

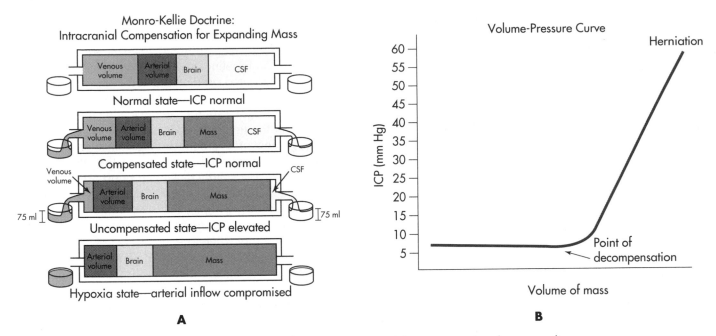

Figure 11-4 A, Monro-Kellie doctrine: Intracranial compensation for expanding mass. The volume of the intracranial contents remains constant. If the addition of a mass such as a hematoma results in the squeezing out of an equal volume of cerebrospinal fluid *(CSF)* and venous blood, the intracranial pressure *(ICP)* remains normal. However, when this compensatory mechanism is exhausted, there is an exponential increase in ICP for even a small additional increase in the volume of the hematoma, as shown in B, volume-pressure curve. (Data from Narayan, R.K. "Head Injury," In Grossman, R.G., and Hamilton, W.J., eds. *Principles of Neurosurgery.* New York: Raven Press, 1991: 267.)

oxygenation. This injury is called **amputation or avulsion.** Initially bleeding may be severe, but the body's defense mechanism causes the vessels around the site to constrict, and the blood loss may become minimal. Local trauma can break apart the clots or interrupt the spasm, and bleeding will reoccur.

The longer the extremity is without oxygen the less likely it will be that the amputated portion can be replaced successfully. Cooling the amputated body part—without freezing it—will reduce the metabolic rate and help to prolong this critical time.

Compartment Syndrome

Compartment syndrome occurs when a structure in an enclosed space is deprived of blood supply because the vessels have been compressed to the point where they cannot supply adequate oxygen to prevent anaerobic metabolism.

When cells are deprived of oxygen, they become anoxic. When cells become anoxic, they swell. When cells swell, they impinge on the structures that surround them. When these structures are vessels, the lumen is reduced in size. When the size is reduced, the blood flow is less; when the blood flow is less, the cells are deprived

of oxygen; and on, and on, and on. The cycle repeats itself.

Two types of material exist in the body: those that are compressible and those that are not. Hollow tubes and spaces that connect to the outside of the compartment are compressible because the fluid can be squeezed out or simply not allowed to enter. In the skull this is called the Monro-Kellie doctrine (Figure 11-4). In the abdomen and extremities it is called a compartment syndrome. In the thoracic compartment it is called a tension pneumothorax or a cardiac tamponade. Although the outcome in each body region may differ, the physiology is the same.

Any space occupying mass in a closed compartment in the extremity, such as a large hematoma, will reduce the amount of space that can be occupied by other things in this space. The most common occurrence is a reduction in the the size of the arteries, capillaries, and veins so that less blood can flow though them. This reduction of blood flow reduces the amount of oxygen delivered to the cells, which produces ischemia and leads to anaerobic metabolism. This causes the cells to swell, which further increases the pressure inside the space and further reduces the flow. The ischemia and anaerobic metabolism worsen, which leads to more swelling and more pressure. At some point in this process the cells began to die. The cells most sensitive to this process are the same in other parts of the body (brain cells) The peripheral nerves are an extension of the brain and therefore are the first to feel the effects of the ischemia.

This condition is cyclic, and if not recognized and corrected it can be an emergent situation. This syndrome also compromises the tissue distal to the injury, and the distal tissue does not receive the nutrients it requires.

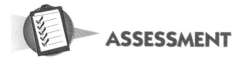

ASSESSMENT

MECHANISM OF INJURY

Mechanism of injury is one of the most important things the EMT should assess. As stated earlier, the EMT is the person on the scene who should be aware and look for evidence of what happened before, during, and after the incident and events that led to its occurrence. Not only should the EMT ask questions of bystanders, family, and the patient, but the EMT should also look around and evaluate the scene. If a car was involved, how much damage was sustained by the car? Are there any skid marks on the street? For a stab wound, how big was the knife? Was the knife wound made by a man or a woman? How far was the fall? All of this information is very important for understanding the patient's injuries, and the information must be collected and documented by the EMT (see Chapter 1: Kinematics of Trauma).

GROSS ASSESSMENT

Primary assessment addresses the most important life-threatening conditions that the EMT can evaluate and treat. If the patient has no life-threatening injuries, the EMT should proceed to the secondary assessment.

In the secondary assessment, the EMT should visually assess for swelling, lacerations, abrasions, hematomas, color, movement, and deformity. The EMT should feel for pulses, temperature, crepitation, and movement. It is also important to listen. If the patient is conscious, question him or her about sensation, pain, and mechanism of injury, and ask the patient to describe how the pain feels. Voluntary movement of the extremities tests for neurologic and muscular involvement.

Lacerations may bleed a little or a lot. As noted previously, pressure is the best method of control initially. Hemorrhage contained within the skin will produce swelling and ecchymosis (bruising). Hematomas and deformity may indicate a closed fracture. Pain indicates potential serious injury unless there is a loss of sensation to that area from nerve injury.

Pulses, movement, and sensation are an important part of the initial and ongoing assessments. Lack of pulses, movement, and/or sensation indicate a lack of blood flow or neurologic defects. An initial assessment is performed to establish a baseline and identify initial injury. Reassessment repeated on multiple occasions is performed to identify changes.

Crepitus is both a sound and the feeling the bones can make when the fractured ends rub together. It is caused by the grating of the bone ends against one another. Crepitus can be elicited by palpating the site of injury and sounds like a snap, crackle, and pop. Another analogy is the popping of bubble packing. Although this feeling of bones grating against each other is frequently noted during the assessment of the patient, it can produce further injury. Therefore, once it is noted, additional and repetitive steps to produce it should not be used. Crepitus is a distinct sound and feeling that is not easily forgotten.

Auscultation assists in locating a fracture: Placing a stethoscope on the symphysis pubis and percussing over the patella will detect sound when the bones are intact, but none when a fracture is present.

It is virtually impossible to rule out a fracture by physical examination in the field, regardless of the examiner's skill level. Many fractures can be asymptomatic, especially immediately after the injury when the muscles may contract and hold the bone ends together. Many times sprains or strains can present signs and symptoms identical to those of a fracture. In addition, the patient may be distracted from the presence of a fracture by the presence of other injuries, or the patient may be unconscious and unable to inform the EMT of the extent of his or her pain or injuries. The presence of a fracture can only be ruled out by appropriate radiographic evaluation of the injured part. Therefore, if in doubt, treat the injury as a fracture.

ARTERIAL HEMORRHAGE

External arterial bleeding should be identified during the primary assessment and controlled after the airway and breathing are stabilized. This type of bleeding can usually be assessed easily, but sometimes there is difficulty when blood is hidden under the patient and/or in heavy or dark clothing. All clothing should be removed. The EMT cannot assess what cannot be seen. Continued swelling of an extremity is potentially a hematoma and is indicative of internal arterial hemorrhage.

External hemorrhage that has occurred prior to the arrival of EMS personnel can be estimated by taking a few seconds to scan the surrounding area and visualize the amount of blood present. Estimation of blood loss becomes more difficult if the patient has been moved from the site of injury or when blood has been (1) concealed by waterproof or dark-colored clothing, (2) absorbed through the surface the patient is lying on, or (3) washed away in water or by rain. Overt signs of blood loss may not always be apparent.

The EMT should rapidly assess the potential blood loss caused by extremity trauma. This will help the EMT evaluate the potential of blood loss that will lead to decreased perfusion and shock. Such advance knowledge will prepare the EMT for the possibility of systemic deterioration and indicate initial steps to prevent its occurrence. *Life-threatening hemorrhage and shock, regardless of the source, should be immediately identified and managed as part of the primary assessment.*

OPEN AND CLOSED FRACTURES

Open fractures may be easy to locate on a trauma patient (Figure 11-5). These injuries can be associated by bleeding. Bone ends may or may not be visible. Any open wound near a possible fracture should be considered an open fracture and treated as such. Pulses, movement, sensation, and color should be initially assessed and reassessed continuously as with any fracture.

Closed fractures are usually accompanied with swelling and hematomas. Crepitus may or may not be present. Pulses, movement, sensation, and color must be assessed and reassessed continuously for changes.

Strains and sprains may appear like a closed fracture. Since these injuries can only be differentiated by radiorophy, treat strains and sprains as if they are closed fractures.

JOINTS AND DISLOCATIONS

Dislocations of all bony injuries are the most easy to discover during physical examination (Figures 11-6 and 11-7). This injury usually involves a great deal of pain to the patient. Pain and deformity usually are the initial findings. Gentle examination will identify that the bones on

either side of the joint are out of position. Attempted motion of the joint will usually produce pain and may not be possible since the bones are locked by the abnormal relationship. Hematomas are not usually found with dislocations since the joint has only minimal blood supply. The exception is the knee. The close proximity of the popliteal artery and the strong attachments of this vessel to the femur and the tibia make it vulnerable to damage.

PELVIC FRACTURE

One of the major complications with a pelvic fracture is bleeding (Figures 11-8 and 11-9). Because of the amount

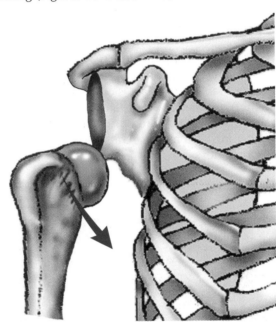

Figure 11-6 A dislocation is a separation of a bone from a joint. (From McSwain, N.E. *The Basic EMT.* St. Louis: Mosby, 1997.)

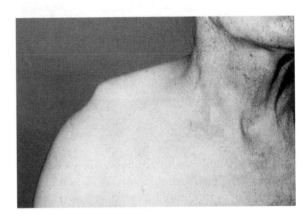

Figure 11-7 Dislocation of the acromioclavicular joint. (From London, P.S. *A Colour Atlas of Diagnosis after Recent Injury.* London: Wolfe Medical Publications, Ltd., 1990.)

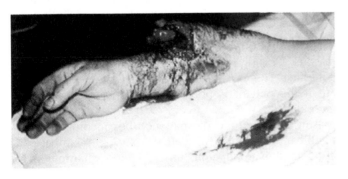

Figure 11-5 Open fracture. (From London, P.S. *A Colour Atlas of Diagnosis after Recent Injury.* London: Wolfe Medical Publications, Ltd., 1990.)

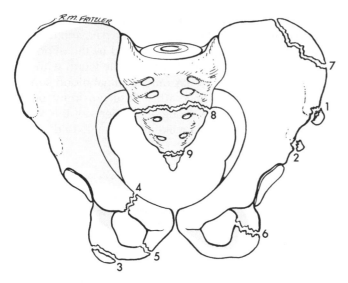

Figure 11-8 Fractures of individual pelvic bones. *1,* Avulsion of anterosuperior iliac spine; *2,* avulsion of anteroinferior iliac spine; *3,* avulsion of ischial tuberosity; *4,* fracture of superior pubic ramus; *5,* fracture of inferior pubic ramus; *6,* fracture of ischial ramus; *7,* fracture of iliac wing; *8,* transverse fracture of sacrum; *9,* fracture of coccyx.

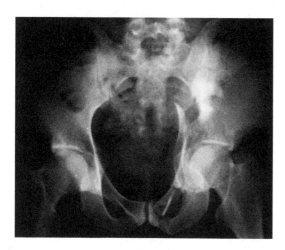

Figure 11-9 Pelvic radiograph demonstrating a complex comminuted fracture of the left hemipelvis. (Courtesy Riverside Methodist Hospitals, Columbus, Ohio.)

of space within the pelvic cavity, a lot of hemorrhage may occur with few external signs of difficulty. The first indication of difficulty may be the onset of shock. Therefore, patients with pelvic fractures should be closely observed for the development of shock, and the precaution of IV access should be obtained as soon as practicable.

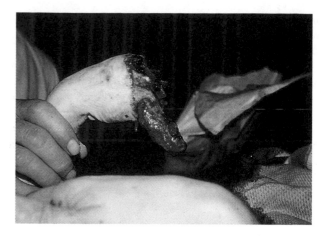

Figure 11-10 Hand with a nearly amputated thumb and amputated fingers. (From London, P.S. *A Colour Atlas of Diagnosis after Recent Injury.* London: Wolfe Medical Publications, Ltd., 1990.)

AMPUTATIONS

Amputations are evident to the EMT as he or she approaches the scene (Figure 11-10). This type of injury receives a great deal of attention from bystanders, and the patient may or may not know the extremity is missing. Psychologically this injury must be dealt with cautiously. If the patient does not know the extremity is missing, to tell him or her about the injury on scene may or may not be beneficial. The patient may not be ready to deal with the loss of a limb and should be told by someone after being stabilized. The patient needs to be told of the amputation in a controlled environment, and the scene of an incident is not a controlled environment. Effort must be made to try and locate the missing extremity. The hospital staff may be able to reattach the extremity. With the advances of modern medicine, it is often possible to reattach the extremity and regain function. Even if it is not possible to regain complete function of the extremity, partial function may be regained. Because of the psychologic trauma of the loss of a limb, even if function will not be regained, the hospital personnel may feel the limb should be replaced for cosmetic reasons. Do not get sidetracked; the ABC steps must be done first. The look of an amputation may be horrifying, but if the patient is not breathing, the loss of limb is secondary.

Amputations may or may not be accompanied by significant bleeding. The patient may complain of pain distal to the amputation; this is called **phantom pain.** Phantom pain is the sensation that pain still exists after an extremity is removed. The reason for phantom pain is not understood completely, but it may be because the brain does not realize the extremity is not present. The brain sends a message to the limb and does not get an answer, so the brain assumes the limb is experiencing pain.

COMPARTMENT SYNDROME

Any injury to an extremity has the potential to cause a compartment syndrome. Signs and symptoms of compartment syndrome are: (1) pain greater than expected that typically increases by passive stretching of the involved muscles, (2) decreased sensation or functional loss of the nerves distal to the injury, and (3) tense swelling of the involved area. The 6 P's are the most important signs to assess: for (1) pain, (2) pulselessness, (3) paralysis, (4) paresthesia, (5) pallor, and (6) puffiness. A palpable distal pulse usually is present in a compartment syndrome. Since nerves are the most sensitive part of the body, one of the first signs of compartment syndrome is paresthesia of the web space. The web space is the space between the thumb and the first finger, and the space between the first and second toes. If the patient has no feeling in this space, the EMT should be suspicious of compartment syndrome. Weakness or paralysis of involved muscles and loss of pulses in the affected extremity are late signs of compartment syndrome.

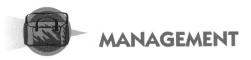 ## MANAGEMENT

The following priorities must be considered and followed at all times when managing a patient with extremity injuries:

First: Manage any life-threatening conditions.
Second: Manage any limb-threatening conditions.
Third: Manage all other conditions (if time allows).

Adherence to these priorities does not imply that extremity injuries are to be ignored or that injured extremities should not be protected from further harm. It does mean that in multisystem trauma patients with extremity injuries that are not life threatening, abbreviated general measures are used to care for the extremity injuries. This will allow the EMT's main focus to remain on those injuries and conditions that directly threaten the patient's life. The easiest and fastest way to accomplish abbreviated care of extremity injuries is to correctly immobilize the patient onto a longboard.

Patients with life-threatening conditions in addition to extremity trauma must have their critical injuries prioritized. This allows for essential lifesaving intervention to be provided where and when it will be most beneficial to the patient. This may mean abbreviating the care of specific extremity injuries so the focus can

remain on those conditions that are life threatening to the patient.

GROSS MANAGEMENT

Patients with life-threatening extremity trauma (hemorrhage) but no other critical problems should be identified during the primary assessment. These patients should have appropriate interventions, including management of shock and rapid transport to the facility that can best treat their condition.

In patients with no life-threatening injuries or conditions, extremity trauma can be located and managed during the secondary assessment.

If an extremity is under abnormal stress because of the patient's position or pathologic angulation, an attempt should be made to straighten the extremity. This will mean moving the extremity back to a normal, relaxed, anatomic position. Having the extremity back in a normal position will help with splinting and normal circulation.

An injured extremity should be moved as little as possible. The primary objective of splinting is to prevent movement of the body part. This will help to decrease the patient's pain and prevent further soft tissue damage. To effectively immobilize any long bone in an extremity, it is necessary to immobilize the entire limb. To do this, it is necessary to manually support the injured site while immobilizing both the joint and bone above (proximal to) and the joint and bone below (distal to) the injury site.

The general management for suspected fractures includes the following steps:

- Stop any bleeding and treat for shock.
- Support the area of injury.
- Immobilize the injured extremity including the joint above and the joint below the injury site.
- Reevaluate the injured extremity after immobilization for changes in distal neurovascular function.

Three points are important to remember when applying any type of splint:

1. Pad rigid splints to help adjust for anatomic shapes and to help increase patient comfort.
2. Remove jewelry and watches so they will not inhibit circulation as additional swelling occurs.
3. Assess neurovascular functions distal to the injury site before and after any splint is applied and periodically thereafter.

Splints: Equipment and Methods

A wide variety of splints and splinting materials are available to the EMT. They include rigid splints, formable splints, and traction splints.

A **rigid splint** cannot be changed in shape (Figure 11-11). This requires that the body part be positioned to fit the splint's shape. Examples of rigid splints include board splints (wood, plastic, or metal) and inflatable "air splints." This group of splints also includes the longboard.

Formable splints (Figure 11-12) can be molded into various shapes and combinations to accommodate the shape of the injured extremity. Examples of these include vacuum splints, pillows, blankets, cardboard splints, wire ladder splints, and foam-covered moldable metal splints.

Traction splints (Figure 11-13) are designed to maintain mechanical in-line traction to help realign fractures. Traction splints are most commonly used to stabilize femur fractures.

ARTERIAL HEMORRHAGE

A major arterial hemorrhage usually can be easily detected unless it is an internal hemorrhage. In general, open hemorrhages are controlled by using direct pressure first, then elevation and pressure points. Extremity trauma is no different. For direct pressure, once a dressing is ap-

plied, do not take it off. If the bleeding goes through the first dressing, simply place another dressing on top of the first one without moving it. If a fracture is associated with the gross bleeding, the extremity should be realigned and splinted while direct pressure is applied to the open wound. Hopefully, this procedure will also help control the bleeding.

In the case of an internal hemorrhage, direct pressure applied to the outside of the body over the area of suspected injury will help the bleeding, just as it would for an open wound. For an extensive pelvic or lower extremity injury, use of the PASG may help facilitate the direct pressure. The garment should be filled with enough air to control the hemorrhage, usually to the maximum of the device. Do not be concerned about compartment syndrome until the PASG or air splint has been inflated for more than 4 to 6 hours.

OPEN AND CLOSED FRACTURES

Fractures can be open or closed. The first consideration in open fractures is to control hemorrhage and to treat for shock. Open wounds should be covered with a sterile pressure dressing and pressure applied to further control bleeding. Then the limb should be adequately immobilized. In the case of open femur fractures, a sterile dressing should first be applied to the wound and then a traction splint used to straighten the extremity and to stabilize the fracture. If the bone ends return into the wound, the outcome will not be altered, as long as the physician caring for the patient recognizes what happened. It is the EMT's responsibility to properly inform the physician and other hospital personnel of the initial condition of the wound and any changes that occurred due to its management in the field. It is also the responsibility of the EMT to properly document this information on the run report.

Both open and closed fractures can be immobilized with the use of rigid or air splints. Rigid splints are easier

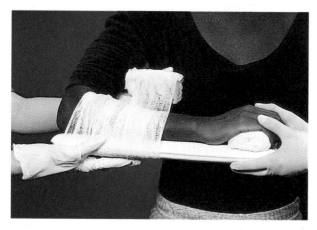

Figure 11-11 Rigid splint. (From Stoy. *Mosby's EMT Basic Textbook.* St. Louis: Mosby, 1996.)

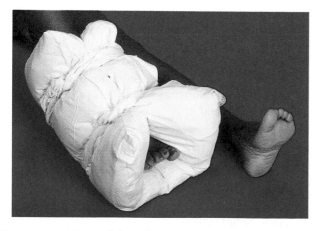

Figure 11-12 Formable splint. (From Stoy. *Mosby's EMT Basic Textbook.* St. Louis: Mosby, 1996.)

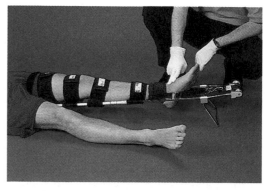

Figure 11-13 Traction splint. (From Stoy. *Mosby's EMT Basic Textbook.* St. Louis: Mosby, 1996.)

to use because once an air splint is inflated, it cannot be deflated or inspected further by the EMT. Padding must be used with a rigid splint to insure that no movement inside the splint is allowed. If a pulse is not detected where once it could be detected, the injury becomes more of a priority. Ice packs may be used to decrease swelling and pain.

Strains and sprains should be managed just like fractures since the EMT is not able to differentiate the injuries on scene.

JOINTS AND DISLOCATIONS

As a general rule, joints and dislocations should be splinted in the position found. If a pulse is not detectable, the joint may be manipulated to try to return blood flow. This manipulation will cause the patient a great deal of pain, so prepare the patient before moving the extremity. Ice packs may be used to decrease pain and swelling.

Any splint that is available to splint the injury in the position found may be used. The EMT may be forced to improvise with the equipment on hand to splint the injury. Documentation of how the injury was found and of presence of pulses, movement, sensation, and color before and after splinting is very important.

PELVIC FRACTURES

Pelvic fractures, especially if hemorrhage is suspected, can be difficult to manage. Not only is bleeding a concern, but it is difficult to move a patient with such an unstable fracture. If the patient is not suspected of having a hemorrhage, the best way to stabilize the fracture may be with a scoop stretcher and padding. The PASG can be very useful in maintaining integrity of the pelvis with or without a suspected hemorrhage.

AMPUTATION

Amputation represents yet another special problem. Amputated parts should be rinsed with sterile normal saline (when available), placed into a plastic bag, and kept cool during transport to the hospital. They *should not* be soaked or placed in water or saline, placed directly on ice or ice packs, or cooled with dry ice. Do not delay transport of the patient in order to locate the missing amputated part. If the amputated part cannot be readily found, law enforcement or other responders should be left at the scene to search for it. When the amputated part is being transported in a separate vehicle from the patient, make sure there is a clear understanding as to where the patient is being transported. Also make sure the group left behind understands how to deal with the amputated part once it is located. The receiving emergency department should be notified as soon as the part is located and transportation of the part should be initiated as soon as possible.

COMPARTMENT SYNDROME

Compartment syndrome can be definitively managed only in the hospital. In the field it should be managed like a fracture. Proper documentation of the position found and presence or absence of pulses, movement, sensation, and color must be reported to the hospital and documented on the run report.

FEMUR FRACTURES

Femur fractures represent a special consideration because of the musculature of the thigh. The thigh muscles have tremendous strength and commonly cause closed femur fractures to present with overriding bone ends. This can be a major contributing factor to hypovolemic shock due to the creation of a "third space" for hemorrhage. The pain created by the overriding bone ends can also be a contributing factor to shock.

The application of traction, both manually and by the use of a mechanical device, will help promote tamponading of internal third-space bleeding and decrease the patient's pain. Contraindications to the use of a traction splint include the following:
- fractured pelvis
- hip injury with gross displacement
- any significant injury to the knee
- avulsion or amputation of the ankle and foot

In a patient whose overall condition does not allow time for use of a traction splint, use of the pneumatic antishock garment will generally be indicated. Applying manual traction to the injured extremity while inflating the PASG will often produce adequate stabilization of the femur fracture and help to control any bleeding. The leg of the PASG that covers the fractured femur should be inflated to full pressure. The inflation of the rest of the garment should follow usual procedures and indications. In addition, if mechanical traction is also felt to be necessary and time allows, the traction splint should be placed *over* the PASG. Any traction device placed under the PASG can produce a space between the patient's extremity and the garment. This in turn will permit an internal capsule to form, resulting in trapped blood, soft tissue damage, or circulation compromise.

IMPAIRED OR ABSENT CIRCULATION

Impaired or absent circulation at the injury site or distal to it will place the extremity in jeopardy. After stabilizing all life-threatening conditions or injuries, the next priority is to correct any condition that threatens an extremity. Slight repositioning of the extremity toward extension will often reinstate circulation and is not time consuming. Avoid moving the extremity to the extreme range of either full extension or full flexion. If one or two attempts do not restore circulation, it is unlikely that continued attempts will prove successful. In such cases it is safer and more prudent to splint the limb as it lies and rapidly transport the patient to the nearest appropriate hospital. Be sure that the receiving facility understands the patient's condition.

• •

• Summary •

The management of patients with extremity trauma varies, based on an evaluation of the priority of a particular patient's extremity injuries compared with all of that patient's other injuries and conditions.

In patients with multisystem trauma, attention is directed to the primary assessment and to the finding and management of all life-threatening injuries, including internal or external hemorrhage in the extremities. These patients should be rapidly secured to a longboard in a normal, supine, anatomic position. This will efficiently stabilize all injured extremities. It will also allow the EMTs to focus their efforts on meeting the patient's critical needs. Care of individual injuries that are not life threatening in multisystem trauma patients often cannot be provided until the patient's systemic condition is stabilized. The EMT should not be distracted from life-threatening conditions by the gross appearance of any noncritical injuries or by the patient's request for management of them.

Patients with only noncritical isolated injuries represent another category. The initial priority is to establish that the patient truly does not have multisystem trauma. Only after the patient has been fully assessed and found to have only simple injuries without any systemic implication can management be provided in the normal prescribed way. When the mechanism of injury indicates sudden violent changes in motion, multisystem trauma, or spinal trauma, potential systemic decline must be anticipated. The patient's age, physical condition, and past medical history must also be included in the evaluation for potential systemic decline.

Scenario Solution

The findings for this scenario are interesting. At first Lisa appears to be cooperative and pleasant although in some pain. Her only complaint is that of the midshaft femur. As time goes on she becomes confused and agitated. A clue to the underlying progression of this scenario are the patient's vital signs. While they do not paint the picture of decompensated shock, they do suggest the compensatory mechanism is working to maintain homeostasis. As the shock becomes more profound, the patient's level mentation begins to worsen. As we know up to 500 cc of blood can be lost when the femur is fractured; however, this does not explain the level of shock that is present. A reevaluation of the patient's status is in order. Transport considerations may change, reflecting the ongoing shock state. A move away from traction splinting and to the PASG may be indicated depending on the reassessment of vital signs. The cornerstone to the treatment of this patient is a reassessment of Lisa's current status. If indicated, aggressive treatment for shock should begin and transportation to an appropriate facility initiated without further delay.

Review Questions

Answers provided on page 333.

1 A 35-year-old man falls off a 10-foot ladder. Based on this information, which injuries would you attend to first?
   A fractured femur
   B angulated wrist
   C C-spine precautions
   D hip fracture

2 Which signs and symptoms are most important when dealing with musculoskeletal injuries?
   A pulses, movement, and sensation
   B capillary refill, clubbing, and blanching
   C pain, color, and sensation
   D numbness, tingling, and capillary refill

3 What condition would you assess for when dealing with a crushing injury?
   A infection
   B degloving
   C compartment syndrome
   D absence of mobility

4 The driver of a vehicle involved in a head-on collision is your patient. What injuries would you suspect if damage was noted to the dashboard?
   A fractured wrist
   B lumbar spine injury
   C ankle fracture
   D pelvic injury

5 Your patient is a 70-year-old female complaining, "I've fallen and I can't get up." She denies pain; however, she is unable to lift her leg. Your assessment shows shortening of the left lower extremity, with external rotation. What injuries do you suspect?
   A femur fracture
   B C-spine injury
   C dislocated patella
   D hip fracture

CHAPTER OBJECTIVES

CHAPTER 12

Thermal Trauma: Injuries Produced by Heat and Cold

At the completion of this course the student will be able to:

- List basic criteria for assessing burn severity.

- List two life-threatening injuries resulting from burns that require prehospital treatment.

- List five signs that indicate inhalation injury and possible respiratory sequelae after a burn injury.

- Define the rule of nines for adult and pediatric patients.

- List key assessment and management elements for chemical and electrical burns.

- Identify and differentiate between critical and noncritical hyperthermia.

- List the major elements of management of hyperthermia from different causes.

- Define superficial and deep frostbite and explain the management of each.

- Identify and detail the management of patients in primary and secondary hypothermia.

- Explain the difference between immersion and submersion hypothermia and the management of each.

Scenario

A 25-year-old male has full and partial thickness burns involving both legs from his toes to midthigh. A 30-year-old female has walked out of a burning building in severe respiratory distress. An elderly male is found unresponsive, in a snowdrift with slow, shallow respirations and a weak, slow, carotid pulse. A marathon runner is found wandering around off the course, confused, diaphoretic, and barely ambulatory. On a day with temperatures well below freezing, a homeless woman complains of numb lower extremities with no sensation in the feet and ankles.

This chapter covers a wide range of possibilities caused by thermal trauma. By the end of this course you will be able to address each of the scenarios just presented.

Thermal trauma includes a variety of different injuries and conditions. For discussion purposes these are divided into two main categories: *heat* and *cold.* Each of these is further divided into *localized* (cutaneous) conditions, such as burns or frostbite, and *systemic* conditions, such as hyperthermia or hypothermia, that produce a generalized effect on the entire body.

Within the heat category are even more divisions, reflecting the differences between burn injuries (from both thermal and nonthermal sources), those conditions in which body temperature is elevated, and those which are prompted by heat but in which the body temperature itself is not elevated.

The cold category includes frostbite, hypothermia, and immersion and submersion injuries.

This chapter also includes discussion of the different priorities necessary for the management of thermal trauma patients. For example, the severely hypothermic patient requires rewarming in the hospital setting before any other significant treatment is provided; the burn patient with multisystem trauma is treated first for trauma and any systemic burn-related deficits, and only secondarily for the actual surface burn injuries. The heat exhaustion or heat stroke patient is treated more in the context of his or her environment than for specific injuries.

HEAT-RELATED CONDITIONS AND INJURIES

Burn trauma is the fourth leading cause of trauma deaths, preceded only by vehicular accidents, penetrating trauma, and falls. The types of burns vary depending on the age group involved. For instance, scalds from hot liq-

uids are more often found in toddlers, whereas flame burns are most frequently seen in the older child. Industrial burns from liquids or caustic agents are most common in adults.

Associated injuries account for a significant part of the morbidity and mortality of thermal injuries. Inhalation pulmonary pathology is the major cause of death. Chemical injury to the lung tissue and toxic by-products of combustion are both prime contributors to pulmonary pathology.

Elderly patients may have a number of other existing conditions that can complicate their care. Reduced vital organ function, decreased resistance to infection, and atherosclerotic vascular disease make age a major factor in burn management. The patient's age in years over 50 and under 2 plus the percentage of body surface with deep partial-thickness (second-degree) and full-thickness (third-degree) burns provide an estimate of burn mortality.

CUTANEOUS HEAT INJURIES (BURNS)

Heat coagulates protein. This is the primary mechanism of injury with burns. Low levels of heat for a long period of time or high heat for a short time that have equal calorie exchange produce the same result. Cooking an egg is an excellent analogy to what happens to tissues with a burn injury.

The priorities of care for burn victims follow the same principles and priorities as for any trauma patient:
- First, stop the burning process (thermal or chemical).
- Next, use the A B C D E method for assessment and management.
- Finally, provide specific care for individual wounds (burns).

A large number of patients who die as a result of thermal injuries do so because they have inhaled carbonaceous by-products of combustion, have inhaled toxic gases, or have been in a hypoxic environment for a sustained period of time—rather than from their burn injuries. Often these effects may not present with alarming signs and symptoms immediately postinsult. It is essential that the EMT recognize the probability of such associated conditions and provide a high FiO_2 and assisted ventilation as necessary.

A victim of a fire who has been in a confined area for any length of time must be considered to have carbon monoxide (CO) in his or her blood as well as pulmonary and systemic problems that can be caused by toxic inhalation. Such patients, regardless of contradictory findings during the primary and secondary assessment, must be considered unstable and must be transported to an appropriate hospital without delay, with $FiO_2 \approx 0.85$.

Burn trauma often includes other nonthermal injuries resulting from falls, jumping, or being struck by falling objects. In some cases these related injuries can be more serious and present a greater risk to life than the burns. *Assume the presence of such associated injuries in all burn patients until they can be ruled out by a thorough primary and secondary assessment.*

Anatomy and Physiology

The skin, the largest organ of the body, is composed of three tissue layers: the epidermis, dermis, and subcutaneous tissue. The *epidermis,* which is the outermost layer, is made up entirely of epithelial cells with no blood vessels. Underlying the epidermis is the thicker *dermis,* made up of a framework of connective tissues containing blood vessels, nerve endings, sebaceous glands, and sweat glands. The *subcutaneous layer* is a combination of elastic and fibrous tissue as well as fat deposits, and this layer is also known as the *superficial fatty fascia* (Figure 12-1).

The skin serves many functions for the body, the most important being to form a protective barrier against the outside environment, which helps in preventing infection. The skin also prevents fluid loss and helps regulate body temperature. The dermal layer contains nerve endings that convey impulses between the brain and the body. When thermal injuries occur to skin tissue, many or all of these functions are either destroyed or severely impaired. This protective layer must have adequate perfusion with red blood cells and other nutrients to survive. Heat, in addition to coagulating the protein, can compromise this blood flow.

An understanding of the surface area of the various regions of the body will be of great assistance in the estimation of the relative size of the area that is burned. This determination will in turn assist in the decision of the amount of fluid replacement needed for the patient. The percentage of the body's total surface area represented by each part or region of the body varies with the size of that region. This percentage also varies as the individual develops in size from an infant to a fully mature adult. An approximate estimation can be made by using the rule of nines (Figure 12-2). Although this is not completely

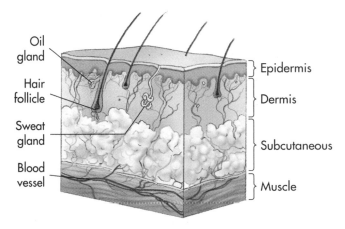

Figure 12-1   The skin is composed of three tissue layers—epidermis, dermis, and subcutaneous—and associated muscle. Some layers contain structures such as glands, hair follicles, blood vessels, and nerves. The depth of the burn determines the portion of these organs involved.

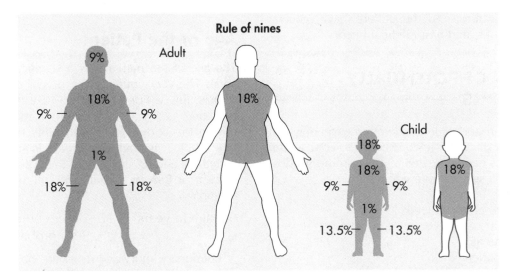

Figure 12-2   Determining the amount of burn involved is a major consideration in the resuscitation of the burn patient. The rule of nines is a fairly accurate and simple approach to this determination.

accurate, it is close enough for determining fluid replacement needs, estimating mortality, and computing other components of burn therapy that use body surface area (BSA) as a factor.

In an adult, each arm's surface area is estimated to be 9% of the total body surface area, and the front and back of the torso are each 18%. The total surface area of the entire torso, front and back, is 36%. Each leg is 18%. The head is 9% and the genital area is 1%. (Note that all but the last are multiples of 9.) In a child (3 to 9 years old), the arms, front and back of the torso, and genitalia are all estimated to be the same percentage as in the adult. However, in a child under 3, due to the relatively larger size of the head and smaller size of the legs, the percentage for the head is increased to 18% and the percentage for each leg is decreased to 13.5%. (It may be helpful to remember that compared with an adult, 4.5% is subtracted from each leg and the combined 9% is added to the head.) For smaller burns the hand can be used as a scale (palm = 1% BSA).

Pathophysiology

Human skin will show no apparent damage when exposed to higher than normal temperatures (up to 104° F [40° C]) even for relatively long periods of time. However, when exposed to much higher temperatures for shorter lengths of time or only moderately higher temperatures for longer periods of time, tissue destruction occurs. The same temperature/time principle is true for exposure to varying degrees of cold.

Thermal injuries also differ with regard to location, extent, and depth. Heat injury to the hands, feet, genitalia, or face and burns that completely encircle body areas are considered to have high priority. Other key factors to be considered are inhalation injuries, length of exposure, core body temperature, and the patient's age, general health, other injuries, and past medical history.

EVALUATION OF POTENTIALLY CRITICAL BURNS

Seven factors are important in the determination of which burn patients are critical, which ones need to go to a burn center, which ones can be treated by the community hospital, and what the survival rate will be:

1. Depth of the burn
2. Body surface area involved
   a. Total area
   b. Critical areas
3. Age of the patient
4. Pulmonary injury
   a. Smoke inhalation
   b. Toxic by-products
5. Associated injuries

6. Special considerations
   a. Chemical
   b. Electrical
   c. Carbon monoxide
7. Preexisting disease (past medical history)

Depth

The first step in the evaluation of the burn itself is a visual examination to determine depth (Figure 12-3). Such an assessment is only an estimate, as the full extent of the injury may not be apparent for several days.

superficial burns (first-degree burns)
- injury to the epidermis only
- red, inflamed skin, painful to touch
- generally no field treatment required

partial-thickness burns (second-degree burns)
- injury to both the epidermis and dermis
- skin presents with reddened areas, blisters, or open, weeping wounds
- patient complains of great deal of pain
- significant fluid loss occurs with subsequent shock

full-thickness burns (third-degree burns)
- injury to the epidermis, dermis, and subcutaneous tissue (possibly deeper)
- may look charred or leathery
- not painful (although associated second-degree burns will cause pain)
- no capillary refill

Body Surface Area Involved

Using the chart for BSA (see Figure 12-2), the total area of involved skin is estimated. In figuring fluid replacement, only areas of partial- and full-thickness (second- and third-degree burns) are used.

Age of the Patient

The age of the patient has a significant impact on survival. The very young and the very old respond poorly to burn injury. For patients who are more than 50 years old, there is a gradual increase in mortality from burns due to the body's general inability to respond to massive insult. This gradual decrease in survival can be estimated by adding the age of the patient in years to the percent of BSA of partial- and full-thickness burns. For example:

60 (age in years) + 30 (% BSA burned) =
90% probability of mortality

Pulmonary injury and sepsis are the major components that affect the patient's overall outcome. Preexisting medical conditions, which are either diagnosed or undiagnosed prior to admission, adversely affect both of these components. Preexisting medical conditions usually in-

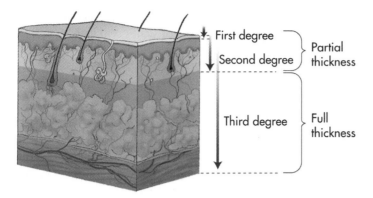

Figure 12-3 Burns are divided into superficial (first-degree), partial-thickness (second-degree), and full-thickness (third-degree) categories. Each level carries different prognostic, diagnostic, and therapeutic implications.

crease with advancing age and are a part of the reason that age is an important factor in determining how critical burn injuries are.

PULMONARY INJURY
Smoke Inhalation

Smoke inhalation injuries account for over half of the deaths each year from burns. Of the 75,000 victims hospitalized for major burns, 30% are treated for smoke poisoning and inhalation injuries.

The upper airway may be injured by direct heat. This is especially true when steam is involved. Air cannot usually conduct enough calories (heat) into the nose and mouth to produce a burn, but water (steam) can.

The smoke particles that are inhaled are the main cause of pulmonary trauma. This type of injury is a form of chemical damage to the cells lining the bronchi and alveoli. If these smoke particles are filtered out and not allowed to reach the lungs, no injury may occur. Wearing some type of mask (even a wet handkerchief) in a house filled with smoke will reduce such injuries significantly. The EMT should not go into a smoke-filled area without adequate protection.

Fluid overload following such an injury further compromises the pulmonary injury. Intravenous fluid therapy should only be used following careful guidelines in the resuscitation of the burn injury patient.

Toxic By-product Inhalation

Much of the long-term lung damage in inhalation injuries is caused by toxic fumes or smoke, since they are full of particles of incomplete combustion. Many of these by-products are highly acidic and cause destruction of the epithelial lining of the bronchi, alveoli, and pulmonary capillaries. Following exposure, initial pulmonary symptoms may not become clinically apparent for 12 to

36 hours. Generally speaking, the earlier the symptoms present, the more severe the damage. Moreover, a variety of toxic, volatile by-products (such as cyanide) may be released when materials such as plastics burn, resulting in inhalation poisoning.

ASSOCIATED INJURIES
Airway Burns

Dry-heat inhalation injuries are usually limited to the upper airway, whereas burns to the lower airway may be caused by steam. Heat, upon entering the air passages, dissipates in the nasopharynx and upper airway, causing burns and inflammation. Airway obstruction secondary to edema may occur within 24 hours. When the potential for losing the airway exists because of the progression of edema, intubation should be performed as early as possible.

Other Associated Nonburn Injuries

What else happened to the patient during the fire? Falls, automobile wrecks, trauma from jumping, and electrical injuries are just a few of the many possibilities. Shock produced directly and only by the burn injury appears late. Early shock is produced by hypovolemia, hypoxia, or some other cause, not the burn. *A burn patient who is displaying signs of shock soon after the injury is most probably not in shock from the burn but from associated injuries that produce hypovolemia or from severe hypoxia due to pulmonary injury.* The mechanism of injury must be reviewed, and other injuries that might cause shock must be assessed.

In burn injuries, as in all trauma, shock occurs when there is a deficiency of circulating blood volume with decreased tissue oxygenation. The body's response to a burn is the formation of edema. Any burn, no matter how small, will produce edema at the burn site. When the burn is greater than 20% BSA, this fluid shifts from the vascular compartment to the tissue (edema). This will produce a gradual decrease in circulating fluid volume that becomes detectable as hypoperfusion of the body tissues with hypotension and other signs of shock. This fluid shift does not become apparent until a large amount has shifted. Such a shift usually requires several hours to become noticeable. Therefore, if a patient is in shock upon the EMT's arrival, it is not from the burn. Hypovolemic shock (indeed, shock of any kind) in the prehospital phase is not secondary to the burn but is caused by another injury.

Evaluation of the circulating blood volume in the severely burned patient may be difficult, and the blood pressure may be unreliable. Tachycardia may be the first indication of impending shock, but it can also be present because of the pain associated with a partial-thickness burn. Manage a burn patient as any other trauma patient would be managed. Upon presentation of the indications of shock, manage the patient as if hypovolemic shock is present. In an elderly patient the possibility of myocardial injury (ischemia) may be present; therefore, do not overload the patient with fluids. Fluid replacement, heat conservation (after the burning process has been stopped), immobilization of possible fractures, hemorrhage control, and supplemental oxygen with a high FiO_2 should be used as indicated.

SPECIAL CONSIDERATIONS
Chemical Burns

A chemical burn occurs when the skin comes in contact with various caustic agents. In most cases, dilution and washing away of the chemical with copious amounts of water is the first step, since the chemical will continue to react until it is completely removed. *Do not waste time:* begin flushing immediately. Do not use neutralizing agents because they may cause further exothermic (heat) injuries from chemical reactions, producing sudden additional heat, additional burning, and further tissue damage. The exact amount of time required for irrigation cannot be predicted. Therefore, flushing should begin at the scene and continue until arrival at the hospital.

The receiving hospital should be notified in advance so that they can be ready to continue irrigation and to prepare a suitable area of the emergency department to contain the washed-off materials. If the identity of the chemical is known, this information should be relayed so the receiving hospital can prepare any special antidotes prior to the patient's arrival.

If the chemical is a dry powder, brushing off as much as possible before flushing will reduce the chemical concentration. While flushing is in progress, the patient's clothes should be removed. Shoes must be removed early to avoid pooling water that contains high chemical concentrations. Care must be taken to avoid runoff or splattering of the EMT or his or her clothing. *The EMT's own safety is paramount. Protective gloves and eye protection are necessary.*

Chemical burns of the eye should be irrigated with large volumes of saline; topical anesthetic agents (such as tetracaine) may be applied if necessary to control eyelid movement. Irrigation should be continued en route to the hospital. Care must be taken to position the patient so that the runoff will not spill into the other eye.

Chemicals that require special treatment are as follows:

- *Dry lime* and *soda ash,* like any powder, should be brushed off, because contact with water will form a corrosive substance. Contaminated areas should not be irrigated unless they are already wet. Large quantities of water should be used if the burning process has already begun.
- *Phenol* is widely used in industry as a cleaning agent. Since it is not water soluble, alcohol should

be used for flushing. Obviously, when alcohol is not available, large amounts of water will suffice.
- *Lithium* and *sodium metal* are substances that react with water, releasing heat and toxic fumes. Therefore, any large chunks remaining in or around the burn must be removed and placed in oil. After this has been done the burn should be washed with copious amounts of water. Irrigation should continue en route to the hospital.

For more exotic chemicals, the EMT should ask medical control to contact the nearest Poison Control Center or CHEMTREC at 1-800-424-9300.

Electrical Burns

The degree of tissue damage in an electrical burn is related to the amount of current involved and the duration of the exposure. The EMT's first priority is to determine if the patient is still in contact with the electrical source. If this cannot be determined with certainty, *do not touch the patient.* An electrocuted EMT only adds to the problems of scene management, adds to the number of patients that must be managed by the remaining EMS personnel, and takes up additional supplies that are needed. Do not attempt to remove the patient from contact with any electrical source unless trained to do so. Electrical burns can cause cardiac arrest. CPR may be required with such patients.

Pathophysiology

Three types of electric injuries occur.

- *Direct contact burns,* with passage of current through tissue, cause extensive areas of necrosis along the current's pathway. Skin is often charred and in some cases has exploded apart. Electrical contact burns may have entry and exit wounds that appear small on the surface. The EMT must assume that there are associated injuries to the nerves, bones, muscles, blood vessels, and other organs along the pathway between the entry and exit points.
- *Arc injuries* occur by arcing of electricity between two contact points close together near the skin. With these injuries the skin can be exposed to temperatures of 4,500° to 5,400° F (2,500° to 3000° C). This may produce significant cutaneous burns. Such injuries can be recognized by the loss or singeing of hair along the arc's pathway. The whole body may be involved.
- *Flash burns* are seen when a victim is too close to an open electrical source. This results in thermal burns, usually to skin unprotected by clothing on the side next to the fire.

Management

Initial management for victims of electrical burns includes lactated Ringer's or normal saline intravenous runs wide open. This will aid in preventing kidney failure by flushing myoglobin, a by-product of muscle damage, through the kidneys. The following are key points to consider with electrical injuries:

- Don't become part of the circuit!
- Anticipate greater tissue damage than is visible externally.
- Examine for associated injuries to bones and internal organs.
- Administer volume replacement, thus protecting the kidneys from tubular necrosis and subsequent shutdown.
- Monitor for possible cardiac arrhythmias.

Carbon Monoxide Poisoning

Carbon monoxide (CO) poisoning should be suspected and treated in all patients who have sustained a thermal injury in an enclosed area, whether the patient presents with symptoms or not. The symptoms of carbon monoxide poisoning include hypoxia with an altered mental state, neurologic deficits, and severe headache. A cherry red color may also be visible; however, this classic sign may be masked by the cyanosis of unoxygenated hemoglobin associated with cardiac or respiratory dysfunction or inhalation of air whose oxygen has been burned away by the fire. In such cases the cherry red color is not visible. It is one of those findings, like crepitus, that is helpful when present but provides no information when absent.

Carbon monoxide, a colorless, odorless, tasteless gas, has been shown to cause no direct trauma to the airway, but has a 200 times greater affinity than oxygen for bonding with hemoglobin. Because the half-life of carboxyhemoglobin is relatively long, all victims with symptoms suggestive of carbon monoxide poisoning should be treated with high concentrations of oxygen. This elevates the partial pressure of arterial oxygen (PaO_2), enhances displacement of CO from the hemoglobin molecule, and improves resaturation of hemoglobin with oxygen. At an FiO_2 of 100%, the carboxyhemoglobin half-life will be reduced from over 4 hours to 40 to 60 minutes. The patient should be rapidly transported to the hospital in the community best able to treat burns. If a burn center is available within a reasonable access time, other hospitals should be bypassed. Patients with very high concentrations (>30) of CO may require hyperbaric oxygen treatment.

PREEXISTING DISEASE

Conditions that exist prior to the onset of the burn injury can compromise the outcome. The conditions that occur during and after the resuscitation of a burn patient, such as sepsis, large volumes of fluid replacement, pulmonary edema, multiple operative procedures, prolonged bed confinement, decreased control of temperature regulatory

mechanisms, and skin grafts, are just part of the recovery from a burn. Any condition such as congestive heart failure, renal failure, hypertension, or atherosclerotic peripheral vascular disease can have a definite negative impact on the patient's prognosis.

CRITICAL INJURIES NEEDING BURN UNIT CARE

Patients with severe burns, injuries to important anatomic parts, and associated injuries or illness need to be treated in a specialized burn unit. This will improve the chances of survival and reduce complications and disabilities. The American Burn Association has developed a list of such injuries:

1. burns complicated by respiratory tract injury
2. all burns of the face
3. burns involving over 30% of the body, regardless of degree
4. third-degree (full-thickness) burns of more than 10% of the body
5. serious caustic substance burns
6. all electrical burns
7. burns with other associated injuries (e.g., fractures)
8. burns occurring in the very young, very old, or patients with serious underlying disease
9. burns of hands, feet, and genitalia (due to potential loss of function and inability to care for self)

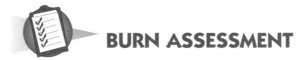

BURN ASSESSMENT

SAFETY, SCENE, AND SITUATION

Upon arrival at the scene of the incident, the situation must be rapidly and thoroughly assessed. Potential safety threats to both patient and crew must be identified and addressed immediately upon arrival. If the fire department has arrived, this determination can come from the chief fire officer. However, *assume nothing—check it yourself*. EMTs should *not* attempt rescues for which they do not have specific training experience and equipment.

Once the patient is in a safe place, the burning process should be stopped to eliminate further injury and tissue damage.

PRIMARY SURVEY (INITIAL AND FOCUSED EXAMS)

During the primary survey, close attention should be paid to the airway, including a search for signs of inhalation injuries: burns of the face and upper torso, singed facial and nasal hairs, carbonaceous sputum, hoarseness, stridor, or burns around the mouth and nose. Smoke poisoning, carbon monoxide poisoning, and respiratory injuries should be considered when the exposure has occurred in a confined space. Once the airway is secure, assessment of the other vital signs should include the pulse rate, respiratory effort, skin color, and level of consciousness. Since the exact amount of pulmonary injury or laryngeal injury cannot be determined in the field, oxygen with a high FiO_2 should be started ($FiO_2 - 0.85$ or greater). Also, any concurrent injuries that may be life threatening should be stabilized at this time.

SECONDARY SURVEY (DETAILED AND ONGOING EXAMS)

With critical patients in a potentially unstable environment, performing a secondary survey (focused physical examination) is inappropriate until both the patient and the environment have been secured from danger. In many cases the only way to ensure a secure environment is to move the patient. Therefore, attention should be paid to critical injuries and to stabilizing the spine. When no critical conditions require attention, and the environment is safe, a thorough head-to-toe examination should be performed rapidly, evaluating the burns and other injuries, pertinent medical history, and allergies (when this information is available). During this time, sites for placement of intravenous lines can be located.

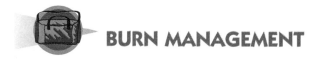 **BURN MANAGEMENT**

AIRWAY AND BREATHING

Due to the high possibility of inadequate oxygenation and impaired circulation, any patient, conscious or unconscious, who has suffered a thermal injury should be treated with supplementary oxygen with a high FiO_2, and the airway and breathing should be monitored for adequacy. Carbon monoxide and cyanide respond to an FiO_2 as close to 1.0 as possible. This should be used during transport whenever the potential of either exists. A stable patient with an intact gag reflex and airway should be given oxygen and should be monitored. Placement of an endotracheal tube should be used as required. Burns that lead to laryngeal problems early have edema from steam or chemical injury. Although management using an endotracheal tube may be required, the edema of the laryngeal structures may allow only one attempt. This attempt should be done by the most experienced person on the scene. The potential for laryngospasm is high in patients with a heat-injured larynx.

In the apneic or hypoxic patient, endotracheal intubation should be achieved early so that positive pressure ventilation can be administered and aspiration prevented.

If the hypoxic patient has a gag reflex, rapid sequence intubation (RSI) should be the first choice. Blind nasotracheal intubation may be required if RSI is not part of the training of the EMTs on the scene. Laryngospasm may result from contact of the device with the cords. Endotracheal intubation in these cases should be done only when necessary and by the most experienced EMT on the scene.

In patients with charred burns that surround the entire chest, expansion of the thoracic cavity may be extremely limited. The restricted chest excursion, caused by lack of elasticity of the burned tissue, results in inadequate tidal and minute volumes. A very small and limited number of these patients may need to have surgical incisions (*escharotomy*) made in the burned tissue to allow better chest excursion. This may need to be done in the field by appropriately trained personnel. If such trained personnel are not available, these patients should be intubated, assisted ventilation with FiO_2 0.85%, and rapidly transported to the nearest hospital that is capable of resuscitating the severely burned victim.

CIRCULATION

In a burn patient with associated injuries, transport of oxygen to the body organs may be diminished because of a decrease in circulatory blood volume due to other injuries. The decreased blood volume that is so commonly associated with burns does *not* happen in the immediate burn period. Usually 6 to 8 hours pass before this type of shock starts to develop. Shock at the scene is most often due to other causes. Management of hypovolemia should include the following measures:

- Intravenous lactated Ringer's (or normal saline) with large-bore catheters and tubing run at desired rate, unless other conditions contraindicate fluids.
- Application of the pneumatic antishock garment when indicated by other injuries. The PASG is *not* the treatment of choice for shock associated with burns.

The unburned arm should be used for intravenous access unless both upper extremities are affected. In this case the intravenous line can be placed through the burned area.

Although many formulas for fluid replacement exist, the Parkland formula serves as a good acute prehospital care guideline because it is not dependent upon laboratory findings. The name comes from Parkland Hospital in Dallas, Texas, where it was developed. This formula indicates that the patient should receive 4 cc of fluid in the first 24 hours for every 1% of second- and third-degree body surface area burned per kilogram of the patient's weight.

$$4 \text{ cc} \times \text{TBSA} \times \text{kg}$$

One-half of this total amount is to be given in the first 8 hours.

$$\frac{4 \text{ cc} \times \% \text{ of } 2nd°/3rd° \text{ BSA burns} \times \text{weight in kg}}{2}$$

$$= \text{fluid replacement in first 8 hours}$$

An example using this method will illustrate the need for early intravenous fluid administration: a 70-kg patient with 50% partial-thickness burns will require 7 liters of fluid in the first 8 hours.

$$\frac{4 \times 50 \times 70}{2} = 7,000 \text{ cc} = 7 \text{ liters}$$

The EMT can use the 8-hour total as the basis for calculating the drip rate that he or she begins in the field.

Many burn centers are now using other acceptable methods of fluid replacement. Every EMT should know and use the method preferred by the treatment facility to which burn patients will be transported.

PAIN RELIEF

The pain experienced by a burn victim is related to the severity of the burn. Third-degree (full-thickness) burns are painless because of the destruction of the nerve receptor endings; however, second-degree (partial-thickness) burns involve a great deal of pain. Because partial-thickness burns are usually associated with full-thickness burns, a patient with full-thickness burns may experience a great deal of pain.

Analgesics such as morphine or nitrous oxide can be used to relieve the pain. Because morphine can cause vasodilation, and both analgesics can induce respiratory depression, they can be dangerous if shock or respiratory problems are present. Their use should be determined by the patient's overall condition, not just the amount of pain. All analgesics must be given intravenously.

Another method of pain relief is cooling the wound with cool, moist sterile pads. There is no evidence to indicate that such therapy produces any pain relief; however, the cooling sensation is sometimes of psychological benefit to the patient. (Tar is about the only material that may still be producing heat on a nontrapped victim when the EMT arrives on the scene. Adding cool, moist pads in such cases to cool the wound and reduce the amount of tissue injury is also not based on any facts.) When using cool, moist sterile pads, they should cover only 10% of the body surface, and for only 10 to 15 minutes at a time. *It must be noted that the preferred method of dressing burns is with **dry sterile dressings**. In the seriously burned patient, the hypothermia brought on by the wet dressings could seriously compromise the patient.*

Since the burn patient's ability to regulate body temperature may be impaired, care must be taken not to contribute to or cause hypothermia. Heat loss through the burned area is a major problem in the management of burn patients. This problem should not be compounded by making the patient severely hypothermic in the field through the use of moist dressings. A shivering patient is too cold—do not allow skin cooling to proceed to this point.

WOUND CARE

The object of wound care in the burn patient is to prevent further damage and infection. Remove all clothing around the burn, but do not pull away any clothing that is stuck to the wound. Wrap the victim in a clean or sterile dry sheet. Avoid any type of dressing that shreds and leaves particles in the wound, and do not apply any ointment or solutions. All burned tissue should be covered with dry dressings. *Do not attempt to open blisters.* They are a protective mechanism. Where active bleeding is present, pressure dressings should be applied and any associated injuries treated before the burn area is covered. However, no debridement should be attempted in the field. *Time is of the essence.* Once the victim is breathing adequately, is not bleeding, and has been treated for shock, he or she should be transported to the appropriate hospital's emergency department for stabilization before transfer to a burn center. Alternatively, the patient should be transported directly to a burn center when one is available within a reasonable transport time.

SUMMARY: BURNS AND RELATED INJURIES

Consider the patient with a major burn just as any other multisystem trauma patient and manage accordingly. Airway maintenance is of prime importance with all burn victims. Aggressive prehospital management of the acutely burned patient may reduce mortality in the two-thirds of burn patients who die annually before reaching the hospital.

The following are major considerations when managing burn patients:

- Do not become a victim yourself: address potential safety threats to crew and patient immediately upon arrival.
- Airway management is the most important consideration for the burn patient. Have all the equipment ready so that intubation, if required, proceeds smoothly.
- All patients suspected of inhalation injuries must receive supplemental oxygen with a high FiO₂.
- The primary cause of shock in the severely burned patient is hypovolemia; shock should be treated

with proper fluid replacement. Shock early on is from other injuries; identify and manage them.

- Most chemical injuries should be irrigated with copious amounts of water.
- Burn patients should be transported without delay to an appropriate facility.
- Avoid hypothermia.

Many of these deaths may be prevented with systematic patient assessment and management by EMTs, based on the pathophysiology of the burn and its etiology. In the severely injured multisystem trauma patient, *first treat the trauma and systemic effects of the burn, then treat the burn.*

SYSTEMIC HEAT INJURIES

Elevated body temperatures, derived externally from the environment or internally from endogenous sources, can cause illness and death by overwhelming the body's ability to dissipate heat. When heat buildup is greater than heat loss, internal body systems begin to malfunction. In certain instances, only rapid intervention by EMS personnel can alter this destructive path. There are three major types or stages of signs and symptoms of systemic heat injuries: heat cramps, heat exhaustion, and heat stroke. These terms do not describe the physiologic changes that occur. However, because of their very common and widespread usage, they continue to be used. The EMT should recognize that these terms are simply names. They are not descriptive of the conditions.

HEAT CRAMPS

Heat cramps usually occur when individuals are at rest but have exercised or performed hard physical labor in hot weather without proper rehydration with fluids and electrolytes. The primary electrolytes lost in such cases are sodium and potassium. Water loss may also add to the onset of heat cramps. Between 15 and 20 grams of sodium can be lost through sweating with heavy muscular activity in hot environments.

Assessment

Patients with heat cramps typically complain of muscle cramping in the lower extremities, back, abdomen, or arms. The muscle will feel tight and hard when palpated, and the pertinent history will probably include physical exertion of some kind.

Management

Immediate management includes removing the patient from the hot environment and gently stretching the mus-

cle to alleviate the cramp. Having the patient drink fluids containing an electrolyte solution usually corrects the problem. Rarely does the patient need intravenous fluids. Care must be taken not to mistakenly eliminate heat exhaustion as a possibility, which may coexist with heat cramps.

HEAT EXHAUSTION

Heat exhaustion results from excessive fluid and electrolyte loss through sweating and lack of adequate fluid replacement when the patient is exposed to high environmental temperatures for a sustained period of time. Activity during such a period of exposure can increase the fluid loss to the point of hypovolemia. The patient's signs and symptoms are those of dehydration. The management is the same.

Assessment

Patients suffering from heat exhaustion may collapse; complain of nausea, lightheadedness, or anxiety; or display signs of confusion. They may feel better while lying down but become very light-headed when they attempt to stand or sit (*orthostatic hypotension*). Their skin usually feels cool and clammy. Profuse sweating is not unusual. Ventilations and pulse rates are rapid, and the pulse may feel thready at the radial artery. Systolic blood pressure may be normal or slightly decreased, and an orthostatic test of vital signs (tilt test) will be positive. The patient's core body temperature may be either normal or slightly elevated.

Management

Management of heat exhaustion is similar to that for any hypovolemic patient, although the patient should be moved into a cool environment rather than a warm one. The patient should be kept in a supine position and have any heavy clothing removed. Lactated Ringer's solution or normal saline should be administered intravenously during transport to the hospital. Proper temperature control and regular monitoring of vital signs during transport are essential.

HEAT STROKE

Heat stroke occurs from a sudden loss of the body's ability to control internal heat dissipation. This can result from two different causes and may be differentiated as classical and exertional heat stroke.

Classical heat stroke is most often seen in the elderly. This age-related problem can be worsened by various types of medications that an elderly person may be taking. Exposure to high room temperatures without benefit of air conditioning is a classic presentation during the hot summer months. This is especially common in large cities where effective home ventilation is either not possible or not used. Elderly patients living on fixed incomes will frequently not use air conditioning because of the cost. They may not open their windows for safety concerns. The EMT's scene assessment will provide information helpful in the identification of this condition.

Exertional heat stroke stems from a combination of high environmental temperature and physical activity, which rapidly elevates internal heat production to the point where the body can no longer regulate heat gain or loss. Under certain conditions when the humidity reaches beyond 75%, the body is no longer able to lose heat by sweating. Athletes who practice in high humidity are very prone to exertional heat stroke. If the condition is not recognized and immediately managed, body temperatures above 106° to 108° F (41° to 42° C) are possible, and death is imminent.

Assessment

Heat stroke patients typically present with hot, flushed skin. They may or may not be sweating depending upon where they are found and whether they have classical or exertional heat stroke. The blood pressure may be elevated or diminished, and the pulse is usually tachycardic and thready. Level of consciousness can range from altered to unconsciousness, and seizure activity may also be present. The key clues for the EMT to separate heat stroke from one of the other heat-related conditions are the elevation in body temperature and level of consciousness.

Management

Heat stroke is a true emergency. The higher the temperature and the longer the patient remains with an elevated internal temperature, the more destructive and deadly the condition can become. High core (and thus, brain) temperatures are much more destructive when combined with advancing age. Levels that can be tolerated by a pediatric patient often cannot be tolerated by an adult.

Management consists of rapidly cooling the patient with whatever means are available. Ice water poured directly over the patient is the fastest method of cooling. If ice is not immediately available, cool water or alcohol should be used. Cooling should begin prior to transport. Some of the steps that can be taken include removing heavy clothing, placing the patient in an air-conditioned ambulance, and pouring bottled irrigation fluids over the patient. Fanning the patient will promote evaporation of heat. Ice packs should be placed in the groin, axillae, and around the neck. In cases when the transport time is extended, the need to cool the patient even justifies stopping at a store or commercial establishment to acquire more ice.

COLD-RELATED CONDITIONS AND INJURIES

Cold injuries differ from burns in that, although the skin is involved in both situations, pulmonary complications predominate as associated problems with burn patients while changes in core temperature and reduced circulation are the primary associated complications with cold injuries. The clinical conditions of cold injuries often are not as dramatic as with heat trauma, neither in rapidity of onset nor as immediately visible diagnostic clues. The extent of injury to the skin and underlying tissue may be much more superficial with a cold-related condition than that produced by a similar appearing burn. Prolonged exposure and moisture are the usual causative factors in cold injuries.

PHYSICS AND PHYSIOLOGY

Heat loss is due to the transfer of heat (calories) from one body to another body, or from one body into the atmosphere. Caloric exchange occurs through several mechanisms: convection, conduction, evaporation, and radiation.

Convection: Air currents blowing across the torso, head and neck, and extremities remove heat and lower the body's temperature.

Conduction: Direct heat exchange takes place from one body or surface into another. The second body can be the environmental air, a solid surface, or a liquid that directly touches the patient.

Evaporation: Changing a liquid into a gas requires calories. Evaporation of a liquid from the surface of the skin removes calories from the patient as the liquid is converted into a gas.

Radiation: Energy in the form of heat radiates in waves through the air or through another medium, in this case radiating from the patient and warming other objects around it. Unlike conduction, direct contact is not present.

Although caloric loss can occur through more than one of these routes at the same time, usually a combination of factors exists.

Forty percent of the caloric loss of the body takes place from the head and neck. Awareness of this high heat-loss area can help the EMT, both in protecting him- or herself and in effectively treating the patient affected by cold temperatures or in trying to reduce the core temperature of a hyperthermic patient.

CUTANEOUS CONDITIONS OF COLD

Cold injuries to the skin are generally isolated to such body areas as the fingers, toes, hands, feet, face, and ears—places where there is a significant ratio difference between surface area and blood volume circulating through the body part. These body parts are also more exposed and farther away from the core temperature zone of the trunk, making them more susceptible to cold injuries. The most common injury to these areas is frostbite.

Anatomy, Physiology, and Pathophysiology

Frostbite is the actual freezing of body tissue as a result of exposure to freezing or below-freezing temperatures.

The human's normal response to lower than desirable temperatures is to reduce blood flow to the skin surface and thereby reduce heat exchange with the environment. This is accomplished by vasoconstriction of peripheral blood vessels in an attempt to shunt warm blood to the body's core to maintain normal body temperature. Reducing this blood flow greatly reduces the amount of heat delivered to the distal extremities.

The longer the period of exposure, the more that blood flow is reduced to the periphery. The body conserves core temperature at the expense of extremity and skin temperature. The heat loss from the tissue becomes greater than the heat supplied to that area. In cases of below-freezing temperatures when the extremities are left unprotected, the intracellular and extracellular fluids can freeze. This results in the formation of ice crystals that cause damage to local tissues in the exposed areas. Blood clots may also form, further impairing circulation to the area. Drug use, alcohol intoxication, and wet clothing can also contribute to the development of frostbite.

The assessment of any patient who has been in below-freezing temperatures without proper clothing and shelter should always include a particular examination of those body parts that are most susceptible to frostbite. Hydrocarbon fluids, such as gasoline, can cause immediate frostbite when spilled onto exposed skin in below-freezing temperatures due to rapid evaporation and conduction. Frostbite can also immediately result from warm moist skin contacting extremely cold metal due to rapid conduction.

Types of Frostbite

Frostbite is divided into two types: superficial (or "frost nip") and deep. *Superficial frostbite* is less severe than deep frostbite. With superficial frostbite the patient will feel slight pain or a burning sensation in the affected extremity, which later develops into numbness. The skin of the affected area will appear grayish or yellow. When digital pressure is applied to the area, the tissue below the discolored extremity will feel soft and malleable like normal tissue.

Deep frostbite develops if the patient does not recognize or react to the numbing sensation of the extremity. If the freezing of the tissue is allowed to continue, the affected area becomes more waxy-looking in appearance. When the nerve endings become frozen, the numbness and pain stop. The frozen parts are hard, and they will not be pliable when the affected tissue is compressed. The longer the extremity is allowed to remain frozen and the lower the temperature of the environment, the more severe the injury will be. The severity of deep frostbite cannot be fully determined until the frozen body part has thawed and the body allowed to begin to repair the damage. Frostbitten extremities may continue to improve gradually over a period of several days to several weeks. Early excision is not the correct treatment for frostbite.

Assessment and Management

The prehospital assessment of superficial frostbite is usually accomplished through a combination of recognizing the environmental conditions that prevail; considering the patient's chief complaint of pain or numbness of a digit, hand, foot, or facial area; and observing a discolored patch of the skin in the same area. Gentle palpation of the area can determine if the underlying tissue is compliant or hard when compressed. The patient with superficial freezing will usually complain of increased discomfort during the manipulation of the frostbitten area. The frozen tissue in cases of deep frostbite will be hard, and usually is not painful when touched or compressed.

The immediate treatment is to remove the frostbite patient from the cold environment into a heated area. Patients with superficial frostbite should be treated by placing the affected area against a warm body surface (such as covering the patient's frostbitten ears with warm hands, or placing affected fingers into the armpits). Superficial frostbite should be warmed at normal body temperatures only.

The prehospital care for deep frostbite should consist of appropriate shelter, supportive care, and early transport to an appropriate hospital. The patient can be given something warm (and nonalcoholic) to drink if it is available, depending upon his level of consciousness and other injuries. Tobacco use (smoking or chewing or using nicotine pads) should be prohibited since nicotine causes further vasoconstriction.

Attempts to begin rewarming of deep frostbite patients in the field can be hazardous to the patient's eventual recovery and is not recommended unless long transport times are involved. Rewarming of deep frostbite should be accomplished in a controlled hospital setting for the following reasons:

- The rewarming of the extremity should be a rapid immersion process, using consistent water temperatures of 102° to 108° F (38.5° to 42° C).

- The rewarming process is an extremely painful event for the patient. Intravenous analgesics are usually required for pain relief.
- If rewarming attempts have been started and for some reason the extremity is allowed to refreeze, gangrene can set in and the extremity or a part of the extremity may have to be amputated (do no harm).

As mentioned earlier, the severity of deep frostbite injuries is determined after the thawing process is completed. Frostbite is categorized into four degrees of severity similar to the categorization of burns. Superficial frostbite is first degree. Fourth degree frostbite, the most severe, develops gangrene shortly after thawing.

If rewarming has been initiated prior to EMS arrival, the affected body parts should be gently elevated to reduce swelling. The individual digits should be carefully separated with cotton to reduce skin irritation and to decrease the chance of the digits sticking together. If blisters have formed on the extremity, they should be left intact and not punctured. While transporting a patient once rewarming has begun, do not allow the thawed part to refreeze. Pain relief may be necessary during transport.

SYSTEMIC CONDITIONS OF COLD

The most common systemic cold injury or condition is *hypothermia.* Hypothermia is defined as the condition in which the core body temperature is below 95° F (35° C) when using a rectal thermometer placed at least 15 cm into the rectum. Unlike frostbite, hypothermia can occur in environments with temperatures well above freezing. Hypothermia can affect healthy individuals who are placed into adverse conditions unprepared *(primary hypothermia),* or develop secondary to the patient's existing illness or injury *(secondary hypothermia).* If unrecognized or improperly treated, hypothermia can be fatal—in some cases within 2 hours. There is a 50% mortality rate in cases of secondary hypothermia caused by complications of other injuries, as well as in severe cases where the core body temperature is below 90° F (32° C).

Anatomy, Physiology, and Pathophysiology

There are many variables that can promote hypothermia in humans. Environmental conditions can lower an individual's core body temperature to the point where their mental status has become affected by the hypothermia. In such cases they must rely on others to recognize their condition. If unrecognized and untreated, death may be imminent.

As the body's core temperature falls below 95° F, heart rate, respiratory drive, blood pressure, and cerebral blood flow all begin to decrease. Skeletal muscles begin to shiver in an attempt to produce heat, at first subtly and then more violently. This eventually ceases and the muscles become stiff as the core temperature drops below 90° F. Due to decreased cardiac output and increased oxygen deficit caused by the shivering, cellular hypoxia develops with increased lactic acid production and eventual metabolic acidosis. Incontinence, called "cold diuresis," occurs at this time.

Central nervous system (CNS) impairment progresses from initial confusion to stupor and eventually to coma. The pupils become fixed and dilated. Atrial fibrillation develops and may continue between 90° F and 83° F (32° C and 28° C). When the core temperature reaches 82° to 80° F (28° to 25° C), physical stimulation of the heart causes ventricular fibrillation. The stimulation could be caused by CPR or possibly by rough handling of the patient on the part of the EMT. Core temperatures below 80° F (25° C) usually bring death, as respiratory and cardiac functions fail in combination with the development of ventricular fibrillation and pulmonary edema.

However, do not assume the patient is dead until he or she is warm yet still has no signs of life (ECG, pulse, respiration, and mental function).

Severity and Exposure

The severity of hypothermia is determined by the core temperature of the body at its lowest reading. It is classified into two divisions: *mild,* a core temperature of 90° F (32° C) and above, or *profound,* a core temperature below 90° F (32° C).

The duration of exposure that contributes to the hypothermic condition is divided into three categories:

acute: exposures of up to 1 hour
subacute: exposure times from 1 hour to a day
chronic: exposure times of more than a day

The significance of exposure time deals with the difference between the core and the peripheral body temperatures. The longer the patient is exposed, the closer the core temperature becomes to the peripheral skin temperature. With minimal exposure time prior to rewarming, serum glucose levels remain within normal to slightly above normal limits, permitting adequate aerobic metabolism to occur. With normal cellular metabolism, lactic acid production and acid base balance remain within normal limits.

As exposure time lengthens, as in subacute and chronic conditions, the core temperature more closely approaches the peripheral body temperature. When this occurs, hypoglycemia and acidosis begin to develop, and continued aerobic metabolism is threatened. Although the exact length of exposure is significant, it is important to remember that any patient can develop profound hypothermia in a very short time span.

Hypothermic Situations

EMS personnel will encounter hypothermia patients in many different settings and situations. Four broad categories are used to describe the settings.

1. **Immersion hypothermia** occurs when an individual is placed into a cold environment without preparation or planning. Someone who has fallen through the ice in a pond or river is immediately placed in danger of hypothermia. The driver of a stalled automobile who attempts to walk in freezing rain and wind can be a victim of hypothermia. Near-drowning victims in waters 70° F (21° C) or less also fall into this category. These situations are usually acute hypothermia settings.

2. **Submersion hypothermia** is a combination of both hypothermia and hypoxia. Wilderness experts and the United States Coast Guard have shown remarkable results in resuscitating cold water near-drowning patients. Successful resuscitation without neurologic impairment has occurred in cases of cold water submersion of up to 66 minutes. The mammalian diving reflex, which involves instinctive breath holding, vital function slowing, and blood shunting to the body's core, is credited with enabling these patients to survive. Cold water is also thought to protect the central nervous system from the otherwise damaging effects of cerebral hypoxia.

Several factors may influence the outcome of a cold water submersion patient. These include age, length of submersion, water temperature, amount of struggle, water purity, quality of CPR and other resuscitative measures, and any associated injuries or illnesses the patient may have.

Age: The large number of successful infant and child resuscitations in the United States and Europe has been well documented. It is believed that the smaller mass of a child's body cools faster than an adult's, thus permitting fewer harmful by-products of anaerobic metabolism to form and causing less irreversible damage.

Submersion time: Obviously, the shorter the length of submersion, the less chance there is for cellular damage due to hypoxia. EMS personnel should attempt to obtain the most accurate information concerning submersion time. However, rescue and resuscitation efforts should be initiated regardless of the length of submersion.

Water temperature: Water temperatures of 70° F (21° C) and below are capable of inducing hypothermia. The colder the water, the better the chance of survival. This is probably due to decreased harmful anaerobic metabolism when the body is quickly chilled.

Struggle: Submersion victims who struggle less have a better chance of being resuscitated (unless, of course, their struggling efforts are successful enough to avoid drowning). Individuals who are intoxicated by drugs or alcohol usually struggle less and usually recover once revived. Less struggle means less muscle activity, which translates to less heat (energy) production and to less vasodilation. These in turn cause decreased muscular oxygen deficits (decreased deficits mean less CO_2 and lactic acid production), and thus cooling is speeded up.

Cleanliness of the water: Patients generally do better after resuscitation if they were submerged in clean water rather than in muddy or contaminated water. There appears to be no difference in survivability between freshwater and saltwater submersions.

Quality of CPR and resuscitative efforts: Patients who receive adequate and proper CPR, combined with proper rewarming and advanced life support measures, generally do better than patients for whom one or more of these items was substandard. Immediate initiation of CPR is a key factor for submersion hypothermia patients.

Associated injuries or illness: Patients with an existing injury or illness, or who become ill or injured in combination with the submersion, do not fare as well as otherwise healthy individuals.

The preceding list of factors that appear to contribute to a submersion patient's chances of successful recovery is based on ongoing research. Every submersion patient should have full resuscitation efforts made, regardless of the presence or absence of any of these factors. A patient should be warm and dead before resuscitation is terminated.

3. **Field hypothermia** involves a protracted exposure to the elements, usually by healthy individuals participating in outdoor sports and adventure activities. Skiing, backpacking, hunting, climbing, and other outdoor sports enthusiasts can become overexposed to the cold temperature and placed in danger of hypothermia.

4. **Urban hypothermia** can sometimes be missed because of the possibility of a more common illness or injury. A variety of acute and chronic medical conditions may make the patient more susceptible to hypothermia. In turn, the underlying hypothermia may hamper the effectiveness of normal treatment modalities. Hypothermia should be suspected in all the following cases:

- newborns and infants
- alcohol-related illness/injury
- drug use/overdose (to include both recreational drug abuse and certain prescription drugs; e.g., beta blockers and sedatives)
- cocaine-induced hypothermia
- all elderly patients, regardless of obvious injury or illness
- diseases such as hypothyroidism, heart disease, and diabetes
- burn patients
- malnutrition

- homeless individuals who are underclothed and/or in shelters

A typical situation in which hypothermia may not be suspected is a cool, rainy day with a temperature of 60° F (15° C). The patient "sleeping off" a heavy alcohol intake, wearing wet clothing, and lying on cool pavement or a sidewalk is a perfect situation for unrecognized severe hypothermia.

Assessment

There should be a high index of suspicion for hypothermia even when the environmental conditions are not highly suggestive (wind, moisture, cold, etc.). Rectal temperatures are not commonly assessed in the field nor widely used as a vital sign in most prehospital systems. Ambulances usually only carry a standard-range oral or rectal (for infants) thermometer, which only reads to 94° F (34.4° C). If hypothermic temperatures are to be obtained, a low-range rectal thermometer is necessary.

The best assessment tool an EMT can use when suspecting hypothermia is muscular shivering and the patient's level of consciousness. Mildly hypothermic patients (core temperature higher than 90° F) will have an altered level of consciousness and usually show signs of confusion, slurred speech, altered gait, and clumsiness. They will be slow in their actions and are usually found in a nonambulatory state—sitting or lying. They will be shivering. This condition may be misinterpreted by law enforcement and EMS personnel as drug or alcohol intoxication.

When the core temperature falls below 90° F (32° C), profound hypothermia is present and the patient will probably not complain of feeling cold. Shivering will be absent and the level of consciousness will be markedly decreased, possibly to the point of unconsciousness and coma. Pupils will react slowly or may be dilated and fixed. Palpable pulses may be diminished or absent, and the systolic blood pressure may be low or unable to be determined. Respirations may have slowed to as little as one or two breaths a minute. The ECG may show atrial or ventricular fibrillation.

Management

Prehospital care of the hypothermic patient consists of preventing further heat loss, gentle handling of the patient, initiating rapid transport, and beginning rewarming in certain patients.

Prevention of further heat loss includes moving the patient to the warm ambulance or to a warm shelter if the patient is to be air evacuated. Wet clothing should be removed by cutting to avoid unnecessary movement and agitation of the patient. Cover the patient with warm blankets. If the patient is conscious and alert, warm sweet fluids can be given by mouth. Intravenous fluids warmed

to 104° F (40° C) should be administered if the intravenous line can be begun without unduly agitating the patient. *Do not give the patient cold (room temperature) fluids.* This fluid is below body temperature and will make the patient colder than he or she currently is. These two forms of therapy are minimal at best for rewarming, and common sense should decide whether fluid (orally or intravenously) are worth the risks of aspiration, coughing, and painful stimuli. Applying hot packs and massaging the patient's extremities should be avoided.

Rewarming of the extremities, or other methods that increase peripheral circulation before central rewarming can occur, can increase acidosis and hyperkalemia and can actually decrease the core temperature. This will complicate resuscitation and may precipitate nonresponsive ventricular fibrillation.

The phrase "they are not dead until they are warm and dead" was coined specifically for the hypothermic patient. All efforts to resuscitate the patient should be continued until actual brain death can be determined with the core temperature in the normal range.

In the more profoundly hypothermic patient, gentle handling is of utmost importance. If an ECG is available, cardiac monitoring should be used to assess electrical activity. If palpable pulses are absent, this is the only way the EMT will be able to determine whether CPR is warranted. *If the ECG shows any kind of organized electrical cardiac rhythm, do not start CPR regardless of the absence of a palpable pulse.* CPR usually will precipitate ventricular fibrillation in such patients. If ventricular fibrillation is present, normal CPR should be initiated and continued until the patient has been transported and rewarmed at the hospital. In contrast, patients who are submersion victims should be treated like any other drowning victim with immediate CPR (if the patient is apneic and pulseless) and full advanced cardiac life support procedures.

The patient with profound hypothermia may be bradycardic, but airway adjuncts such as oral airways, esophageal obturator airways (EOA), and endotracheal tubes should not be used unless ventricular fibrillation is verified by ECG and CPR has been started. Oxygen can be provided by mask, but its usefulness is questionable. It may be of more benefit if the oxygen can be warmed.

In the profoundly hypothermic patient, defibrillation and conventional advanced cardiac life support drug therapy may not be beneficial because of the depressed core temperature. Some EMS protocols allow for one defibrillation attempt for ventricular fibrillation, followed by basic cardiac life support measures until the patient is rewarmed at the hospital.

In the rare event that rewarming is attempted in the field because of the inability to transport a patient (severe blizzard or other disaster), the patient should be placed in a bathtub or similar-size container full of warm water (104° F or 40° C). The extremities should be left out of the water so that the body's core will warm first. This will help to avoid "after drop," which results when the extremities warm more quickly than the core and vasodilate, causing central hypotension and promoting ventricular fibrillation. This type of rewarming is a last-ditch effort. Central rewarming in a hospital setting is the preferred method.

• Summary •

Cold and heat injuries can result from environmental conditions and underlying medical conditions. They can cause both localized and systemic complications for the patient and present situations that can threaten life and limb. Proper recognition, assessment, and management by prehospital personnel can limit the danger cold and heat injuries may cause and lower the morbidity and mortality of these emergencies. In certain cases of hypothermia, basic treatment modalities in the field are more productive for the patient than aggressive actions and therapies. Proper assessment of the environmentally ill patient can make the difference in resuscitation and long-term recovery.

Scenario Solution

A 25-year-old male has full and partial thickness burns involving both legs from toes to midthigh. This case represents a common problem: a patient presents with obvious, horrific looking injuries, and the prehospital provider is drawn immediately to those injuries, thus failing to find other more life-threatening conditions. Proper management for this patient would first involve evaluation of the scene for safety, and if safe, the next action would be to stop the burning process. Next, the A B C D E format of assessment and management must take place. Following the initial assessment and treatment, specific care for the burn can take place. In this case, burn care would involve covering with dry, sterile dressings, initiation of IV therapy, if applicable, and pain relief if hemodynamically stable. Transport to a burn center if available is indicated.

A 30-year-old female has walked out of a burning building in severe respiratory distress. This case represents the need for aggressive assessment and management of breathing problems associated with structure fires. This patient presents with no burn trauma, but instead severe respiratory distress secondary to inhalation of by-products of combustion. Treatment of this patient would include primary assessment and management of all life-threatening conditions. The breathing problems that this patient is experiencing would be addressed during this survey. Oxygen at 100% should be started, and ventilations should be supported if needed. Advanced airway management may be indicated.

An elderly man is found unresponsive in a snow drift, with slow, shallow respirations and a weak, slow carotid pulse. This case represents a typical presentation of a hypothermic patient. Because the elderly are more susceptible to the extremes of temperature ranges, care for this patient would include primary assessment and treatment of life-threatening problems. In the hypothermic patient, vitals signs may be altered but can still provide acceptable oxygenation to the tissue. This patient should be handled with care because rough movement could induce ventricular fibrillation. The patient's clothes, if wet, should be removed, and the patient wrapped to prevent any further heat loss. Transport to an appropriate facility should be carried out expeditiously but carefully. Alerting the receiving facility early will allow time to prepare the necessary equipment and personnel.

A marathon runner is found wandering off course, confused, diaphoretic, and barely ambulatory. This case represents situations that develop in high heat environments. This patient is experiencing heat exhaustion. Treatment should follow the primary assessment, including placing the patient in a cool environment, keeping the patient supine, and starting an IV line of normal saline or lactated Ringer's, if possible.

On a day with below-freezing temperatures, a homeless woman complains of numb lower extremities with no sensation in the feet and ankles. This patient suffers from severe frostbite, which is commonly seen in urban areas. Treatment of this stable patient consists of removing the patient from the cold environment and transportation to medical attention. Rewarming should not be started in the field unless prolonged transport times exists.

Review Questions

Answers provided on page 333.

1 The proper way to dress most burn injuries prehospital is to use:
   A moist dressings
   B dry sterile dressings
   C water soluble gels
   D Silvadene

2 The biggest concern with electrical burns is:
   A the wick effect
   B tissue loss
   C entry and exit wounds
   D cardiac arrest

3 The first step in treating heat-related emergencies is to:
A remove the patient from the environment
B administer cold IV fluids
C apply ice packs
D apply wet sheets

4 Cold-water drowning victims are suffering from the effects of both hypoxia and:
A Immersion hypothermia
B Submersion hypothermia
C Urban hypothermia
D Field hypothermia

5 A burn covering the face and the entire anterior surface of both arms would have a TBSA of:
A 50%
B 35%
C 13.5%
D 9.5%

CHAPTER OBJECTIVES

CHAPTER 13

Initial Care and Resuscitation of the Child

At the completion of this course the student will be able to:

- Identify the unique differences in injury patterns for children.

- Demonstrate an understanding of the special importance of managing the airway and restoring adequate tissue oxygenation in pediatric patients.

- Identify the quantitative vital signs for children.

- Demonstrate an understanding of management techniques for the variety of injuries found in pediatric patients.

- Calculate the Pediatric Trauma Score.

- Identify the signs of pediatric trauma suggestive of child abuse.

Scenario

You are called to respond to a report of an injured child at a playground. On your arrival, you find a group of children and adults surrounding a 5-year-old girl who has apparently fallen from a "jungle gym" from a height of about 8 feet onto a concrete surface.

The adults present state that they did not witness the fall but that the child reportedly lost her balance and fell, first striking her chest on the apparatus then landing directly on her head. They report that the child was unconscious for about 10 minutes immediately following the fall.

Your initial evaluation reveals a child who is lethargic and does not respond appropriately to commands. Her RR equals 10. The pupils are equal and reactive. Her pulse is 160, and BP is 70 systolic. Her skin is cool, and capillary refill is significantly prolonged. There is an abrasion on the left lateral chest over the lower ribs, and the child moans when the abdomen is palpated. There is an obvious deformity of the left wrist. When you ask, you are told the patient's mother is en route. The babysitter asks that you wait for the mother.

- What are the management priorities in this patient?
- What are the most likely injuries in this child?
- What is the most appropriate destination for this child?

Injury is the most common cause of death for the American child. Tragically, 20% to 40% of these deaths may be preventable. Just as with all other aspects of pediatric care, proper assessment and management of the injured child requires a thorough understanding of the unique characteristics of childhood growth and development.

Good pediatric care is far more than simple application of adult principles to a smaller person. Children have common patterns of injury and unique physiologic responses and special needs based on their size, maturity, and psychosocial development. To ignore these requirements is to invite disaster.

This chapter will first describe the special characteristics of the pediatric trauma victim and then will review optimal trauma management and its rationale. Although it is important to understand the unique characteristics of pediatric injury, it is essential to remember that basic life support measures following the standard A B C D E method are the same for every patient, regardless of his or her size.

THE CHILD AS A TRAUMA VICTIM

DEMOGRAPHICS OF PEDIATRIC TRAUMA

There are many unique characteristics that must be addressed when considering the child as a trauma victim. The incidence of blunt (instead of penetrating) trauma is highest in the pediatric population. Although recent analysis of the National Pediatric Trauma Registry (NPTR) continues to identify blunt trauma as the most common mechanism of injury over the last 4 years, penetrating injury has increased to almost 15% of cases. The consequences of penetrating trauma are relatively predictable, but there is greater potential for multisystem injury from blunt mechanisms.

Falls are the most common cause of injury (39%) and occur most frequently in children less than 5 years old. Vehicular related trauma (38%) is the next most common mechanism. According to statistics, injury is accidental in 87% of cases, sports related in 4% of cases, and the result of assault in 5%. Multisystem involvement is the rule rather than the exception; therefore, all organ systems must be assumed to be injured until proven otherwise. Although there may be minimal external evidence of injury, potentially significant internal derangement of every major organ must be assumed until ruled out by definitive assessment or careful follow-up evaluation.

KINEMATICS OF PEDIATRIC TRAUMA

The child's size produces a smaller target to which linear forces from fenders, bumpers, and falls are applied. Because of diminished body fat, increased elasticity of connective tissue, and close proximity of multiple organs, these forces are not dissipated as well as in the adult and therefore disperse more energy to multiple organs. Because the skeleton of a child is incompletely calcified and contains multiple active growth centers, it is more resilient. It is, however, less able to absorb the kinetic forces applied during a traumatic event and may allow significant internal derangement with apparently minor external injury. For example, although rib fractures are uncommon, pulmonary contusion is common.

THERMAL HOMEOSTASIS

The ratio between a child's body surface area and body volume is highest at birth and diminishes throughout infancy and childhood. This means that there is relatively more surface area through which heat can be quickly lost. As a result, thermal energy loss becomes a significant stress factor in the smaller child. Although this may not be life threatening by itself, it frequently provides additional stress to the child who may be hypotensive and in severe pain. Severe hypothermia will frequently initiate irreversible cardiovascular collapse.

PSYCHOSOCIAL ISSUES

The psychologic ramifications of caring for an injured child can also present a major challenge. Particularly with the very young child, regressive psychologic behavior may result when stress, pain, or other perceived threats intervene in the child's environment. The child's ability to interact with unfamiliar individuals in strange surroundings is usually limited and makes history taking and cooperative manipulation extremely difficult. An understanding of these characteristics and a willingness to cajole and soothe an injured child will frequently be the most effective means of achieving good rapport and obtaining a more comprehensive assessment of the child's physiologic state. Additionally, the child's caretakers or parents frequently have needs and issues that must be addressed to successfully care for the child. In many cases they should be considered a second patient.

RECOVERY AND REHABILITATION

Another problem unique to the pediatric trauma victim is the effect that injury may have on subsequent growth and development. Unlike the anatomically mature adult, the child not only must recover from the injury but also must continue the process of normal growth and development. The effect of injury on this process—especially in terms of long-term disability, growth deformity, or abnormal subsequent development—cannot be overestimated. Children suffering even minor injury may have prolonged disability either in cerebral function, psychologic adjustment, or organ system disability. Recent evidence suggests that as many as 60% of children with severe multiple trauma have personality changes and 50% are left with subtle cognitive or physical handicaps. Additionally, pediatric trauma can substantially impact siblings and parents, resulting in a high incidence of family dysfunction, including divorce. The cost of correcting these problems can be staggering and lifelong.

The effect of inadequate or inappropriate care in the immediate posttraumatic period may have consequences, not only on the child's survival but also, and perhaps more importantly, on the quality of the child's life for years to come. Major organ injury may exist in the face of minimal external signs. A high index of suspicion and clinical common sense should prompt transport of the child to an appropriate hospital for a more thorough evaluation whenever there is any possibility of severe injury.

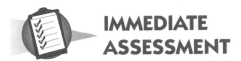

IMMEDIATE ASSESSMENT

In terms of death and disability, the ultimate result of care for the injured child is largely determined by the quality of care rendered in the first moments after injury. During these critical minutes, a systematized approach based on the A B C D E method and use of a well-understood protocol is the best defense against overlooking an injury that may be rapidly fatal or that may cause unnecessary morbidity. As in the adult, the three most common causes of immediate death are hypoxia, overwhelming central nervous system (CNS) trauma, and massive hemorrhage. Lack of expedient triage and transport to the most appropriate center for treatment can compound any or all of these problems.

HYPOXIA

The first priority of initial management is always the establishment of a patent airway. Confirming that the child has an open and functioning airway does not preclude the need for assisted ventilation and supplemental oxygen, especially where central nervous system injury or hypoperfusion may be present. Injured children can rapidly deteriorate from labored breathing and tachypnea to a state of total exhaustion and apnea. Once an airway is established it is essential that rate and depth of ventilation be evaluated to confirm adequate alveolar ventilation. If alveolar ventilation is not adequate, merely providing excessive concentration of oxygen will not prevent ongoing cellular hypoxia.

Adequate oxygenation is especially critical to the initial care of a closed head injury. The patient may be densely obtunded and yet have excellent potential for good functional recovery if cerebral hypoxia can be avoided. If at all possible, patients who require airway manipulation management should be hyperoxygenated with mask O_2 prior to initiation of any attempt at intubation. In many cases this very basic maneuver may be all that is necessary to begin reversal of hypoxia and improve the margin of safety when intubation is performed.

BRAIN INJURY

Recent animal studies indicate that the pathophysiologic changes that follow trauma to the central nervous system begin within a matter of minutes. It becomes obvious, then, that early adequate resuscitation is the key to increased survival of children with a central nervous system injury. Although a certain percentage of CNS injuries will be overwhelmingly massive and relentlessly fatal, many children present with central nervous system injuries that are made more severe by subsequent hypoperfusion or ischemia. Adequate oxygenation and ventilation are extremely critical in the management of closed head injuries. Even densely comatose children may recover if they do not develop cerebral hypoxia.

A recent analysis of pediatric brain injury documented that, for given degrees of injury severity as measured by the Abbreviated Injury Scale (AIS), children have a lower mortality and higher potential for survival than their adult counterparts. With the introduction of an extracranial injury in association with the cerebral injury, however, the child's survival curve matches that of the adult. This illustrates the potentially negative impact of associated injury on outcome from CNS trauma. These findings certainly emphasize the importance of adequate initial resuscitation and stabilization to improve the outcome from central nervous system injury.

Children with closed head injury frequently present with a mild degree of obtundation or sensory dullness, and they may have had a sustained period of unconsciousness that is not always recorded during initial evaluation. A history of loss of consciousness is one of the most important prognostic indicators of potential CNS injury. This should be investigated and recorded for every case. Likewise, complete documentation of baseline neurologic status, including the following, is important:

- response to sensory stimulation
- pupillary reaction
- motor function

These are essential steps in initial pediatric trauma care. Central nervous system injury is a pathophysiologic continuum that begins as an initial depolarization of the intracranial neurons and then proceeds along a recognizable course of secondary edema and hypoperfusion. The absence of adequate baseline assessment makes ongoing follow-up and evaluation of intervention extremely imprecise and difficult.

Attention to detailed history taking is especially important in cases of potential cervical spinal cord injury. Since the child's skeleton is incompletely calcified and has multiple active growth centers, there may be minimal or no radiographic evidence of a mechanism of injury that may have caused a stretch or contusion of the cord.

Transient neurologic deficit may be the only indicator of potentially significant cervical spinal cord injury.

HEMORRHAGE

Most pediatric injuries do not cause immediate exsanguination. Unfortunately, children who do sustain injuries with major blood loss die within moments or are dead on arrival at the hospital. The majority of injured children requiring emergency care have multiple organ injuries with at least one component associated with blood loss. This hemorrhage may be extremely minor as in cutaneous lacerations or contusions, or it may be potentially life threatening, as from a ruptured spleen, lacerated liver, or avulsed kidney.

As in adults, the injured child compensates for hemorrhage by increasing systemic vascular resistance at the expense of peripheral perfusion. Blood pressure alone is an inadequate marker for shock. Ineffective organ perfusion is a more appropriate indication of shock and is evidenced by a decreased level of consciousness, diminished skin perfusion (decreased temperature, poor color, and delayed capillary refill), and decreased urine output. Unlike the adult, however, the early signs of hemorrhage may be subtle and difficult to identify. Tachycardia may be caused by hypovolemia or may be the result of fear or pain. Moreover, the normal heart rate of a child varies with age. Poor peripheral perfusion may be the result of hypotension, hypothermia, or both. If the early subtle signs are missed, the child may lose so much circulating blood volume that compensatory mechanisms fail. In this case, cardiac output plummets, organ perfusion disappears, and the child plunges into uncompensated and usually fatal shock. Therefore, it is essential that every child sustaining blunt trauma have vital signs carefully monitored in order to detect those subtle signs. Inadequate resuscitation could result in profound cardiovascular collapse at some time after the injury.

A major reason for the rapid transition to uncompensated shock is the gradual loss of red blood cell mass. Restoration of shed blood with crystalloid solutions will provide a transient increase in blood pressure but the solutions will dissipate as the fluid leaks across capillary membranes. The net effect is that circulating volume will be gradually replaced with increasingly dilute red blood cell mass, which has virtually no oxygen-carrying capacity. The EMT must constantly assess the child in light of this possibility and must assume that any child who requires more than one 20 cc/kg bolus of crystalloid solution may be indeed following this path of physiologic self-destruction.

A common error in the initial evaluation of the injured child is the tendency to over-resuscitate the patient once venous access has been secured. In the face of minimal bleeding, normal vital signs, and an essentially stable hematocrit, a bolus of 20 cc/kg can artificially dilute the hematocrit by 3 to 4 points and thereby introduce potential error in the diagnosis of hemorrhage. Given the high incidence of closed head injury with associated blunt trauma and the relatively low incidence of severe hemorrhagic shock, it becomes obvious that gross fluid over-resuscitation of a child with a closed head injury may be more detrimental than effective. It may actually worsen evolving cerebral edema. Careful assessment of the child's vital signs and even more compulsive evaluation of the effect of therapeutic intervention must therefore be the EMT's primary consideration in evaluating and treating the child in the immediate minutes after injury.

TRIAGE

The severely injured child must be transported to a hospital that has the equipment and personnel appropriate for care of the pediatric trauma victim. The decision as to which child requires this level of care must proceed from a careful and rapid evaluation of the entire child. Overlooking potential additional organ system injury and inadequately stabilizing the patient are the two most common problems encountered in this area. For this reason, the Pediatric Trauma Score (PTS) has been developed to provide a reliable and simple protocol for assessment and to provide numeric quantitation that is predictive of outcome in regard to morbidity and mortality. Scoring is based on six readily available clinical indicators including patient size, airway status, level of consciousness, systolic BP, fractures, and presence of cutaneous injuries. The Pediatric Trauma Score has been shown to be an effective triage tool and is applicable in the field as well as in emergency centers functioning as referring hospitals in larger trauma networks.

 ## INITIAL ASSESSMENT

The small size of the pediatric patient, the diminished caliber and size of the vascular system, and the unique anatomic characteristics of the airway frequently cause the standard procedures used in basic life support to be extremely challenging and technically difficult (Table 13-1). The immediate availability of appropriately sized equipment is essential for successful initial management of the injured child. Attempting to place an overly large intravenous cannula or an inappropriately sized endotracheal tube may cause more harm than good to the patient. For this reason, Broselow et al. have de-

vised a Resuscitation Tape. The tape allows for rapid identification of a patient's size with a correlated estimation of weight, size of equipment to be used, and appropriate dosages of potential resuscitative drugs. Effective pediatric trauma resuscitation mandates the availability of appropriately sized laryngoscope blades, endotracheal tubes, nasogastric tubes, Foley catheters, chest tubes, blood pressure cuffs, oxygen masks, bag-valve-mask resuscitators, and other associated equipment.

AIRWAY

The primary goal of initial resuscitation of the injured child is restoration of adequate tissue oxygenation as quickly as possible. Oxygenation and circulation are as essential to the injured child as they are to the adult. In this regard, standard principles of airway control, breathing, and circulation are no differently addressed in the child than they are in the injured adult. As always, the first priority of assessment and resuscitation is the child's airway. The smaller the child, the greater the disproportion between the size of the cranium and midface, and the greater the propensity of the posterior pharyngeal area to "buckle" as the relatively large occiput forces passive flexion on the cervical spine. As a result, a child's airway is best protected by a slightly superior anterior position of the midface known as the sniffing position in the nontrauma patient. In the trauma patient the neck must be kept in-line to prevent the hyperflexion at C5–6 and hyperextension at C1–2 that occurs with the sniffing position. Careful attention to airway maintenance of this position is especially important in the obtunded child whose level of consciousness is waxing and waning. Moreover, in providing initial immobilization of the child with support of the cervical spine, the size disproportion of the occiput must be a

 Table 13-1 Height and weight range for pediatric patients

Group	Age	Range of mean norms	
		Height (average)	Weight (average)
Newborn	Birth– 6 weeks	51–63 cm	4–5 kg
Infant	7 weeks– 1 year	56–80 cm	4–11 kg
Toddler	1–2 years	77–91 cm	11–14 kg
Preschool	2–6 years	91–122 cm	14–25 kg
School age	6–13 years	122–165 cm	25–63 kg
Adolescent	13–16 years	165–182 cm	62–80 kg

consideration. Provide adequate padding under the torso so that the cervical spine is indeed maintained in a straight line rather than forced into slight flexion because of the occiput. As in the adult, initial management must include cervical spine immobilization. Care must be taken when elevating the child's chin to avoid manually compressing the soft tissues of the neck and trachea. Once manual control of the airway has been achieved, an oropharyngeal airway can be placed if no gag reflex is present. This type of airway device must be carefully and gently inserted parallel to the course of the tongue rather than turned 90° or 180° in the posterior oropharynx as in the adult. Use of a tongue blade to depress the tongue may be helpful.

The child's larynx is smaller than an adult's, has a slightly more anterocaudad angle (forward and toward the feet), and is frequently more difficult to visualize for direct cannulation. Despite this, the most reliable means of ventilation in the child with airway compromise remains direct orotracheal intubation. Nasotracheal intubation requires blind passage around a relatively acute posterior nasopharyngeal angle and might cause severe bleeding or even inadvertent penetration of the cranial vault. In the absence of appropriate intubation equipment, bag-valve-mask (BVM) ventilation with 100% oxygen is an acceptable alternative. The child whose craniofacial injuries cause upper airway obstruction should be considered for immediate needle cricothyroidotomy through which high-flow oxygen (FiO_2) can be delivered through a Y connector in cycles of 1 second on (inhalation) and 3 seconds off (exhalation). This is only a temporary measure and must be converted to more definitive airway support either via tracheostomy or surgical cricothyroidotomy as soon as safely possible.

Rapid Sequence Intubation

Many trauma centers and increasing numbers of prehospital providers are using rapid sequence intubation (RSI). Rapid sequence refers to a protocol for sedation and paralysis prior to intubation. The steps in the process of RSI include preoxygenation with 100% FiO_2. In a spontaneously breathing patient, this can be with a nonrebreather mask. In the apneic or hypoventilating patient, use a period of BVM ventilation along with the Sellick maneuver to avoid insufflating the stomach.

All children undergoing endotracheal (ET) intubation should receive atropine sulfate to keep the heart rate high since heart rate is the major determinant of perfusion in children. After preoxygenation, sedation is given. A short-acting barbiturate such as thiopental is standard, but in hypotensive patients short-acting benzodiazepines or other agents may be used. This is followed by muscle paralysis with rapid-onset, short-acting agents such as succinylcholine. Patients in whom succinylcholine is contraindicated (increased intracranial pressure [ICP], increased intra-orbital pressure, muscle disease, or recent burns) may need alternative non-depolarizing muscle relaxants. Intubation then is performed with cricoid pressure maintained until tube position is confirmed.

Some studies suggest that tube confirmation by auscultation alone can be unreliable and an alternative method such as direct visualization, end tidal CO_2 or an ETT detector device be used as a supplement. However the use of an end tidal CO_2 device has also been found to be unreliable when used as the sole method of tube placement confirmation. Saturation with O_2 is another adjunct that may assist in confirming endotracheal location of the tube.

As in the adult, endotracheal intubation must include careful attention to the cervical spine. The head must be maintained in a neutral position by a second EMT while careful laryngoscopy and endotracheal intubation are performed. The narrowest portion of the pediatric airway is the cricoid ring, so an uncuffed endotracheal tube should always be used in infants and toddlers. Appropriate size can be readily assessed by evaluating the diameter of the child's fifth finger or the diameter of the patient's external nares. A slight amount of cricoid pressure (the Sellick maneuver) will frequently bring the anterior structures of the child's larynx into better view and will passively obstruct the esophagus. This diminishes gastric insufflation and ensures accurate cannulation of the trachea.

A common error that occurs during intubation of children under emergency circumstances is an overly aggressive insertion of the endotracheal tube causing right mainstem bronchial intubation. Because of this, careful auscultation of the chest must be performed as soon as the endotracheal tube is placed and must be periodically reevaluated to ensure that the tube's position is appropriate. In addition to confirming the presence of the endotracheal tube above the carina, auscultation will also confirm breath sounds bilaterally and rule out the possibility that a tension pneumothorax or other primary pulmonary injury has occurred. The child with a compromised airway and a primary pulmonary parenchymal injury who is successfully intubated may be in greater jeopardy for the development of a tension pneumothorax as a result of a more efficient delivery of tidal volume to the tracheobronchial tree. *It is absolutely essential that careful auscultation be a reflex maneuver performed immediately and periodically thereafter to document both the presence of breath sounds and the overall status of ventilatory function.*

BREATHING

As in all trauma patients, the significantly traumatized child needs an FiO_2 of 0.85 to 1.00. This is accomplished by use of supplemental oxygen and an appropriately sized pediatric mask. When hypoxia occurs in the small child, the body compensates by increasing the breathing rate (tachypnea) and by a strenuous increase in ventilatory effort, including increased thoracic excursion efforts and the use of accessory muscles in the neck and abdomen. This increased effort can produce severe fatigue, resulting in ventilatory failure. Respiratory distress can rapidly progress from a compensated ventilatory effort to ventilatory failure, then respiratory arrest, and ultimately cardiac arrest secondary to the respiratory problem.

Evaluation of the child's level of ventilation with early recognition of distress and the provision of ventilatory assistance are key elements in the management of the pediatric trauma patient. The normal ventilatory rate of infants and children less than 4 years old is 2 to 3 times that of adults (Table 13-2).

Tachypnea with signs of increased effort or difficulty may be the first manifestations of respiratory distress and/or shock. As the distress increases, additional signs and symptoms will include shallow breathing with minimal chest movement. Breath sounds may be weak or infrequent and air exchange at the nose or mouth will be reduced or even minimal. The ventilatory effort will become more labored and may include the following:

- head bobbing with each breath
- gasping or grunting
- flared nostrils
- stridor or snoring
- suprasternal, supraclavicular, and intercostal retractions
- use of accessory muscles of neck and abdomen
- distension of the abdomen when chest falls (seesaw effect between the chest and abdomen)

The effectiveness of the child's ventilation should be evaluated using the following indicators:

Exchange
- rate and depth (minute volume) and effort

Auscultation
- breath sounds confirming depth of exchange
- wheezing, rales, or rhonchi indicate a problem and inefficient alveolar oxygenation

Skin color and color of mucosa
- pink: adequate respiration
- dusky, gray, cyanotic, or mottled indicates insufficient oxygen exchange

Mental status
- overly anxious, restless, or combative: possible early signs of hypoxia
- lethargy, lowered level of consciousness, or unconsciousness: probable advanced signs of hypoxia

A rapid evaluation of ventilation can be made using the rate (particularly tachypnea), effort (degree of labor, nostril flaring, accessory muscle use, retraction, seesaw movement), auscultation (air exchange, bilateral symmetry, pathological sounds), skin color, and mental status as primary indices. Central (rather than peripheral) cyanosis is a fairly late and often inconsistent sign. Visualization of cyanosis requires that the patient have at least 5 grams of unoxygenated hemoglobin.

In the child initially presenting with tachypnea and increased ventilatory effort, a subsequently decreasing respiratory rate and apparent lessening in effort may actually be indicative of exhaustion and further reduced ventilation. This sequence should not be misinterpreted as always being a sign of improvement.

Children with diminished air exchange (minute volume) or those who are in acute ventilatory distress should be provided with ventilatory assistance. Such patients will not benefit materially from only receiving high-percentage supplemental oxygen, since their main problem is one of volume rather than oxygen percentage in the inspired air. Assisted or provided respiration in apneic children is best provided using a bag-valve-mask device. Use of the correct mask size is essential for obtaining a proper mask seal. It is also essential in providing the proper tidal volume and in ensuring that hyperinflation (resulting in gastric distension) or barotrauma does not occur.

When obtaining a mask seal in infants, caution must be used to avoid compressing the floor of the mouth, as this will push the tongue back into the airway and against the soft palate. Care must also be taken to avoid any pressure on the uncalcified soft trachea. One or two hands can be used to obtain a mask seal. Excessive delivered

Table 13-2 Respiratory rates for pediatric patients

Group	Age	Breaths/min	Suspect possible ↓ in minute volume and need for ventilatory assist with BVM
Newborn	birth–6 weeks	30–50	↓ 30 or ↑ 50
Infant	7 weeks–1 year	20–30 ⎫	
Toddler	1–2 years	20–30 ⎪	↓ 20 or ↑ 30
Preschool	2–6 years	20–30 ⎬	
School age	6–13 years	(12–20)–30 ⎭	
Adolescent	13–16 years	12–20	↓ 12 or ↑ 20

volumes and excessively high pressures within the pharynx must be avoided, as either will result in producing gastric distension. Gastric distension may result in regurgitation or may prevent adequate ventilation by limiting diaphragmatic excursion.

Once ventilation has been initiated, the bag-valve-mask should be supplemented with an oxygen reservoir and be attached to high-flow oxygen to ensure an FiO_2 of 0.85 to 1.00. Because the child's airway is so small, initial and periodic suctioning may be necessary. In infants, who are obligate nose breathers, suctioning of the nostrils should be included.

Changes in a child's respiratory status can be subtle, and breathing effort can rapidly deteriorate until ventilation is inadequate and hypoxia occurs. Breathing should be carefully evaluated as part of the initial primary survey, and then carefully rechecked periodically to ensure its continued adequacy.

CIRCULATION

The survival rate from immediate exsanguinating injury is very low in the pediatric population. Fortunately, however, the incidence of this type of injury is also very low. Injured children usually present with at least some circulating blood volume and respond appropriately to expeditious volume replacement. As in assessment of the airway, it must be emphasized that a single measurement of heart rate or blood pressure does not equate with physiologic stability. Close monitoring of vital signs is absolutely essential to prevent hypotension and shock. The normal ranges for pulse rate and blood pressure for different age groups are presented in Tables 13-3 and 13-4 and will be helpful guidelines for the EMT.

If the initial assessment suggests severe hypotension, the most likely cause is blood loss—either through a major external wound (readily observable), an intrathoracic wound (identifiable by diminished ventilatory mechanics and auscultatory findings), or loss of blood from a major intra-abdominal injury. Since blood is not a compressible medium, blood loss from a major intra-abdominal injury will frequently produce abdominal distension and increasing abdominal girth.

Vascular Access

Fluid replacement in a child with severe hypotension or frank shock must deliver adequate fluid volume to the right atrium as directly as possible to avoid fur-

Table 13-3 Pulse rates for pediatric patients

Group	Age	Beats/min	Assume a serious problem exists (bradycardia or tachycardia)
Newborn	birth–6 weeks	120–160	↓100 or ↑150
Infant	7 weeks–1 year	80–140	↓ 80 or ↑120
Toddler	1–2 years	80–130 ⎫	↓ 60 or ↑110
Preschool	2–6 years	80–120 ⎬	
School age	6–13 years	(60–80)–100 ⎫	↓ 60 or ↑100
Adolescent	13–16 years	60–100 ⎬	

Table 13-4 Blood pressure in pediatric patients

Group	Age	Expected mean for blood pressure*	Lower limit of systolic BP
Newborn	Birth–6 weeks	74–100 mg Hg ⎫ 50–68 mm Hg	
Infant	7 weeks–1 year	84–106 mm Hg 56–70 mm Hg ⎬	↓70 mm Hg
Toddler	1–2 years	98–106 mm Hg 50–70 mm Hg	
Preschool	2–6 years	98–112 mm Hg 64–70 mm Hg ⎭	
School age	6–13 years	104–124 mm Hg ⎫ 64–80 mm Hg	↓80–90 mm Hg
Adolescent	13–16 years	118–132 mm Hg 70–82 mm Hg ⎬	

*The top numbers represent systolic range; the bottom numbers represent diastolic range.

ther reducing cardiac preload. Thus, the most appropriate initial site for intravenous access is above the diaphragm and should first be attempted at the antecubital fossa. In the absence of adequate venous access at this location, the saphenous vein at the ankle should be considered. Despite the fact that this latter location provides fluid replacement at a distal point below the diaphragm, the ready availability of this vessel usually ensures reliable vascular access.

In the unstable, or potentially unstable, patient, attempts at peripheral access should be limited to two attempts in 90 seconds. If access is unsuccessful, central access via intraosseous infusion in the child under 7 years old is indicated. Percutaneous cannulation of the external jugular or saphenous cutdown are other possibilities.

Intraosseous infusion can provide an adequate alternative site for volume replacement in injured children. Certainly this is an effective route for infusion of medication and recently has been documented as an equally effective means to provide high-volume fluid resuscitation (Box 13-1).

Cannulation of the femoral vein is contraindicated due to the risk of thrombosis and circulatory compromise of the leg.

Placement of a subclavian catheter in the injured child should be performed only under the most controlled circumstances within the hospital and should not be attempted in the prehospital setting.

Vascular access should be obtained in any child needing fluid replacement. The establishment of a "to keep open" (TKO) intravenous "lifeline" in anticipation of the potential need for fluid replacement, however, represents a prehospital problem without an easy answer.

In adults, such an intravenous line is established if any chance of its need exists. Because of the possibility of evolving shock and the child's potential to decompensate rapidly, there would appear to be a greater indication for TKO intravenous lines in children. However, this is offset by the fact that starting an intravenous line in children can be extremely difficult and time consuming for the EMT and may add to the child's psychologic trauma.

The determination of which pediatric patients should have an IV access line started is dependent on transport times and local trauma protocols. If the EMT is unsure, or if the EMT has any suspicion that fluid replacement has become indicated during transport, he or she should contact medical direction for concurrence in obtaining IV access.

Fluid Therapy

As in the adult, Ringer's lactate is the initial resuscitation fluid for the hypovolemic child. Since the length of time a crystalloid fluid remains in the vascular system is so short, a 3:1 ratio of crystalloid fluid to blood lost must be

followed. As in the adult, signs of significant hypotension develop with the loss of approximately 25% of the circulating volume. Thus, an initial resuscitative bolus should reflect approximately 25% of the standard circulating volume in the pediatric patient. This calculates to be approximately 20 cc/kg. Considering the 3:1 ratio, it becomes obvious that a bolus of 50 to 60 cc/kg is required to achieve adequate and rapid initial replacement in response to significant volume loss. Any child who does not show a response after receiving the second or third 20 cc/kg bolus is severely bleeding and will need blood as soon as possible. The crystalloid bolus may temporarily restore cardiovascular dynamics as it transiently fills and then leaks from the circulatory system. Until red blood cell mass is replaced and oxygen transport restored, however, the basic process of cellular hypoxia will continue unchecked.

Injured children usually present in one of three ways: normotensive, hypotensive, or rapidly decompensated shock. Most demonstrate very little evidence of blood loss and hypotension. With the high incidence of potential head injury, it becomes obvious that volume replacement must balance restoration of adequate circulating

---

Box 13-1   Intraosseous Infusion

The easiest site for intraosseous infusion is the anterior tibia, just below the tibial tuberosity. After preparing the skin antiseptically and securing the leg adequately, choose a site on the anterior portion of the tibia, 1 to 2 cm distal and medial to the tibial tuberosity. Specially manufactured intraosseous infusion needles are optimal for the procedure, but spinal or bone marrow needles also may be used. Spinal needles that are 18 to 20 gauge work well because they have a trocar to prevent the needle from being obstructed as it passes through the bony cortex into the marrow. Any 14 to 20 gauge needle can be used in an emergency. Place the needle at a 90° angle to the bone and advance it firmly through the cortex into the marrow. Evidence that the needle is adequately within the marrow includes:

1. a soft "pop" and lack of resistance after the needle has passed through the cortex
2. aspiration of bone marrow into the needle
3. free flow of fluid into the marrow without evidence of subcutaneous infiltration

Consider intraosseous infusion of fluid, blood, and medication during the initial minutes of resuscitation if percutaneous venous cannulation has been unsuccessful. Because the flow rate is limited, the intraosseous route alone will seldom be sufficient.

volume against fluid overload with its potentially detrimental effect on evolving cerebral edema.

Children who present in hypovolemic shock and respond to large amounts (50 to 60 cc/kg in 20 cc/kg boluses) of crystalloid resuscitation need blood replacement as soon as possible. As a result of the crystalloid bolus, these patients frequently regain adequate cardiac output. However, the resulting circulating volume has minimal oxygen-carrying capacity. Continuing hypoxia induces a cellular shift to anaerobic metabolism which presents as a significant lactic acidosis. *These children must be aggressively resuscitated and must be transported without delay to the hospital in order to be transfused with red blood cells.* Only under these circumstances will they have even the slightest chance of surviving their hemorrhagic injury.

A major consideration in the assessment of the pediatric victim is the concept of compensated shock. Because of their increased physiologic reserve, children with hemorrhagic injury will frequently present with only slightly abnormal vital signs. Initial tachycardia not only may be the result of hypovolemia but also may be the effect of psychologic stress, pain, and fear. Moreover, a very small patient may have a systolic blood pressure that, while considered alarmingly low for an adult, may be within the normal range for a healthy child. All injured children must be monitored continuously with close ordered observation of blood pressure, heart rate, ventilatory rate, and overall central nervous system status. The child with hemorrhagic injury can maintain adequate circulating volume by increasing his or her peripheral resistance to maintain mean arterial pressure. If initial resuscitation is inadequate, circulating volume will eventually diminish to a point below which increased peripheral resistance can maintain arterial pressure. The concept of evolving shock must be of prime concern in the initial management of the injured child and is a major indication for transport to the hospital and proper physician evaluation of even minor appearing injuries.

The EMT must always remember the priorities of the A B C D E method. If a child is alert enough to be managed without an airway, it is highly unlikely that a massively exsanguinating lesion is present. Any injury more severe will first require establishment of an airway and then an intravenous line, which can serve as an emergency portal of entry for the LEAN drugs (lidocaine, epinephrine, atropine, and Narcan). Moreover, a rapidly placed intravenous line will save precious minutes and provide a quick site for fluid infusion.

DISABILITY
Neurologic Assessment

Once initial assessment, airway control, and fluid resuscitation have been accomplished, attention can be addressed to a thorough examination of the entire child. The overall guidelines for this are based on a high index of suspicion—until proven otherwise—that every major organ system has been injured. The initial examination must include an assessment of neurologic status. While the child's level of consciousness (using AVPU) remains a reliable prognostic indicator of the severity of any central nervous system deficit, this assessment must be expanded to include PEARRL, orientation and mentation, motor function, and sensory perception. (Refer to Chapter 2 for a review of AVPU and PEARRL.) The Glasgow Coma Scale is an excellent guideline for assessment of neurologic status. It should be repeated frequently and used to document progression or regression of neurologic status during the post-injury period. (Refer to Chapters 2 and 8 for a review of the Glasgow Coma Scale.)

Primary Survey

The initial physical examination of the child follows the standard assessment protocol. The thorax must be evaluated with special consideration of potential cardiac or pulmonary contusions, both of which may be worsened by overly aggressive fluid resuscitation. Since the increased resiliency of a child's ribs may have allowed transmission of significantly greater energy to underlying thoracic organs, there may be an extensive pulmonary contusion with no external signs. Because trauma patients frequently have full stomachs, the possibility of pulmonary aspiration must always be considered. This is especially true for children who are obtunded or who have posttraumatic seizure activity.

Although rib fractures are rare in childhood, they are associated with a high risk of death. Even if a rib fracture is an isolated injury, it should be viewed by the EMT as an indicator of severe trauma. The risk of mortality increases with the number of ribs fractured.

Examination of the abdomen must focus on distension, tenderness, discoloration, or presence of a mass. Careful palpation of the iliac crests may suggest an unstable pelvic fracture and increase suspicion for possible retroperitoneal or urogenital injury.

Finally, each extremity must be palpated to rule out deformity, diminished vascular supply, or neurologic deficit. The child's incompletely calcified skeleton with its multiple growth centers increases the possibility of epiphyseal disruption. Accordingly, any area of edema, pain, tenderness, or diminished range of motion should be carefully evaluated and suspected as being fractured until ruled out by radiographic examination at the hospital. In adults and children alike, a missed orthopedic injury in an extremity has little impact on mortality, but it may have a major long-term effect on deformity and disability.

ASSESSMENT OF QUANTITATIVE VITAL SIGNS AND QUANTITATIVE NORMS

The term "pediatric" or "child" includes a vast range of physical development, emotional maturity, and body sizes. The approach to the patient and the implications of many injuries vary greatly between an infant at one end of the spectrum and an adolescent at the other end.

In most anatomic and therapeutic dosage considerations, the child's weight (or specific height/length) serves as a more accurate indicator than does exact chronologic age. As mentioned earlier, Table 13-1 describes the average height and weight for healthy children of varying ages and is a helpful tool for the EMT.

Additional information on normal findings can be found in the Pediatric Advanced Life Support (PALS) text published by the American Heart Association and the Advanced Pediatric Life Support (APLS) course produced by the American Academy of Pediatrics and the American College of Emergency Physicians.

The acceptable ranges of quantitative vital signs vary for the different ages within the pediatric population. Adult norms cannot be used as guidelines in smaller children. In an adult a ventilatory rate of 30 would be tachypneic and a pulse rate of 120 would be tachycardic. Both would be considered alarmingly high and would be significant pathologic findings. The same findings in an infant, however, may be well within the normal ranges.

Studies in the pediatric literature and lists in various pediatric texts may not be consistent, displaying the normal ranges for different age groupings. As an additional complication, in a child who has been injured and for whom the EMT has no previous history of normal vital signs, a conservative approach dictates viewing borderline signs as if they are pathologic—even though in that individual child they may be physiologically acceptable. To aid the EMT in evaluating vital signs, the guidelines in Tables 13-2, 13-3, and 13-4 will be helpful.

It must be noted that these tables represent ranges into which the findings of most children in these age groups will fall. They do not define the limits of good health, they only describe the ranges that are statistically common.

Being able to remember all of these numbers is unrealistic for the EMT who treats pediatric patients as a small percentage of his or her total runs. It is more practical to keep a handy reference guide, both in the ambulance and in the pediatric resuscitation kit. Copies of the tables in this text can be made and used for that purpose. (Permission to duplicate these tables for such use is herein granted to EMS services.) Alternately, several commercially available items exist to serve as rapid references for pediatric vital signs and equipment size. These include the Resuscitation Tape devised by Broselow et al. and several slide rule–type plastic scales.

It may also be helpful to use the following guideline formulas to estimate the expected finding for any age:

Weight

$$\text{Weight (kg)} = 8 + (2 \times \text{child's age in years})$$

Systolic blood pressure

$$\text{Systolic BP (mm Hg)} = 80 + (2 \times \text{child's age in years})$$

Total vascular blood volume

$$\text{Blood volume (cc)} = 80 \text{ cc} \times \text{child's weight in kilograms}$$

As in adults, it is important to note that the quantitative vital signs—though important—are only an additional piece of information in making an assessment. It is essential to remember how rapidly a child can deteriorate into either critical respiratory difficulty or decompensated shock. The EMT should not assume that a pediatric trauma victim is stable just because the vital signs are presently within acceptable ranges. Instead, they must be used in the context of all of the findings. The EMT must ascribe equal value to the mechanism of injury, the qualitative findings, and the quantitative vital signs in evaluating potential problems.

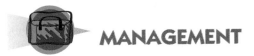

MANAGEMENT

The key to pediatric trauma survival is a good rapid assessment followed by appropriate aggressive management.

AIRWAY, VENTILATION, AND CIRCULATION

As in the adult, the immediate priority and focus is on airway management, ventilation, and circulation. The relatively large tongue and more anterior position of the airway make small children more likely to have an airway obstruction than adults. A patent airway should be ensured and maintained with suctioning, manual maneuvers, and airway adjuncts along with proper spine protection throughout. The airway adjuncts of choice in patients with an absent gag reflex are the oropharyngeal airway and—if advanced personnel are available—visualized orotracheal intubation.

Minute volume and ventilatory effort must be carefully evaluated. Due to the child's potential for rapid deterioration from hypoxia to ventilatory arrest, the EMT should promptly consider assisted ventilation if he or she observes dyspnea and increased effort. This assisted ventilation should be provided using a properly sized bag-valve-mask with a reservoir and high-flow oxygen to provide an FiO_2 of between 0.85 to 1.00. In patients who do have an adequate minute volume, supplemental oxygen should be provided by mask (with a goal of FiO_2 of 0.85 to 1.00).

Circulation and perfusion need to be carefully evaluated. The pediatric vascular system is commonly able to maintain a normal blood pressure until severe collapse occurs, at which point it is often unresponsive to resuscitation. Therefore, fluid resuscitation should be started whenever signs of compensated hypovolemic shock are present, and especially in those patients who present with decompensated shock. Therapy begins with lactated Ringer's or normal saline in 20 cc/kg boluses.

Remember that for pediatric trauma patients who display any signs of hemorrhagic shock or hypovolemia, key factors to survival are blood replacement and rapid initiation of transport to a suitable facility.

At present, use of the pneumatic antishock garment in children is limited to patients who can be properly fitted into either a pediatric or adult garment. In most cases, this latter group could be considered "almost-adult size" children, and PASG use follows the same indications and contraindications as for adults. Use of the PASG should be limited to children who can be properly fitted into the garment (pediatric or adult size) without the need to modify either the garment or the standard methods of application (see Chapter 6).

The most frequently cited caution regarding the use of a PASG on pediatric patients is the possibility of the abdominal section overlapping the lower ribs. When the abdominal section is inflated in such cases, this invariably provokes ventilatory compromise and significant respiratory distress.

No present studies indicate any benefit from PASG usage on children. In the absence of specific studies, use of the garment on a child smaller than the general size for which the garment has been designed (pediatric or adult size) must be assumed to be potentially dangerous and should not be attempted. Alternatively, use of the garment on a patient whose body size is large enough should not be withheld simply because the patient is chronologically still a child.

HEAD INJURY

Head injury continues to be the most common cause of death in the pediatric population. Of the fatalities listed in the first 40,000 patients in the National Pediatric Trauma Registry, 89% had a central nervous system injury as either the primary or secondary contributor to mortality. Although many of the most severe injuries are treatable only by prevention, there are initial resuscitative

measures that may at least lessen the serious consequences of the child's central nervous system injury. Again, the premise of adequate oxygenation, ventilation, and circulation must be addressed and must be the primary consideration.

In the child with a head injury, hyperventilation with adequate oxygenation must be considered as soon as the signs and symptoms of increased intracranial pressure (ICP) and impending herniation are suggested. From the moment of injury, the reflex responses occurring within the closed cranial vault are partially related to perfusion pressure, tissue oxygenation, and evolving edema. Thus, any child who presents with signs and symptoms of impending herniation such as unilateral dilated pupil, hypertension, or bradycardia should be considered for hyperventilation as soon as possible. This is easily achieved in the sensory-depressed or comatose child by initial airway control, ventilation with a bag-valve device via either mask or endotracheal tube, and supplemental oxygen providing an FiO_2 of 0.85 to 1.0.

Initial assessment of the level of consciousness is a rapid and reliable prognostic exercise. Regardless of the outcome of the neurologic evaluation on the first examination, any child sustaining potential head injury may be susceptible to cerebral edema and hypoperfusion. This can result from even the most minor trauma. Every child who presents with even a transitory loss of consciousness must be assumed to have sustained a significant level of mechanical trauma to the brain stem and reticular activating system.

Even if the level of consciousness returns to normal, careful observation should be considered to rule out the possibility of evolving secondary dysfunction as a result of cerebral edema or a space-occupying lesion in the form of a subdural or epidural hematoma. Because head trauma is frequently the most severe and life-threatening injury, the probability of an injured child requiring an immediate CT scan for assessment of the central nervous system is quite high. Therefore a careful Glasgow Coma Scale baseline and transport to a suitable facility without delay are paramount to successful management of these children.

SPINAL TRAUMA

The indication for spinal immobilization in a pediatric patient—as in adults—is based on the mechanism of injury; the presence of other injuries suggesting violent or sudden movement of the head, neck, or torso; or the presence of specific signs of spine injury, such as deformity, pain, or neurologic deficit. As with adult patients, the correct prehospital management of a suspected unstable spine is manual immobilization, use of a properly fitting cervical collar, and immobilization of the patient to a rigid device so that the head, neck, torso, pelvis, and legs are maintained in a neutral in-line position. This must be achieved without inhibiting ventilation, the ability to open the mouth, or any other required resuscitation.

It is important to note that when most small children are placed on a rigid surface, the relatively larger size of the child's head posterior to the spinal column will result in moving the head into a flexed position. Such padding as is necessary should be placed under the torso to elevate it enough to allow the head to be in a neutral position. The padding should be continuous and flat from the shoulders to the pelvis and extend to the lateral margins of the torso to ensure that the thoracic, lumbar, and sacral spine are on a flat, continuous, stable platform without movement. It is also important to pad between the lateral sides of the child and the edges of the board to ensure that no lateral movement occurs when the board is moved or if the patient and board need to be rotated to the side to avoid aspiration of vomitus.

A variety of new pediatric immobilization devices are becoming available and should be evaluated and considered by EMS services. The EMT must practice and be familiar with the required adjustments when immobilizing a child with adult size equipment. Vest devices designed for adult use should not be used on children with body sizes smaller than an adult's. Any modified use may not provide proper immobilization or may produce dangerous or otherwise deleterious side effects. The EMT must also be familiar with the techniques of immobilizing a young child in a car safety seat.

THORACIC INJURIES

As mentioned earlier, the extremely resilient rib cage of a child with its incomplete calcification provides a means where energy transferred through the thoracic cage to the intrathoracic organs is frequently less reduced and more potentially devastating than in the adult population. As a result, the child may have significant organ injury, disruption of vascular anatomy, or simple contusion without manifestation of even the slightest degree of skeletal abnormality on external examination.

A high index of suspicion is the key to diagnosis of these injuries. Every child sustaining trauma to the chest and torso should be carefully monitored for signs of respiratory difficulty and shock. Even if no distress is present, the child should be transported without delay to a suitable facility for radiographic chest examination and careful evaluation of cardiopulmonary and ventilatory function. Radiologic evidence of pulmonary contusion has been found in children who, other than having a history of blunt torso trauma, are completely asymptomatic.

Being aware of this potential problem requires the EMT to provide continuous careful monitoring of the child's fluid status to ensure prevention of gross intra-

venous fluid overload. It is also important to remember that, unlike adults, *rib fractures in children are associated with a high risk of death*. Even if they are an isolated injury, one or more fractured ribs should be viewed by the EMT as an indication of the presence of multisystem trauma, even in the absence of other apparent signs.

Finally, the possibility of a cardiac contusion in children who suffer blunt thoracic trauma must be considered. When transporting a child who has sustained a high-impact blunt thoracic injury, EMTs should monitor cardiac rhythm once they are en route.

The key items in managing thoracic trauma involve the A B C D E method, careful attention to ventilation, and timely transport to an appropriate facility.

ABDOMINAL INJURIES

Because of the increased size of the torso relative to the extremities in children, abdominal injuries continue to be an extremely common problem. As has been discussed, the presence of blunt trauma to the abdomen; an unstable pelvis; post-traumatic abdominal distension, rigidity, or tenderness; or otherwise unexplained levels of shock must be assumed to be associated with possible intra-abdominal hemorrhage.

The key elements in management include fluid resuscitation, supplemental oxygen to provide a high FiO_2, and rapid initiation of transport to an appropriate facility with continued careful monitoring en route.

EXTREMITY TRAUMA

In comparison to the adult, the child's skeleton is actively growing and consists of a large proportion of cartilaginous tissue and metabolically active growth plates. The collateral ligaments holding the skeleton together are frequently stronger and better able to withstand mechanical disruption than the bones to which they are attached. As a result, children with skeletal trauma frequently sustain major deforming forces prior to developing fractures or disruptions of their bony skeleton.

Primary joint disruption from injury other than penetrating injury is uncommon in comparison to disruption of the diaphyseal or epiphyseal segments of bone. Fractures involving the growth plate must be carefully identified and managed in a manner that will ensure not only adequate healing but also prevention of subsequent displacement or deformity as the child grows. The association of vascular injuries with orthopedic injuries must always be considered in children, and the EMT should carefully evaluate the distal pulse.

In pediatric patients with an isolated extremity injury, it is important for an EMT to assume that even a seemingly minor skeletal injury requires hospital treatment. Because the potential for unrecognized growth plate injury or vascular disruption may result in subsequent impaired limb growth and deformity, such injuries require careful examination and evaluation at the hospital. Often the presence of a potentially deforming injury can be ruled out only by radiologic study or, when there is the slightest suggestion of a decrease in distal perfusion, by arteriography.

In the child with more than just isolated extremity injuries, as with adult patients, the EMT must focus on the essentials and not be distracted from potentially life-threatening injuries by the apparent gross deformity sometimes associated with extremity injury. Uncontrolled hemorrhage represents the sole life-threatening condition associated with extremity trauma. In multisystem pediatric and adult trauma patients alike, the initiation of transport to an appropriate facility without delay after the primary assessment, resuscitation, and rapid packaging have been completed remains paramount in reducing mortality. In such cases, even though the patient is packaged and moved prior to a secondary examination, proper immobilization on a longboard supports and splints any extremity fractures—known, unknown, or missed.

TRIAGE

Because timely arrival at an appropriate hospital may be the key element in survival, triage is an important consideration of management.

The tragedy of preventable pediatric traumatic death has been documented in multiple studies reported over the past three decades. As many as 53 out of 100 pediatric trauma deaths could be classified as preventable. These statistics have been one of the prime motivations for the development of regionalized pediatric trauma centers where continuous high-quality, sophisticated care can be provided.

In some areas, both pediatric trauma centers and adult trauma centers exist. If there is only a small delay, the pediatric multisystem trauma patient benefits from the initial resuscitation capability and definitive care available at a facility specialized in treating traumatized children. For many locations, however, the nearest specialized pediatric trauma center is hours away. In such places, the seriously traumatized child should be transported to the nearest adult trauma center. In areas where no specialized pediatric trauma center is nearby, personnel working in adult trauma centers are experienced in the resuscitation and treatment of both adult and pediatric trauma victims. In areas where neither are readily close, the EMT should transport the seriously injured child to the nearest appropriate hospital (for trauma victims) according to local protocols.

In many areas, the problems of distance have been surmounted by the availability of a medical helicopter that responds directly to the field. This option often makes it possible to deliver advanced trauma care in the field and allows transport to a higher level facility in situations where—if only ground transport were available—this level of care and facility availability would be unrealistic in terms of the time required. Where helicopter response and advanced care transport are available, this option should be included in the triage scheme.

Review of over 15,000 records in the National Pediatric Trauma Registry (NPTR) indicates that 25% of children are injured severely enough to require triage to a designated pediatric trauma center. Objective identification by the EMT of the one patient in four who does require appropriate triage to such a facility is essential for improved survival from pediatric injury.

PEDIATRIC TRAUMA SCORE

As mentioned previously, the Pediatric Trauma Score (PTS) was developed specifically as a triage tool for pediatric trauma victims. It consists of a categorization system where six components of pediatric injury are each graded and then added together to produce a score that is predictive of injury severity and potential for mortality. The system is based on an analysis of pediatric injury patterns and is designed to provide a protocol checklist that will ensure that all the major factors relative to outcome from pediatric injury are considered in the initial evaluation of the child. It is different from the Revised Trauma Score (RTS), which only considers vital signs (blood pressure, respiratory rate, Glasgow Coma Scale). The PTS is intentionally designed as a checklist that addresses the six factors critical to outcome from injury in the pediatric patient (Table 13-5).

In evaluating a patient with the PTS size is the first consideration because it is readily observed and is a major consideration in the infant/toddler group where mortality from injury is highest. Airway is assessed not only as a functional status, but also as a description of what type of care is required to provide adequate management.

The most important factor in initial assessment of the central nervous system is level of consciousness. Because children frequently sustain very transient loss of consciousness during an injury, the obtunded (+1) grade is applied to any child with loss of consciousness—no matter how fleeting. This grade identifies the patient as likely to develop potentially fatal yet frequently treatable intracranial sequelae secondary to head injury.

Systolic blood pressure assessment is arranged primarily to identify those children in whom evolving preventable shock may occur (51 to 90 mm Hg systolic

Table 13-5 Pediatric Trauma Score: category definitions

Component	+2	+1	−1
Size	child/adolescent >20 kg	toddler 11–20 kg	infant <10 kg
Airway	normal	assisted: O_2, mask, cannula	intubated: ETT, EOA, cricothyroidotomy
Consciousness	awake	obtunded lost consciousness	coma unresponsive
Systolic blood pressure	>90 mm Hg good peripheral pulses, perfusion	51–90 mm Hg carotid/femoral pulse palpable	<50 mm Hg weak or no pulses
Fracture	none seen or suspected	single closed fracture anywhere	open or multiple fractures
Cutaneous	no visible injury	contusion, abrasion laceration <7 cm not through fascia	tissue loss any GSW/stab through fascia

The Pediatric Trauma Score is primarily designed to function as a checklist. Each component can be assessed by basic physical examination. Airway evaluation is designed to reflect intervention required for effective care. An open fracture is graded −1 for fracture, and −1 for cutaneous injury. As clinical observation and diagnostic evaluation continue, further definition and reassessment will establish a trend that predicts severity of injury and potential outcome.

blood pressure; +1). Regardless of size, a child whose systolic blood pressure is below 50 mm Hg (−1) is in obvious jeopardy. On the other hand, a child whose systolic blood pressure exceeds 90 mm Hg (+2) probably falls into a better outcome category than a child with even a slight degree of hypotension. If the appropriately sized blood pressure cuff is not available, the systolic pressure is assessed as +2 if radial or pedal pulse is palpable, +1 if only carotid or femoral pulse is palpable, and −1 if no pulse is palpable.

Because of the high incidence of skeletal injury in the pediatric population and its potential contribution to mortality and disability, the presence of a fracture is included as a component. Finally, open wounds—both as an adjunct to common pediatric trauma patterns, as well as an injury category that includes penetrating wounds—are considered in computing the Pediatric Trauma Score.

By nature of its design, the PTS serves as a straightforward checklist that ensures that all of the components that are critical to initial assessment of the injured child are considered. It can be used by prehospital providers, as well as by physicians and in facilities other than pediatric trauma units.

As a predictor of injury, the PTS has a statistically significant inverse linear relationship with patient mortality. There is a threshold score of 8, below which injured children should be triaged to an appropriate pediatric trauma center. These are the children in whom the potential for preventable mortality and morbidity is greatest.

THE BATTERED/ABUSED CHILD

Child abuse is a significant cause of childhood injury. It is critical that EMTs consider the possibility of child abuse when circumstances warrant.

In many jurisdictions, EMTs are legally mandated reporters if they identify potential child abuse. Generally, reporters who act in good faith are protected from legal action by the reported party.

An EMT should suspect abuse if he or she notes any of the following scenarios.

1. A discrepancy exists between the history and the degree of physical injury.
2. A prolonged interval has passed between the time of the injury and when medical care is actually sought.
3. A history of the injury is inconsistent with the developmental level of the child. For example, a history indicating that a newborn rolled off a bed would be suspect since newborns are developmentally unable to roll over.

Certain injury types also suggest abuse such as the following:

1. multiple bruises in varying stages of resolution
2. bizarre injuries such as bites, cigarette burns, or rope marks
3. sharply demarcated burns or scald injuries in unusual areas

Reporting procedures vary from state to state, so EMTs should be familiar with the appropriate agencies that handle child abuse cases in their location. The need to report abuse is emphasized by data suggesting that up to 50% of abused children who are released back to their abusers subsequently die of further abuse episodes.

• Summary •

1. The initial and continuing prehospital care of the injured child requires application of standard trauma life support principles modified by the unique characteristics of children.

2. Children have the ability to compensate for volume loss longer than adults, but when they exceed their ability to compensate, they deteriorate suddenly and severely.

3. Significant underlying organ and vascular injury can occur without apparent external injury, often with only mild external signs and symptoms.

4. Children with trauma and the following signs should be considered unstable and should be transported without delay to an appropriate facility.
   - difficulty breathing
   - signs of shock or circulatory instability
   - any period of post-insult unconsciousness
   - any significant blunt trauma to the thorax
   - any fractured ribs
   - any significant blunt trauma to the abdomen
   - any pelvic fracture

5. Children with multisystem trauma and a Pediatric Trauma Score less than 8 should, if possible, be triaged to a pediatric trauma center.

Scenario Solution

You correctly identify this child as a victim of multisystem trauma who is in shock. Because of the head injury, you elect to orally intubate and hyperventilate the patient using rapid sequence intubation and appropriate cervical precautions. You correctly identify hypotension and tachycardia, which you assume is related to hypovolemic shock, probably as a result of an intra-abdominal injury, most likely a ruptured spleen. Brief efforts at peripheral venous access are unsuccessful. You begin crystalloid infusion via an intraosseous line.

Because of the nature of the child's injuries, you consult with medical control who agrees that helicopter transport to a more distant pediatric trauma center is more appropriate than ground transport to a nearby community hospital that has no pediatric resources. The patient's mother arrives just as you are transferring care to the helicopter crew.

Review Questions

Answers provided on page 333.

1 Differences in injury patterns for children as compared to adults include all of the following *except:*
   A Bone growth plates are more likely to be damaged than tendons or ligaments.
   B Pulmonary contusions are more common than rib fractures.
   C Spinal cord injuries can occur in the absence of bony vertebral fracture better than children.

2 In managing the pediatric airway, the EMT should consider the following:
   A Cuffed endotracheal tubes are preferred over uncuffed.
   B A good estimate of ET tube diameter is the diameter of the patient's pinky finger.
   C oropharyngeal airways are inserted the same way in adults and children.
   D The Sellick maneuver is contraindicated in children.

3 A good way to estimate normal systolic blood pressure is to use the formula 80 + (2 × child's age in years)
   A True
   B False

4 The primary modifications of the Glasgow Coma Scale for children involve changes in the scoring for which component?
   A eye opening
   B motor
   C verbal
   D cognitive

5 In a pediatric patient who requires vascular access, all of the following are potentially appropriate for prehospital use *except:*
   A autocubital fossa (brachial vein)
   B intraosseous in proximal tibia
   C subclavian vein
   D saphenous vein at the ankle

6 In the child with hypovolemic shock, initial fluid replacement should consist of bolus therapy of D5W at 50 cc/kg.
   A True
   B False

7 Which of the following signs should alert the EMT to potential child abuse?
   A a 4-month-old with a skull fracture that occurred, according to the parents' report, when the child attempted to crawl down the stairs
   B a 12-year-old with multiple bruises in various stages of resolution
   C a 3-year-old with well-demarcated scald burns of the legs and buttocks that reportedly occurred while taking a bath
   D all of the above

8 There is clear data from the literature supporting the benefit of PASG use in children.
   A True
   B False

CHAPTER OBJECTIVES

CHAPTER 14

Special Considerations in Trauma of the Elderly

At the completion of this course the student will be able to:

- Demonstrate an understanding of the differences in the mechanism of injury for the elderly.

- Identify the variables in the pathophysiology of aging.

- Demonstrate an understanding of the special considerations in assessing the elderly.

- Understand the importance of identifying any preexisting medical conditions.

- Demonstrate an understanding of the effects of medications taken by the elderly.

- Communicate appropriately with the elderly.

- Define implied consent and explain the usually limited role of third-party powers in trauma scene decision making.

- Identify the signs and symptoms of abuse and neglect in the elderly.

Scenario

Called to the scene for a man down, you find a 70-year-old man at the bottom of a flight of ten stone steps. He appears lethargic and confused. Skin is pale and dry, respirations 14, pulse 90, BP 118/70. You note many abrasions to his arms and legs, and he groans when you palpate his pelvic area.

- What do you think is going on with this patient?
- What do his appearance and vital signs tell you?
- What will you do for him?

The elderly, generally thought of as persons 65 years of age and older, represent the fastest growing age group in the nation. Gerontologists (medical specialists who study and care for the elderly) divide the term "elderly" into several more specific categories:

- middle age: 50 to 64 years of age
- late age: 65 to 79 years of age
- older age: 80 years of age and older

The elderly currently represent 11% of the population of the United States or approximately 26 million persons. By the year 2030 the elderly will achieve a projected 20% of the U.S. population. As with other common age groups (such as adolescence or middle adulthood), it is difficult to identify an exact starting age. Although there are social and legal distinctions—for example, the age requirements for receiving discounts at movies, stores, and restaurants and the legal age for receiving social security benefits—these do not provide a valuable medical guide. Some people are afflicted with infirmities (such as Alzheimer's disease) at the early ages of 45, 50, or 55; therefore, they will have many of the progressive, interactive physical problems commonly associated with the elderly. However, some octogenarians enjoy such health, mental capacity, and physical ability that they do not exhibit these problems. Retirement is also an inaccurate guide to a person's health, as an increasing number of people either opt to retire early or continue in the work force after they have reached retirement age.

Some problems specific to the elderly are a part of the chronologic aging process and afflict all people as age advances. Other problems are dependent on heredity, lifestyle, and environmental factors that affect different individuals in varying degrees and at different ages.

The elderly present EMS providers with great challenges in emergency medical care management, which are second only to those encountered with infants. The emergency medical management of sudden illness and trauma in the elderly presents different emergency medical care dimensions than in younger patients.

AGING

The aging process causes changes in physical structure, body composition, and organ function, creating unique problems during emergency medical care intervention that must be considered by the EMT (Figure 14-1). In addition, changing patterns of mental health may have an impact on the elderly patient's functioning and activities of daily living (ADL). The mental status of the elderly may be a major factor in determining what emergency medical problems exist. The elderly are also considered at high risk for many mental health problems.

Some older individuals have reached advanced age with minimal medical problems. Others may live with chronic illnesses and are dependent on modern medical means. The latter group may deteriorate more rapidly in an emergency medical situation.

The elderly may be considered more susceptible to disease and injury. When acute illness or trauma strikes, it is often accompanied by a chronic disease. In addition, acute illness and trauma are more likely to alter organ systems beyond those initially involved. For example, an elderly patient who has fallen and fractured a hip may also be suffering from a lung disorder. These situations represent challenges to all EMS providers, particularly when an elderly person is involved in a traumatic event. The following risk factors affecting mortality have been identified for elderly patients:

- over 75 years of age
- living alone
- recent death of a significant other
- recently hospitalized
- inability to hold urine or feces (incontinence)
- immobile
- unsound mind

Because older persons are more susceptible to critical illness and trauma than the rest of the population, the EMT needs to consider a wider range of complications in patient assessment and emergency medical care. As the elderly access medical care via emergency systems (e.g., 9-1-1), EMTs must be capable of rendering care that is different than for patients younger in age.

The range of disabilities experienced by the elderly is enormous, and field assessment may take longer than with younger patients. Difficulties in assessment can be expected as a result of sensory deficits in hearing and vision, senility, and physiologic changes. Trauma deaths are usually associated with:

- blunt trauma (motor vehicle accidents)
- motor vehicle versus pedestrian incidents
- falls
- penetrating trauma (gunshot, knife wounds)

The advances in medicine and the increasing awareness of healthier lifestyles during the last several decades have resulted in a significant increase in the percentage of

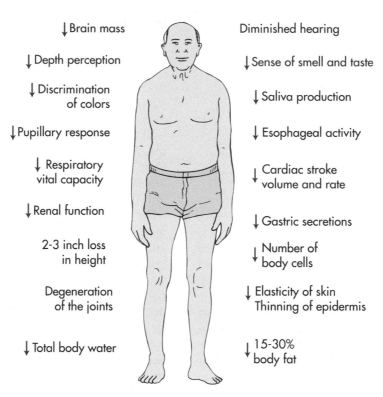

↓ Brain mass

↓ Depth perception

↓ Discrimination
of colors

↓ Pupillary response

↓ Respiratory
vital capacity

↓ Renal function

2-3 inch loss
in height

Degeneration
of the joints

↓ Total body water

Diminished hearing

↓ Sense of smell and taste

↓ Saliva production

↓ Esophageal activity

↓ Cardiac stroke
volume and rate

↓ Gastric secretions

↓ Number of
body cells

↓ Elasticity of skin
Thinning of epidermis

↓ 15-30%
body fat

Figure 14-1 Changes caused by aging.

the population that is over 65 years of age. Although trauma has its highest frequency in young people and geriatric emergencies are most commonly medical in nature, a growing number of geriatric calls result from or include trauma. Trauma is currently the fifth leading cause of death in the elderly, and trauma deaths in this age group account for 25% of all of the trauma deaths nationwide.

Progress in recent years has not only increased adult life expectancy but has also affected the quality of life and therefore the range of physical activities performed at older ages. As more people live longer and enjoy better health in their older years, more of them will travel, drive, and continue active physical pursuits that will result in an associated increase in geriatric trauma in the future. Many who could retire choose to continue working, whether motivated by need, the desire to maintain a productive social pursuit, or simply because they desire a different career. Often these people continue to work in spite of a health problem or advancing age.

Recent social changes have increased the number of older people living in independent housing, retirement communities, or in a variety of assisted-living opportunities rather than in nursing homes or other more guarded and limited environments. This suggests a probable increase in the incidence of simple household trauma, such as falls, in the elderly. The past few years have also seen an increase in geriatric victims of crime in the home

and on the streets. Older people are often singled out as "easy marks" and can suffer substantial trauma from crimes of seemingly limited violence—such as purse snatching—when they are struck, knocked down, or when they fall.

The EMT should include the special considerations outlined in this chapter in the assessment and management of any trauma victim who is 65 years or older, who physically appears elderly, or who is middle aged but has any significant medical problem(s) commonly associated with the elderly.

MECHANISM OF INJURY

Falls are the leading cause of trauma death and disability in the elderly. Approximately 9,500 of these victims die each year, and of the larger majority that survive falls, a significant number require hospitalization.

Motor vehicle trauma is the second leading cause of trauma death in the geriatric population. An elderly patient is five times more likely to be fatally injured in a car crash than a younger driver, even though excessive speed is rarely a causative factor found in the older age group.

Pedestrian accidents, such as being struck by a car, and burns are also common mechanisms of elderly trauma that can result in mortality, serious injury, and disability.

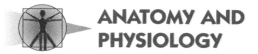

ANATOMY AND PHYSIOLOGY

THE AGING PROCESS: INTRODUCTION

The human body is constructed for a long-distance journey. The main organs—brain, heart, lungs, and liver—are remarkably strong and hardy. Aging, or senescence, is a natural biologic process and is sometimes referred to as a process of biologic reversal that begins during the years of early adulthood. At this time, organ systems have achieved maturation and a turning point in physiologic growth has been reached. The body gradually loses its ability to maintain homeostasis (the state of relative constancy of the body's internal environment), and viability declines over a period of years until death occurs.

The fundamental process of aging occurs at the cellular level and is reflected in both anatomic structure and physiologic function. The period of old age is generally characterized by frailty, slower mental processes, impairment of psychologic functions, diminished energy, the appearance of chronic and degenerative diseases, and decline in sensory acuity. Functional abilities are lessened and the well-known superficial signs and symptoms of older age appear, such as skin wrinkling, changes in hair color and quantity, osteoarthritis, and slowness in reaction time and reflexes.

The aging process occurs in all the body systems; however, discussion here is limited to the major systems.

RESPIRATORY SYSTEM

Respiratory function declines in the elderly and occurs partly as a result of the inability of the chest cage to expand and contract and also in part from a stiffening of the airway. The increased stiffness in the chest wall is associated with a reduction in the ability to expand the chest wall and a stiffening of cartilagenous connections of the ribs. As a result of these changes, the chest cage is less pliable. With these declines in the efficiency of the respiratory system, it takes more exertion for the elderly to carry out ADL. The alveoli become smaller and more shallow, reducing the alveolar surface. A reduction of the number of cilia (hair-like processes that propel foreign particles and mucous from the bronchi) predisposes the elderly to problems from inhaled particulate matter. Elderly people exposed over a long time to particle-laden air have difficulty removing material from the lungs. Oxygen uptake is decreased by the occlusion of the already reduced alveolar surface.

Another factor in decreased compliance of the chest wall is change to the spinal curvature. The curvature changes accompanied by an anteroposterior hump (as seen in osteoporosis patients) often lead to additional respiratory difficulty (Figure 14-2). Changes affecting the diaphragm also contribute to respiratory problems. In part due to stiffening of the rib cage, older people rely more on diaphragmatic activity to breathe. This increased reliance on the diaphragm makes the older person especially sensitive to changes in intra-abdominal pressure. Thus, a supine position or an overly-filled stomach from a large meal may provoke respiratory insufficiency. Obesity also plays a part in diaphragm restriction, especially when fat distribution tends to be central.

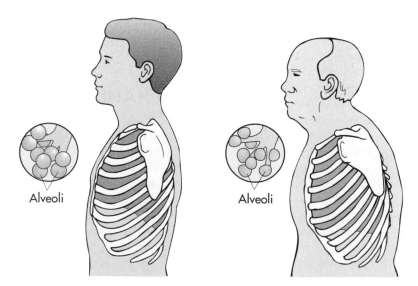

Figure 14-2 Spinal curvature can lead to an anteroposterior hump, which can cause respiratory difficulties. Reduction in the size of the alveoli can also reduce the amount of oxygen that is exchanged in the lungs.

As the lung loses its elasticity, it empties less completely on expiration so that the elderly person breathes at higher lung volume levels.

Decreased responsiveness to hypoxia and a high concentration of carbon dioxide in the blood (hypercarbia) may occur. This situation is often aggravated by drugs (e.g., salicylates used in making aspirin) or sedatives. The ability to acquire and deliver oxygen to the cells is also decreased.

TEETH

Tooth decay, gum disease, and injury to teeth result in the need for a variety of dental prostheses. The brittle nature of capped teeth, fixed bridges, or loose, removable bridges poses a special problem of possible foreign bodies that can be aspirated and obstruct the airway.

In patients who have a large number of teeth that are absent or have been replaced by removable dentures, changes occur in the shape of the mandible and maxilla. These changes often make it difficult to obtain a good mask seal for ventilation.

CARDIOVASCULAR SYSTEM

Diseases of the cardiovascular system are the major cause of death in the elderly. Cardiovascular disease accounts for over 3,000 deaths per 100,000 persons over 65 years of age. The cardiac emergency situations that are most consequential in the care of geriatric patients are:

- acute chest pain
- arrhythmias
- coronary artery disease
- pericarditis
- thoracic aortic dissection

Physical Changes of the Cardiovascular System

Age-related decreases in arterial elasticity lead to increased peripheral vascular resistance. The heart and blood vessels rely greatly on their elastic, contractile, and distensible properties to function properly. With aging, these properties decline, and the efficiency of the cardiovascular system to move circulatory fluids around the body decreases. The arteries undergo structural changes due to an increase in smooth muscle and fibrous tissue (collagen). The intima (the innermost coat of blood vessels) thicken.

Arteriosclerosis is the name given to a group of diseases characterized by the thickening and loss of elasticity of arterial walls. It is caused by an accumulation of fibrous tissue, fatty substances (lipids), and/or minerals.

Atherosclerosis is a narrowing of the blood vessels—a condition in which the inner layer of the artery wall thickens while fatty deposits build up within the artery. These deposits, called plaque, protrude above the surface of the inner layer and decrease the diameter of the internal channel of the vessel. One result of this narrowing of the diameter of the arteries is hypertension (high blood pressure), a condition that affects one out of six adults in the United States. The calcification of the arterial wall reduces the ability of the vessels to change size in response to endocrine and central nervous system stimuli. The lowered circulation can adversely affect any of the vital organs and is a common cause of heart disease.

Another risk associated with narrowing and eventual obstruction of the coronary arteries is heart attack (myocardial infarction). Risk factors for heart attacks are smoking, hypertension, high blood cholesterol levels, and a family history of premature coronary death or early death from myocardial infarction.

With age, the heart itself shows an increase in fibrous tissue and size (myocardial hypertrophy). Under stress, overall performance may be affected, demonstrated by a decrease in heart rate and cardiac output. A major result of the aging process as it affects the heart is reduced capability to respond to critical incidents. During incidents of acute illness or trauma, the ability of the heart to respond is a factor of concern in resuscitation efforts.

Even without specific heart disease, advancing age produces some congestive heart failure. The aging heart demonstrates decreases in rate, strength of contraction, compliance, valvular efficiency, and stroke volume. All of this reduces cardiac output. The net result is reduced circulation, pulmonary edema, and reduced blood oxygen levels.

In the elderly trauma victim, this reduced circulation contributes to cellular hypoxia. The result is cardiac arrhythmias, acute heart failure, or even sudden death. The ability of the sympathetic defense mechanisms to compensate for blood loss or other causes of shock is significantly lowered in the elderly due to a diminished inotropic (cardiac contraction) response to catecholamines.

The reduced circulation and circulatory defense responses coupled with increasing cardiac failure produce a significant problem in managing shock in the elderly. Fluid resuscitation needs to be carefully watched because of the reduced compliance of the cardiovascular system and the often "stiff" right ventricle. Care is required to guard against both continued hypotension and fluid overload in these patients who commonly have very delicate homeostasis.

NERVOUS SYSTEM

As individuals age a decrease occurs in brain weight and in the number of neurons or nerve cells. The weight of the brain reaches its peak at approximately age 20 (1.4 kg or 3 lb). By age 80 the brain loses about 100 grams (about

3½ ounces). The speed with which nerve impulses are conducted along certain nerves also decreases. Despite these decreases only small effects on behavior and thinking result. Reflexes are slower, but not to a significant degree, and compensatory function is usually adequate.

The elderly may learn more slowly than the young, but once materials are learned, retention is good. General information and vocabulary abilities increase or are maintained, while skills requiring mental and muscular activity (psychomotor ability) may decline. The intellectual functions involving verbal comprehension, arithmetic ability, fluency of ideas, experiential evaluation, and general knowledge tend to increase after age 60 in those elderly who continue learning activities. Exceptions are those who develop senile dementia and other disorders like Alzheimer's disease.

The normal biologic aging of the brain is not a predictor for diseases of the brain. It is important, however, that emergency medical personnel consider that the decreases in the cortical structure of the brain may be involved in mental impairment. As changes occur in the brain, behavioral problems may result from memory, personality changes, and other reductions in brain function. These changes may involve the need for some form of mental health service; about 10% to 15% of the elderly require professional mental health services.

SENSORY CHANGES
Eye and Ear

One elderly person in four has hearing problems, and more than one in ten suffers impaired vision. Men tend to be more likely to suffer hearing problems. Both genders have a similar share of eye-related problems. Overall, approximately 28% have hearing problems and 13% have visual problems.

Vision

Loss of vision is considered a problem at any age, and for the elderly, it may be even more problematic. Reliance on the sense of sight to carry on the activities of daily living is essential. The ability to read directions, for example, on a prescription vial, needs little elaboration for the possible disastrous effects from a misreading.

The elderly experience decreases in visual acuity, ability to differentiate, and night vision. The decreases are mainly the result of defects in the renewal of cells that occur in all body systems. Since abnormal molecules are not degraded as rapidly as in a younger body, the effects of aging begin to appear. The lens of the eye is particularly affected.

The cells of the lens of the eye are incapable of restoration to their original molecular structure. One of the destructive agents over years of exposure is ultraviolet radiation. Eventually, the lens loses its capability to increase in thickness and curvature. The result is almost universal far-sightedness (presbyopia) in persons over 40 years of age.

As a result of changes in various structures of the eye, it is more difficult for the elderly to see in dimly lit environments. Decreased tear production leads to dry eyes as well as to itching, burning, scratchiness, and the inability to keep the eyes open for long periods of time.

Cataracts refer to any impenetrability of light rays (opacity) in the lens. In a cataract, the compression of the lens leads to gradual opacity, as a glass of water to which milk is added, drop by drop. The milky lens blocks or distorts light entering the eye and blurs vision.

Hearing

Hearing loss is a serious disability in the elderly and contributes to a lack of well being and inability to carry on ADL. Almost all parts of the auditory system undergo changes with age.

Other factors that affect hearing loss should be observed when taking the focused medical history. These factors may include hereditary, metabolic, and vascular changes as well as other systemic tumors affecting the ear and central nervous system. Some of the factors that can produce or result in a hearing deficit include:

- trauma
- diabetes
- vascular lesions
- middle ear disease
- barotrauma
- hypertension
- benign bony growths
- arteriosclerosis
- accumulation of ear wax

The role of environmental noise is not altogether clear but is suspected, especially in men, as being a factor of considerable impact.

Ringing in the ears (tinnitus) is associated with a number of conditions and should not be dismissed casually. It should always be considered as symptomatic of a disease or syndrome.

MUSCULOSKELETAL SYSTEMS

Bone loses mineral as it ages. The loss of bone is unequal among the sexes. Bone mass in young adulthood is greater in women than in men. However, bone loss is more rapid in women and accelerates after menopause. The incidence of osteoporosis (increased loss of bone mass) is greater in women as well. Older women have a greater probability of fractures, particularly of the neck of the femur (thigh).

Older persons are sometimes shorter than they were in young adulthood because of dehydration of the vertebral discs. As the discs flatten, a loss of approximately 2 inches in height occurs between the ages of 20 and 70. Contributing to this shortness is kyphosis (curvature of the spine) in the thoracic region. This condition is commonly caused by osteoporosis (Figure 14-3).

As the bones become more porous and fragile, erosion occurs anteriorly and compression fractures may develop. As the thoracic spine becomes more curved, the head and shoulders appear to be pushed forward (see Figures 14-2 and 14-6). If chronic obstructive pulmonary disease particularly emphysema, is present, the kyphosis may be more pronounced because of the increased development of the accessory muscles of breathing.

Osteoarthritis, a form of arthritis in which joints undergo degenerative changes, is characterized by stiffness, deformity, swelling of the joints, and pain. Osteoarthritis usually involves changes in the hands and feet, particularly in the proximal and distal interphalangeal joints, and in the hips and spine (Figure 14-4).

Changes in the contours of the face result from resorption of the mandible, in part because of absence of teeth (edentulism). The characteristic look is an infolding and shrinking of the mouth. The nose and ears are more elongated than in earlier years because of the continuous growth of cartilage (Figure 14-5). The increased tendency to flex the legs makes the arms appear longer even though no change in their anatomic length has actually occurred (Figure 14-6).

As muscles age, loss of muscle mass occurs, estimated to be 30% between years 30 and 80. Deficits that relate to the musculoskeletal system, for example, a decreased ability to flex the hip or knee, predispose the elderly to falls. Muscle fatigue in the elderly can cause many problems affecting movement, falls-being one of the most frequent. Changes in the body's normal posture are common, and changes of the spine make the curvatures become more acute with aging. Some degree of osteoporosis is universal with aging. Because of this progressive bone resorption, the bones become less pliant, more brittle, and more easily broken. The weakening in bone strength coupled with reduced muscle strength caused by less active exercise easily results in multiple fractures even when only mild or moderate forces come to bear. As the normal arthritic process occurs with aging, the range of joint movement becomes more limited.

The cervical spine must be carefully evaluated in all geriatric patients. The narrowed canal and progressive osteophytic disease put these patients at high risk for spinal cord injury with even minor trauma.

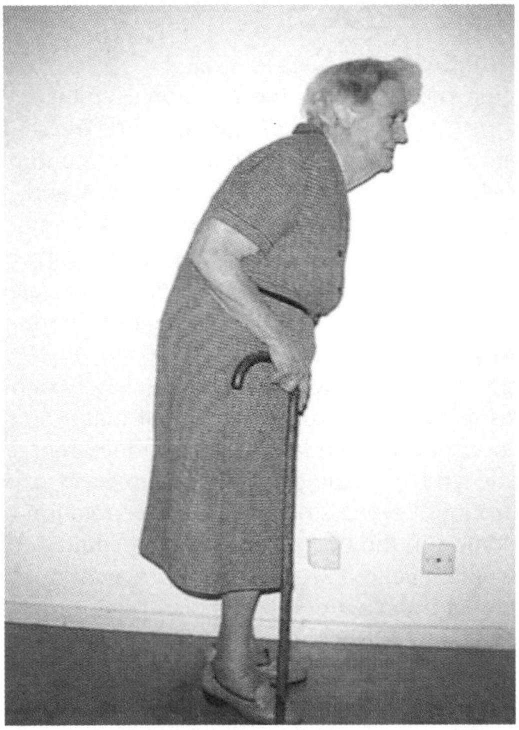

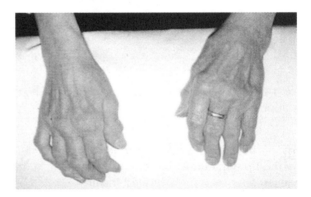

Figure 14-4 Osteoarthritis.

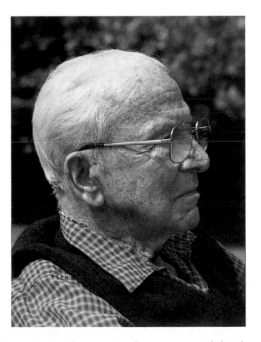

Figure 14-3 Kyphosis, commonly caused by osteoporosis.

Figure 14-5 Changes in the contour of the face.

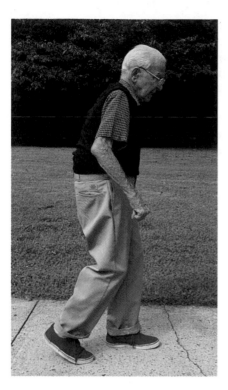

Figure 14-6 Because of the tendency to flex the legs, the arms appear longer.

Any of these musculoskeletal changes can contribute to the multiple fractures that commonly occur in the elderly even after seemingly limited insult.

Skin

As the skin ages, sweat and sebaceous glands are lost. Loss of sweat glands reduces the body's ability to regulate temperature. Loss of sebaceous glands, which produce oil, makes the skin dry and flaky. Production of melanin (the pigment giving color to skin and hair) declines causing an aging pallor. The skin thins and appears translucent due primarily to changes in connective tissue. The thinning and drying of the skin also reduce the protectiveness of the body to microorganisms. As elasticity is lost, the skin stretches and falls into wrinkles and folds, especially in areas of heavy use, such as those overlying the facial muscles of expression. Loss of fatty tissue predisposes the elderly to hypothermia and hyperthermia.

RENAL SYSTEM

Changes common with aging include reduced levels of filtration by the kidneys and a reduced excretory capacity. These changes must be considered when administering drugs that are normally cleared by the kidneys. The chronic renal inhibition commonly found in the elderly contributes to a lowering of the patient's overall health and ability to withstand trauma.

IMMUNE SYSTEM

As the immune system ages, its ability to function decreases. A decrease in cell-mediated and humoral responses also results. This, coupled with preexisting nutritional problems common in the elderly, leads to an increased susceptibility to infection. Sepsis is a common cause of late death following severe or even significant trauma in the elderly.

PAIN AND OTHER SYMPTOMATIC RESPONSES

Many elderly patients have conditions such as arthritis that result in constant chronic pain. Living with daily pain can cause an increased tolerance to pain. This, coupled with the fact that many older people are strong-willed and not prone to readily identifying "minor" pain, may result in the patient's failure in identifying areas of injury. In evaluating patients (especially those who usually "hurt all over" or those who have a high tolerance to pain), it is important to locate areas where the pain has increased or where the painful area has enlarged. It should also be noted if the pain's characteristics or exacerbating factors have changed since the trauma occurred.

SUMMARY OF THE AGING PROCESS

The aging process alters the functional efficiency of all organ systems, usually because of a decrease in cell population. Only some of the major systems and portions of the elderly patient's anatomic structures and physiologic functions have been presented in this chapter. Emergency medical management of the elderly patient must necessarily involve a reasonable degree of understanding of the aging process and its impact on mortality and morbidity.

The human body evolves through a variety of physical changes as part of the healthy, normal maturing process from conception to the later years of adolescence. These anatomic and physiologic changes represent a positive and purposeful process of growth and adaptation without deterioration in the body's evolution to adulthood. From adolescence to about 35 years of age, even though "wear and tear" and the aging process occur, the body usually remains relatively unchanged. After age 35, the cumulative effects of living and aging start to cause physical changes, which result in progressive deterioration in the body's ability to function. Proper medical and dental care, attention to healthy diet and activities, and the absence of specific medical problems may delay this process, but they cannot eliminate it.

The process of aging (whether due to an increase in collagen cross-linkage, an autoimmune reaction, the natural history of cell division, or other causes) is manifested by changes in all of the body's organ systems. The following systems and their changes are particularly important for the EMT to consider when dealing with the elderly trauma patient.

IMPACT OF CHRONIC MEDICAL PROBLEMS

As people grow older, along with the general changes associated with normal aging, more medical problems usually occur. Although some individuals reach a very advanced age without any serious medical problem, statistically the older a person becomes the more likely he or she is to have one or more significant medical conditions. Usually, proper medical care and regulation by the patient can control these conditions, avoiding or minimizing their exacerbation into repeated serious acute (often life-threatening) episodes.

The absence of repeated acute episodes does not, however, minimize the chronic and residual effects these conditions produce on the body. A patient who has previously suffered an acute myocardial infarct has permanent heart damage. The resultant reduced cardiac capacity continues for the rest of his or her life, producing an effect not only on the heart but, because of the ensuing chronic decline in circulation, also on the other vital organs.

As a person's age advances, additional separate or related medical problems occur. None are truly isolated since their influence on the body is cumulative. Because they are interactive, their total impact on the body usually is greater than the sum of each pathology's individual effect. As this condition progresses and reduces the quality of the body's vital functions, the individual's ability to withstand the introduction of disease, serious trauma, or even minor trauma is greatly diminished.

Regardless of whether the patient is pediatric, middle-aged, or elderly, the priorities, intervention needs, and life-threatening conditions commonly found as a result of serious trauma are the same. Elderly trauma victims die as a result of the same causes as trauma victims of any age. But, often due to their preexisting physical conditions, the elderly can die from less severe injuries and die more rapidly than younger patients.

SPECIAL CONSIDERATIONS IN ASSESSING THE ELDERLY

The EMT's assessment based on the A B C D E method should basically be the same for trauma patients of all ages. These priorities have been covered in Chapter 2:

Patient Assessment and Management, and do not require repetition here. Some special considerations in assessing the elderly, however, bear mention.

Some findings from the patient assessment must be evaluated based on the generally accepted pathologic boundaries for any adult, regardless of age. For example, elderly patients ventilating at a rate of less than 10 or greater than 30 breaths per minute, similar to any other adult, will not have an adequate minute volume and will require positive pressure–assisted ventilations. But, there are also findings that must be evaluated based upon the age of the patient and degenerative physical factors common to the elderly. In most adults a respiratory rate between 12 and 20 is unimpressive and confirms that an adequate minute volume is present. In a patient of advanced age, however, the reduction in tidal volume capacity and pulmonary function common at such an age may result in an inadequate minute volume even at rates of 12 to 14 or 16 to 20 breaths per minute. Inversely delayed capillary refill is due to normally less productive circulation in the elderly and therefore is a poor indicator of acute circulatory changes in these patients. Some degree of decreased distal motor, sensory, and circulatory ability in the extremities represents a common normal finding in the aged.

Some findings can only be interpreted properly by knowing the individual patient's preincident norms. Expected ranges of normal vital signs and other findings usually accepted as standard (normal) are not normal in every individual, and deviation is much more common in the elderly patient. Although the commonly assumed ranges are broad enough to include most individual adult differences, an individual of any age may vary beyond these norms; such variation should be expected in the elderly. Medication may contribute to these changes. For example, in the average adult, a systolic blood pressure of 120 mm Hg would be considered normal and would generally be considered unimpressive. In the patient who normally has a systolic pressure of 150 mm Hg, however, a 120 mm Hg pressure would be a concern, suggestive of hidden bleeding (or some other mechanism) of such a degree that decompensation has occurred. No quantitative information or other sign should be used in isolation from other findings. However, failing to recognize that such a change occurred or that it is a serious pathologic finding in a particular patient can produce a poor outcome for the patient.

The importance of viewing all of the findings together and maintaining an increased level of suspicion in the elderly cannot be overemphasized. In the elderly, wide differences in mentation, memory, and orientation (to the past and present) can be found. The identification of significant neurologic trauma must be interpreted in light of the individual's preinsult normal status. Unless there is someone on the scene that can describe this status, the patient must be assumed to have a neurologic injury, hypoxia, or both. The ability to distinguish between a patient's chronic status and acute changes is an essential factor to prevent underreaction or overreaction to the patient's present neurologic status as a key index in evaluating his or her overall condition. Unconsciousness, however, remains a grave sign in all cases.

Care must be taken in the selection of questions to determine the elderly patient's orientation to time and place. People who work 5 days a week with weekends off usually know what day of the week it is. If they don't, it is a safe assumption that they have some level of disorientation. For those who no longer work a traditional job and who are often surrounded by others who do not, a lack of distinction between days of the week or even months of the year may not be indicative of disorientation, but only of a lack of "calendar" importance in the structure of their lives. Similarly, people who no longer drive pay less attention to roads, town borders, locations, and maps. Although normally oriented they may not be able to identify their present locale. Confusion or the inability to recall events and details long past may be more indicative of how long ago the events occurred rather than how forgetful the individual is. Similarly, the repeated retelling of events long past and seemingly more attention to the far past rather than the immediate past often simply represent a nostalgic lingering on years and events from what are perceived to be better times in the individual's life. It is important that such social and psychologic compensations not be considered signs of senility or a diminished mental capacity.

SYSTEMIC IMPACT OF ISOLATED SIMPLE TRAUMA

An increasing lack of the body's ability to isolate simple trauma must also be a consideration in assessing and managing the elderly. In healthy adults in their twenties, an isolated hip fracture is rarely associated with systemic decline. In an 85-year-old patient, the same injury can commonly produce a systemic impact resulting in deterioration and life-threatening hypoxia and shock. Although an injury may be considered isolated and unalarming in most adults, the elderly patient's overall physical condition may have lowered the body's normal defenses and its ability to keep the effects of even simple injury localized.

PREEXISTING CONDITIONS

Obtaining pertinent medical history early in the assessment of elderly patients is a high priority. The patient's normal health, its effect on expected findings, and a knowledge of preexisting deficits and infirmities are each important in interpreting findings and identifying those acute changes that are a result of the trauma. An underlying medical condition may be the primary cause of the patient's condition or may even have been the cause of the trauma. Identifying such a condition may be essential, requiring additional treatments, such as glucose for diabetic patients beyond those simply suggested by the patient's injuries. When an elderly patient is the driver in a motor vehicle accident or the victim of a fall, it is easy to make the assumption that advanced age, eyesight, or another normal condition of elderliness was the cause.

Judgments surrounding the seriousness of the patient's condition and stability must include past medical conditions even if they are not presently acute or symptomatic. For example, a patient with a simple isolated ankle fracture but with a history of unstable angina must be considered highly unstable. In such cases transportation should be rapidly initiated without delay, before the stress and simple trauma exacerbate the angina and deterioration occurs.

MEDICATION

Knowledge of the patient's medications may also represent key information necessary in understanding the trauma assessment or in determining prehospital care. For example, the use of Inderal® or some other beta-blocker may explain a patient's present bradycardia. In this situation an increasing tachycardia as a sign of developing shock may not occur. The lack of warning usually produced by an increasing pulse rate along with the drug's obstruction of a key part of the body's normal sympathetic defense mechanisms can result in masking the true level of the patient's circulatory deterioration. Such patients can rapidly decompensate, seemingly without warning. Medications such as antihypertensives, anticoagulants, beta-blockers, and hypoglycemic agents may profoundly influence the response of patients to trauma and to resuscitation.

GENERAL FACTORS IN TRAUMA ASSESSMENT AND EMERGENCY MEDICAL CARE

In trauma assessment, a number of factors must always be considered.

AIRWAY

The existence of dentures, which is common in the elderly, may affect airway management. Ordinarily, dentures should be left in place because maintaining a seal around the mouth is more difficult without dentures in place. Partial dentures (plates) may become dislodged during the emergency and occlude or partially block the airway; these should be removed in this event.

PREEXISTING PATHOLOGY

Previous disease to both upper and lower airway structures may affect airway management. Elderly patients who have had laryngectomies (partial or full removal of voice box structures), chest surgery, or lateral curvature of the spine may have respiratory difficulty.

CERVICAL SPINE

Protection of the cervical spine, particularly in trauma patients who have sustained multiple system injury, is an expected standard of care. In the elderly this standard of care must apply not only in trauma situations but also in acute medical problems where attempts to maintain airway patency is a priority. Degenerative arthritis of the cervical spine may subject the elderly patient to spinal cord injury from maneuvering the neck, even if there is no injury to the spine. Another consideration with improper or accidental movement is the possibility of carotid occlusion. A carotid occlusion (a blockage of the carotid arteries that supply the brain with blood) could produce anything from an altered level of consciousness to a stroke.

BREATHING
Chronic Obstructive Pulmonary Disease

There is a high prevalence of chronic obstructive pulmonary disease (COPD) in the elderly population. In the presence of COPD, there are some patients whose respiratory drive is not dependent on carbon dioxide levels but on diminished oxygen levels. *Remember: even with a COPD patient, never withhold oxygen from a patient who needs it.*

Lung Volumes

The elderly experience increased stiffness of the chest wall. In addition, reduced chest wall muscle power and stiffening of the cartilage makes the chest cage less flexible. These and other changes are responsible for reductions in lung volumes. Respiratory support may be needed in such cases.

CIRCULATION

Bleeding (hemorrhage) in the elderly is managed no differently than in the young. However, a higher index of suspicion must be maintained for the potential of shock (hypovolemia) when an elderly patient's systolic blood pressure is less than 120 mm Hg.

ALTERED LEVEL OF CONSCIOUSNESS

Besides the usual mechanisms for an altered level of consciousness (LOC), other factors in the elderly must be noted. Most important among these may be the use of medications to help with sleeping disorders, use of antidepressants, or use of medications prescribed for cardiovascular diseases such as hypertension.

CENTRAL NERVOUS SYSTEM

Assessing neurologic deficit in the elderly may be difficult because of preexisting conditions or pathology. It may be quite difficult to decide whether the elderly patient's neurologic deficit is the result of a stroke or if the deficit is a result of the current trauma or illness. Then, too, many medications prescribed for elderly patients may interfere with central nervous system function in times of trauma or acute medical illness. In any event, a rapid neurologic evaluation using the AVPU method is suggested (see Chapter 8). Any decrease in the level of consciousness usually means decreased flow of oxygen to the brain and/or inadequate circulation.

GENERAL CONSIDERATIONS IN ASSESSMENT OF THE ELDERLY

In assessment of acute illness the following factors will be important, after managing urgent life support emergencies (airway, breathing, and circulation [ABC's]). Plan for more than the average time in gathering information and taking a history.

- An important factor in the assessment of the elderly is that the body may no longer respond the same as in younger patients. Typical findings of serious illness such as fever, pain, or tenderness may take longer to develop, thus making it much more difficult to evaluate the patient. In addition, many medications will alter the body response. You will often have to depend on history alone.
- Patience will be necessary, probably more than usual due to conditions of the patient, such as hearing or visual deficits. Empathy and compassion will be essential. Do not underestimate the patient's intelligence merely because communication may be difficult or absent. If the patient has close associates or relatives, ask them to participate in giving information or to stay nearby to help validate information.

- Assessment of the elderly requires using different questioning tactics. Ask for specific information versus general: the elderly tend to respond "yes" to all questions during the assessment process. Asking open-ended questions is a useful tool in evaluating most patients, but sometimes with the elderly it is helpful to provide specific details from which to choose when dealing with a problem. For example, "Describe the pain in your hip" is open-ended. The following questions are more specific and may help the patient provide you with better information. "Is the pain in your hip sharp, stabbing, or dull?" "On a scale of one to five, five being the most intense pain, how would you rate the pain?"

- When assessing an elderly patient, ask precise questions. Asking the patient "What's wrong?" may bring about more answers than needed. If the patient has a history of breathing difficulty (dyspnea), you may need to go further and ask about the changes in his or her breathing difficulty, for example: "Do you have to rest several times when walking to the kitchen?"

- Involve a significant other. With the patient's permission, involving the caregiver or spouse may be necessary to gather valid information. Some elderly may be reluctant to give information without assistance of a relative or support person. Be alert, however, that the elderly patient may not want any other person present for a host of reasons, one of which may be abuse problems. The elderly patient may fear punishment for telling the EMT, in the presence of the abuser, why he or she has multiple bruise marks. There may be some problems that embarrass the elderly patients, and they do not want any family members to know about these. Information from the family, though, may be quite important.

- Pay attention to sensory deficits (hearing, vision, smell, taste, touch, and position). Given the usual presence of these deficits, maintaining eye contact and speaking more slowly than usual and with suitable volume are important in gathering patient information.

- Altered comprehension/neurologic disorders are a significant problem for many elderly patients. These impairments can range from confusion to senile dementia of the Alzheimer type. Not only may these patients have difficulty in communicating with the EMT, but they may also be unable to comprehend or help in the assessment. They may be quite restless and sometimes combative.

- Firmness, reassurance, and clear, simple (and repeated) questioning may be helpful. Often, a family member or friend can be of assistance.

COMMUNICATION

The elderly should not be approached as if they were small children. A common mistake by healthcare professionals in the prehospital and emergency department settings is to treat the elderly in this way. Often, well-meaning relatives are so aggressive in reporting the events for an elderly loved one that they take over as the respondent to the EMT's inquiries. In such a situation it is easy to overlook the fact that the clinical impression and history are from someone other than the patient and may not be correct. Not only does this increase the danger of obtaining poor, inaccurate information through a third party's impressions and translation, but it also discounts the patient as a mature adult.

Proper adult interaction with the patient is essential in obtaining good information, establishing rapport between the EMT and the patient, and preserving the dignity to which the patient is entitled. Although information from relatives, nursing home personnel, or others may contain important additional information, it should not replace the primary information and responses supplied by the patient. Do not assume that a reduced mental capacity is inherent just because of the patient's age or because a relative/caregiver provided that information. The EMT should be guided by his or her own empirical investigation. Many reasons, with good intentions or with malice, cause those living with or caring for the elderly to deal with them in ways often inaccurate from the standpoint of the elderly person's actual mental capacity.

The following are some practical tips and tools to use and remember when dealing with the elderly.

1. Elderly patients present with a host of common complaints. When assessing a geriatric patient, even during a trauma event, it is helpful to know what the complaints are. (An asterisk indicates the most frequently repeated complaints.)
   - alcoholism*
   - constipation or diarrhea
   - dementia*
   - depression*
   - dizziness, vertigo, or syncope
   - dysphagia
   - dyspnea
   - falls
   - fatigue and weakness
   - headache
   - hearing loss*
   - incontinence or inability to void*
   - musculoskeletal stiffness*
   - poor nutrition; loss of appetite
   - sexual dysfunction
   - sleep disorders*
   - visual disorders

2. *Physical assessment:* After ensuring that the ABC's are managed, the following suggestions will assist the EMT in the physical assessment of the geriatric patient.
   - Pay attention to impaired hearing, sight, comprehension, and mobility capabilities.
   - Make eye contact. The patient may be hearing impaired and be dependent on watching your lips and other facial movements.
   - Shake the patient's hand. Feel for grip strength, skin turgor, and body temperature.
   - Address the patient by his or her last name, unless otherwise told by the patient. Avoid phrases like, "Now, now, dearie, you'll be fine."
   - Minimize noise, distractions, and interruptions
   - Use open-ended questions: "Describe pain in your abdomen, is it . . . ?" Avoid questions like, "Where does it hurt?" as you may get more answers than will be appropriate for the mechanism of injury you are assessing.
   - Observe for:
     behavioral problems or manifestations that do not fit the scene
     dress/grooming. Is it appropriate for where and how you found the patient?
     ease of rising/sitting
     fluency of speech
     involuntary movement, cranial nerve dysfunctions, and difficult respirations
     movement: easy, unsteady, and/or unbalanced
     state of nourishment: well, thin, or emaciated?

3. *Dehydration/feeding:* Remember that there is a decreased thirst response. The kidneys have a problem in meeting the challenge of injury. The kidney's ability to concentrate urine is decreased, leading to dehydration even before injury. Urine output is a poor measure of perfusion in the elderly. There is a decreased amount of body fat (15% to 30%) and total body water.

4. *Thermoregulation:* The elderly are more susceptible to ambient environmental changes. There is a decreased ability to respond to changes, decreased heat production, and a decreased ability to rid the body of excessive heat. Thermoregulatory problems are related to imbalance of electrolytes, e.g., potassium (K) depletion; hypothyroidism, and diabetes mellitus. Other factors include: decreased basal metabolic rate, decreased ability to shiver, arteriosclerosis, and effects of drugs and alcohol. Hyperthermia is affected by cerebrovascular accidents, diuretics, antihistamines, and antiparkinsonian drugs. Hypothermia is affected by decreased metabolism, fat, less efficient peripheral vasoconstriction, and poor nutrition.

5. *Neurologic:* By age 70 there is a 10% reduction in brain mass. The dura mater adheres more closely to the skull resulting in loss of some brain volume. One sequelae of this is a lower frequency of epidural hemorrhage and a higher frequency of subdural hemorrhage. Because of brain atrophy there can be fairly large subdural hemorrhage but minimal clinical finding. The combination of head injury and hypovolemic shock yields greater fatality.

6. *Musculoskeletal:* There is a total decrease in skeletal muscle weight, widening and weakening of bones, degeneration of joints, and osteoporosis. There is an increased probability of fractures with minor injuries and a marked increased risk of fractures to the vertebrae, hip, and ribs.

7. *Cardiovascular:* There is degeneration of heart muscle cells and fewer pacemaker cells. The elderly are prone to arrhythmias due to a loss of elasticity of the heart and major arteries. This is further complicated by widespread use of beta and calcium channel blockers and diuretics. Remember that the maximum pulse rate decreases with age: 230 minus age. It is common following injury for the elderly to present with low cardiac output with hypoxia and to have no lung injury. Cardiac stroke, volume, and rate decrease as does cardiac reserve, all leading to morbidity and mortality of the elderly trauma patient. A geriatric patient with a systole of 120 mm should be considered in hypovolemic shock until proven otherwise.

8. *Respiratory:* Vital capacity is diminished by 50%. Kyphotic changes in the spine (anteroposterior) result in a ventilation-perfusion mismatch at rest. Hypoxia is much more likely a consequence of shock than it is in younger patients. There is a decreased ability for chest excursions. Lower tidal volumes and lower minute volumes are typical. Reduced capillary oxygen and carbon dioxide exchange are significant. Hypoxemia tends to be progressive.

SUMMARY OF ASSESSMENT

A variety of special considerations need to be included by the EMT in the assessment and care of the elderly trauma victim due to pathophysiologic changes caused by aging. Seriously traumatized patients, regardless of age, die of the same conditions and have the same priorities and needs. Due to the consequences of the aging process on physical condition, even healthy elderly trauma victims will commonly experience a more devastating effect than would a younger patient from the same level of multiple trauma.

When possible, early assessment of the elderly needs to include knowledge of the patient's preexisting norms, preexisting deficits and infirmities, and the medications taken in order to provide an understanding of the findings and to allow for the safe ruling out of certain conditions. Trauma, major or minor, may include or be caused by an underlying acute medical emergency requiring special additional treatment or the need to initiate transport without delay.

Triage decisions and the establishment of priorities must include the patient's preinsult overall physical condition, the presence of chronic conditions, and the elderly patient's diminished mental capacity should this be considered as a reliable fact. The patient should be treated with respect even if he or she has a diminished mental capacity; this patient's comments should not be viewed as inconsequential. The EMT should evaluate the veracity of the patient's comments in light of the patient's capacity, and even deal with seemingly bizarre comments or activity without belittling or discounting the patient.

Although examples of elderly patients with a diminished mental capacity are memorable, it is important to place these in a proper perspective. By far the greatest number of elderly trauma patients do not have chronic impaired mental status.

LEGAL CONSIDERATIONS

Several legal distinctions can become issues when giving care to the elderly, and these must be understood by the EMT. In most states, spouses, siblings, children, spouses of children, and parents have no legal standing in making medical decisions for an adult. Persons with power of attorney or court-appointed conservators commonly may have authority over the individual's financial affairs, but they do not necessarily have control over the subject's personal medical decisions. Even court-appointed custodians or guardians may or may not have the power to make medical decisions, depending on the laws of the particular state or local jurisdiction and on the specific charge of their appointment. Only where a guardianship-of-person or a durable power of attorney-for-health-care is specified and clear documentation of such third-party powers is present and furnished to the EMT should such powers be considered to exist.

In the midst of a trauma scene, it is difficult for the EMT to make such a fine legal distinction. Since the ambulance was summoned and a "call for help" was made, the EMT must react on the basis of implied consent in cases of patients who are unconscious or have reduced mental capacity.

Should further clarification be necessary or should anyone attempt to obstruct the EMT's care, the EMT should present the problem to the police officer in charge at the scene. In most states the law provides a protocol for that officer to make a timely "speedy decision" at the scene, and for ensuing clarification to occur later at the hospital when time allows. Be sure to carefully document such events in detail as a part of the run report.

ABUSE AND NEGLECT OF THE ELDERLY

Reports and complaints of abuse, neglect, and other related problems among the nation's elderly are increasing. The exact extent of elder abuse is not known for several reasons. One reason is that elder abuse has been a problem largely hidden from society. Another is that there are varying definitions of abuse and neglect in the elderly. Other obstacles involve the uneasiness or fear of elders or others to report the problem to law enforcement agencies or human and social welfare personnel. The typical victim of elder abuse may be a parent who feels ashamed or guilty because he or she raised the abuser. The abused may also feel traumatized by the situation or fear continued reprisal by the abuser. In some jurisdictions, there is also a lack of formal reporting mechanisms. Some states do not even have a statutory provision requiring the reporting of elder abuse.

The physical and emotional signs of abuse—those of rape, beating, or nutritional deprivation—are often overlooked or perhaps not accurately identified. Older women in particular, are not likely to report incidents of sexual assault to law enforcement agencies. Sensory deficits, senility, and other forms of altered mental status (e.g., drug-induced depression) may make it impossible or extremely difficult for the elderly patient to report the maltreatment.

ABUSE

Abuse is any action by an elderly person's family (any relative); associated persons who have daily household contact (housekeeper, roommate); anyone upon whom the elderly are reliant for daily needs of food, clothing, and shelter; or a professional caretaker, who takes advantage of the elderly's person, property, or emotional state. Abuse of the elder is sometimes called "granny" or parent battering.

PROFILE OF THE ABUSED

The elderly most likely to be abused fall into the following profile:

- over 65 years of age, especially women over 75
- frail
- multiple chronic medical conditions
- demented

- impaired sleep cycle, sleepwalking, or loud shouting during the nighttime
- incontinent of feces, urine, or both
- dependent on others for daily activities of living or incapable of independent living

PROFILE OF THE ABUSER

Because many elderly people live in a family environment and are typically women older than 75 years of age, the emergency medical provider must look to that environment for clues. The abuser is frequently the spouse of the patient or the middle-aged daughter-in-law of the elder who is caring for dependent children and dependent parents, while perhaps holding full or part-time employment. Most of these abusers are untrained in the particular care required by the elderly and have little relief time from the constant care demands of their own family—now complicated by the often less-than-flexible elder.

Abuse is not, of course, restricted to the home. Other environments like nursing, convalescent, and continuing care centers are sites where the elderly may sustain physical, chemical, or pharmacologic harm. Care providers in these environments may consider the elderly to represent management problems or categorize them as obstinate or undesirable patients. The emergency medical care provider should not be astounded—this type of abuse can be gruesome, vulgar, barbaric, or worse than that inflicted upon children. The usual profile of the abuser includes the following signs:

- existence of household conflict
- marked fatigue
- unemployment
- financial difficulties
- substance abuse
- previous history of being abused

CATEGORIES OF ABUSE

Abuse may be categorized as follows:

Physical

- assault
- neglect
- dietary
- poor maintenance of habitat
- poor personal care

Psychologic

- neglect
- verbal
- infantilization
- deprivation of sensory stimulation

Financial

- thefts of valuables
- embezzlement
- failure to notify

CHARACTERISTICS OF PHYSICAL ABUSE

The signs of physical abuse or neglect may be quite obvious, such as the imprint left by an item like a fireplace poker, or subtle, such as undernutrition in the fragile elderly (Figure 14-7). The signs of elderly abuse are similar to those of child abuse.

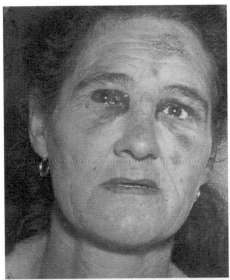

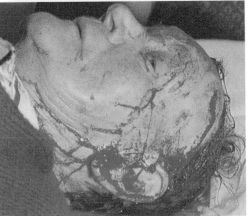

Figure 14-7 Signs of abuse of the elderly. A, Bruising caused by a husband's punch. This woman agreed to go to the hospital only because she was advised to by the police. When about to leave, she mentioned discomfort in her neck. X-rays showed a fracture of the body of C6. B, Wound of the scalp. The scalp is a common site of elderly abuse that often causes hemorrhagic shock. (From London, P.S. *Color Atlas of Diagnosis after Recent Injury.* London: Wolfe, 1990.)

IMPORTANT POINTS TO REMEMBER ABOUT ELDER ABUSE

It is important to remember that many patients suffering abuse are terrorized into making false statements for fear of retribution. In the case of elder abuse by family members, fear of removal from the home environment causes the elder to lie about the origin of the abuse. In other cases of elder abuse, sensory deprivation or dementia may deter adequate explanation. The significance of these assessments is important to uncover pathology as well as to identify abuse that often is not reported by the patient.

In addition to the implicit lifesaving care that must be administered during patient assessment, one of the very significant benefits of a thorough assessment involves reducing further trauma from abuse through its very identification. One of the preventative measures in reducing additional abuse of the elderly is the knowledge of its occurrence uncovered or identified by EMTs. Reporting the abuse may allow for referral and protective services of human, social, and public safety agencies.

Scenario Solution

This patient is in a classic scenario for hip fracture—a common injury in the elderly. We need to be concerned with the fact that he is lethargic and confused with pale skin. We should be thinking about possible complications in the pelvis and associated bleeding. Although his skin condition may not be alarming and his vitals within normal limits, they are not as good as they look. Because of the medications many elderly patients take, they may not become tachycardiac in early shock. They generally have higher blood pressures, so we need to consider any systolic pressure less than 120 as significant. Studies show that even in everyday activity, the elderly often have to breathe much faster than the average person to maintain normal oxygenation. Respiratory rates of 12 and 14 often produce marked hypoxia. Considering the mechanism and patient response, we should immobilize appropriately, secure airway and oxygenation, and be prepared for shock because this patient's vital signs may not be as good as they look.

• Summary •

Chronic medical conditions in the elderly could be exacerbated into an acute emergency, along with the injuries and conditions resulting from the present trauma. Many factors in elderly trauma victims can mask early signs of deterioration, increasing the possibility of sudden rapid decompensation without apparent warning. Even simple isolated trauma can progress to include acute systemic impact and produce potentially life-threatening conditions in the elderly. Aggressive, timely care is particularly important in the treatment of the elderly trauma victim.

The EMT has to take a more wary approach to the elderly trauma patient by assuming that more serious injury may have occurred than is indicated by the presently existing signs and symptoms. The injuries and conditions found will have a more profound effect than in a younger patient, an underlying medical problem may cause additional critical needs, and the elderly patient has greater instability, increasing the possibility for sudden rapid deterioration.

By including these considerations, the EMT will be forewarned, manage more aggressively, and provide better, safer care to older victims of trauma.

Review Questions

Answers provided on page 333.

1 Which of the following affect breathing in the elderly?
A loss of flexibility of the chest wall
B COPD
C previous disease or surgery
D all of the above

2 Which of the following is true of vital signs taken in the elderly?
A In the face of trauma or diminished level of consciousness, anything less than a systolic pressure of 120 is suspicious.
B Vital signs don't change much in adults regardless of age.
C The elderly breathe slower at rates of 10 to 16 breaths per minute
D All of the above

3 The skeletal system in the elderly is:
A mostly cartilage
B more brittle and subject to fracture with seemingly minor mechanisms
C stronger and lighter
D all of the above

4 In trauma, the previous medical history of the elderly, disease, medications, and so on:
A will greatly affect outcomes
B have little effect on outcome
C is unimportant

5 The percentage of the population that will be considered elderly by the year 2030:
A will nearly double
B will be much less
C will be the same

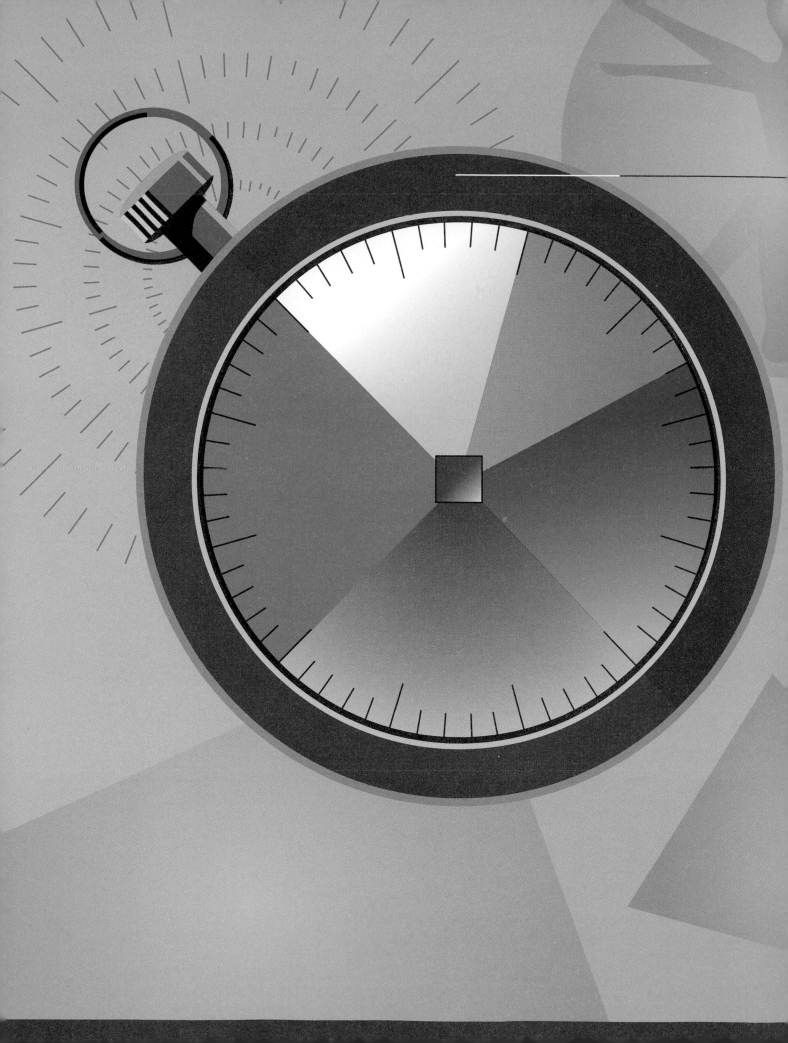

CHAPTER 15

Principles in the Care of the Trauma Patient

In the preceding chapters the assessment and treatment of patients who have sustained injury to specific body systems has been discussed, beginning with the kinematics of trauma and proceeding through the evaluation and resuscitation of seriously injured victims. The majority of the techniques and principles discussed are not new. This text does, however, systematize those practices and establish priorities of patient care that will help reduce permanent injury and mortality in the trauma patients who have sustained injury to multiple body systems. The text is able to present the material through better organization of those actions and interventions that all EMTs have been trained to do, but which are often not done in a truly effective order. By teaching EMTS how to prioritize assessment and management strategies for the multisystem trauma patient, this learned prioritization may lead to better patient outcome. It is important to recognize that while this text has presented the injured patient by individual body system, many patients present with injury to more than one body system, hence the name: multisystem trauma patient. The EMT must effectively recognize and prioritize the treatment of patients with multiple injuries.

The following are the primary considerations in prehospital trauma management:

1. Develop the assessment skills required to recognize actual or potential life-threatening conditions.
2. Establish a priority system that will allow those conditions to be managed in an orderly manner with the most serious patients being managed first.
3. Recognize hypoxia and shock as the most critical of these conditions.
4. Develop a plan of action for the rapid treatment and stabilization of significant injuries.
5. Provide rapid transportation to an appropriate hospital that can quickly manage the patient's conditions.

Upon initial approach of the scene and as field care is provided, the EMT's brain receives input from several senses (sight, hearing, smell, touch). Many of these are simultaneous inputs that must be sorted, placed in the priority scheme of life- or limb-threatening injuries, and used to develop a plan for correct management. This simultaneous input and sorting is recognized as a central component of patient care, but it is a skill that cannot be taught; it must be learned. To help with this learning process, the priority scheme is taught so that the EMT may engage the correct management systems for patient care. It is the premise of the Prehospital Trauma Life Support (PHTLS) program that the EMT can make correct judgments leading toward good outcome only if the EMT is provided with a good base of knowledge. The foundation of the PHTLS program is that patient care should be judgment driven, not protocol driven, hence the detail provided in this course.

Recognizing hypoxia, shock, and hemorrhage depends on the ability to do a rapid, accurate primary assessment. Once recognized, these conditions must be managed aggressively.

Management for **hypoxia** is ensuring adequate oxygen exchange in the lungs and delivery of the oxygenated red blood cells to the tissue cells. This means providing supplemental oxygen as close to 100% ($FiO_2 = 1.0$) as possible. The EMT should remember the following when managing hypoxia:

- A patent airway must be maintained—any obstruction must be cleared.
- Injuries that compromise the integrity of the chest and the ventilatory process must be managed, and the patient must be provided with assisted ventilation if required.
- Procedures must be carried through in such a manner that the ever-present possibility of cervical spine injury is not forgotten or ignored. There are a variety of ways to protect the cervical spine, just as there are a variety of methods to provide airway and ventilatory support.
- The best method for management of each patient condition must be based on that patient's injuries and the EMT's resources.

The critical trauma patient usually needs treatment for both hypoxia and **shock.** For the patient in shock:

- Fluid replacement should be considered, based on the current scientific information available when the patient is seen.
- IV access and fluid resuscitation, *if used,* should be started as quickly as possible.
- Fluid administration *should not* delay transportation to the closest facility where definitive care will be given. This may be accomplished by:
  - starting intravenous lines en route to the hospital when advanced level EMTs are present
  - intercepting an advanced life support service (by air or ground units) when basic EMTs are faced with lengthy transportation time
  - rapid transportation to an appropriate hospital where the IV can be started
- The exact method chosen is, as in airway management, based on the judgment of the EMT and will be determined by the circumstances of each case.

Hemorrhage control is managed:

- temporarily in the field by use of compression dressings (tape, elastic or pneumatic) and/or
- permanently by rapid transportation to a hospital with a medical team ready to move the patient quickly to the operating room

The patient's other injuries must also be **stabilized for transportation.** It is important for the EMT to remember:

- Total "unibody" fracture stabilization is most quickly done by immobilizing the patient to a longboard, thereby splinting the spine and any other fractures—known or as yet unknown—that may be present.

- Once immobilized, the patient needs to be rapidly transported to the hospital. Unless the patient is trapped, there should be no reason for field management of an unstable trauma patient to require more than 10 minutes.
- During transport the patient should be further assessed from head to foot, and additional necessary care should be administered.

The patient must also be continually **reassessed,** since conditions that did not initially appear life threatening can become so in minutes. The flowchart in Figure 15-1 shows key considerations and decisions the EMT faces with the trauma patient.

WHY DO TRAUMA PATIENTS DIE?

In the immediate posttrauma period, trauma patients may die from hypoxia as a result of airway/ventilatory failure, circulatory failure (cardiac or fluid), or brain injury. Subsequently, they may die from the biochemical and pathophysiologic effects of prolonged hypoxia and hypoperfu-

sion, leading to immune system failure (sepsis) or other organ failure (renal, hepatic, pulmonary). If such prolonged anaerobic metabolism can be prevented or reduced, the likelihood of the progression of multiple organ failure (MOF) will be diminished.

Of course, even with the best planned and executed resuscitation, not all trauma victims can be saved. However, with the EMT's attention focused on the reasons for early traumatic death, a much larger percentage of patients may survive, and there may be less residual morbidity than without the benefit of the EMT's correct and expedient field management.

The EMT's efforts at resuscitation must be focused on rapid treatment for hypoxia, hypoperfusion, and hemorrhage control. The initial interventions are aimed only at the restoration of these vital functions and rapid transportation to the appropriate facility to continue the care started in the field and to provide homeostasis. All other treatment of the critical trauma patient is fruitless unless these primary goals are met. Sometimes the most dramatic visible injuries are ignored, and attention is paid only to those conditions that will result in death if they are not managed appropriately and immediately. The management of multisystem trauma patients must be based on resolving the problems that cause death.

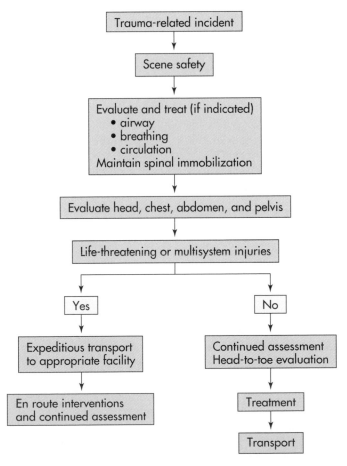

Figure 15-1 Key considerations in treating the trauma patient.

STRATEGIES FOR MULTISYSTEM TRAUMA PATIENT CARE

The key to the prehospital management of the multisystem trauma patient is organizing the knowledge and skills involved into a sound strategy—a plan of attack that can serve as a framework and method for dealing with such patients in a systematic, rapid, and thorough way. Throughout this text such a plan has been presented. It can be outlined briefly as follows:

1. Evaluate the three **S**'s: safety, scene, and situation.
2. Rapidly assess the patient's systemic condition. Evaluate the airway, breathing, and circulation with attention for possible spine injury. Focus on ventilation, shock, hemorrhage control, and spinal immobilization.
3. Provide intervention for these problems as they are found.
4. Reassess vital functions to evaluate the effectiveness of the interventions.
5. Reassess the head, chest, and abdomen to locate potentially life-threatening conditions. Rapidly provide needed interventions for any conditions that are found.
6. Immobilize the patient and expedite transport to the closest appropriate facility.
7. Perform a rapid secondary survey, and provide additional management while en route to the hospital.

Essential to this strategy is the rapid differentiation between patients with multisystem trauma and those with only simple trauma. The needs and priorities of each category are significantly different. All multisystem trauma patients, regardless of apparent stability, must be considered unstable until definitive diagnosis and treatment can be provided in the hospital.

A variety of independent studies published in the past few years have shown that the initiation of transport to a proper facility without delay is one of the key EMT treatments affecting survival in patients with multisystem trauma. The concepts of the golden hour from injury to management and the golden 10 minutes in the field, along with the increasing potential for permanent injury and mortality that results from each delay in definitive care, are universally accepted axioms of current trauma care.

Multisystem trauma patients should be held in the field only for urgent actions that will alter the outcome positively or that are mandated by the scene/situation (e.g., time needed for extrication).

Those steps that the EMT might legitimately take the time to do before beginning transport with such patients include the following:

- establishing scene safety
- rapid assessment (limited to life-threatening conditions)
- emergent interventions

- extrication of the patient
- proper packaging of the patient (longboard, hemorrhage control, spinal immobilization, etc.)

Any trauma patient who currently has, or has demonstrated by history or physical examination, any of the following should be classified and managed as a critical trauma patient:

- lowered level of consciousness
- any period of unconsciousness
- dyspnea
- significant bleeding
- shock (compensated or decompensated)
- incontinence
- significant injury of the head, face, neck, thorax, abdomen, or pelvis
- history of major medical problem
- mechanism of injury that commonly produces significant internal injuries

Only patients without injuries or conditions that are commonly associated with any potential life-threatening impact should be considered and managed as simple trauma patients (i.e., those with an isolated extremity fracture). If any doubt exists, the patient must be considered to have multisystem trauma.

Patients meeting the American College of Surgeons' criteria for physiologic, anatomic, or mechanism of injury for potentially severe injuries should be transported to a trauma center if one is present in the community. It is appropriate to bypass nontrauma centers to reach a trauma center.

In children, pregnant patients, and the elderly, injuries must be considered to be more serious than their outward appearance, have a more profound systemic impact, and have a greater potential for producing rapid devastating decompensation. In pregnant patients, there are at least two patients to care for, the mother and one or more fetus(es), both (or all) of whom may have sustained injury. In children and the elderly, the physical examination can be falsely reassuring and vital signs misleading. Compensatory mechanisms differ from younger adults and may not reveal abnormalities until the patient is profoundly compromised.

Occasionally, problems at the scene can impede the EMT's ability to rapidly initiate transport of the trauma patient. Multiple patient situations, the inability to reach the patient because of external hazards, or the inability of the EMT to extricate the patient from the situation clearly call for alterations in the standard approach to resuscitation. Many lifesaving procedures must be accomplished prior to patient removal. However, once the scene has become safe for the patient and rescuer, or the patient has become available for extrication, all efforts should again be directed at the rapid provision of care for life-threatening injuries and expedient transportation of the patient to a definitive care facility. The needs of the patient must always be the major determinant of the care provided.

Managing multisystem trauma patients is based on ensuring scene safety, rapidly identifying and treating life-threatening problems, and providing expeditious transport to an appropriate receiving hospital (trauma center).

STRATEGY FOR SIMPLE TRAUMA PATIENT CARE

When the EMT's initial assessment indicates that a patient has solely simple trauma, the continued care focuses on a more detailed head-to-toe examination and on the management and stabilization of each injury. Since urgency has been ruled out in such cases, it is prudent to ensure that the injuries have been identified and properly managed prior to moving and transporting the patient to protect the patient from any additional harm. Rapid transportation (lights and siren) should not be used with patients who only have simple trauma since it presents an unwarranted risk of traffic collision and an unnecessary danger of further injury. Although the EMT should take the time needed to identify and treat each injury, this should not be misinterpreted as an invitation to linger. Although no extreme urgency exists, the patient may suffer from undue delay and may, as a result of the simple trauma or of unrecognized injuries, deteriorate if field time is needlessly extended. (See Box 15-1 for key factors in the management of prehospital trauma.)

> **Box 15-1   The Key Dozen Factors in the Management of Prehospital Trauma**
>
> 1. Ensure safety of responders and patient.
> 2. Use rapid assessment to identify systemic deficits and patients with multisystem trauma.
> 3. Provide high FiO_2 to maintain $SpO_2 > 90\%$ to 92%
> 4. Provide airway management and ventilation as indicated.
> 5. Protect normal body temperature (use warm intravenous fluids and inhaled gases, monitor patient compartment temperature, keep patient covered).
> 6. Stop any significant external bleeding.
> 7. Use the pneumatic antishock garment to control pelvic bleeding or use as indicated in individual EMS system.
> 8. Provide basic shock treatment.
> 9. Provide rapid warm fluid replacement en route to the hospital.
> 10. Protect spine and other musculoskeletal injuries by immobilization to a longboard.
> 11. Include significant medical problems or history in assessment and care.
> 12. Rapidly initiate transport to an appropriate facility.

• Summary •

1. Maintaining a focus on priorities is the key to successful management of the multisystem trauma patient, whether there is one patient or many. The information contained in this text serves as a framework for a general approach to the patient.

2. Generally, no more than 10 minutes is necessary or recommended in the field when dealing with the critical trauma patient. If a review of your own recent run reports shows that you are taking more time, try to determine the reason. Can such patients really afford the wasted time at the scene?

3. Providing for the basics of airway, ventilation, and circulation management and adequate immobilization can be done in various ways. The EMT must select the methods that best meet the patient's needs in each circumstance. Is the time in the field being spent efficiently—to rapidly provide needed intervention—or is it wasted through inefficient techniques or by caring for low-priority injuries? We all may occasionally find ourselves being meticulous and tidy when the patient's needs dictate a broader and more sweeping approach.

4. Trauma care:
   - is dependent on the ability to perform a meaningful rapid assessment
   - is dependent on the ability to quickly locate and recognize life-threatening and potentially life-threatening conditions
   - must follow a given set of priorities that establish an efficient and effective plan of action, based on available time frames and any dangers present at the scene, if the patient is to survive
   - must provide appropriate intervention and stabilization
   - must be integrated and coordinated between the field, the emergency department, and the operating room. Each and every provider, at every level of care and at every stage of treatment, must be in harmony with the rest of the team.
   - must have as its goal the provision of definitive surgical care of the critical trauma patient within the golden hour

These basic concepts, rather than new specific skills, are the cornerstone to reducing morbidity and mortality in the critical trauma patient.

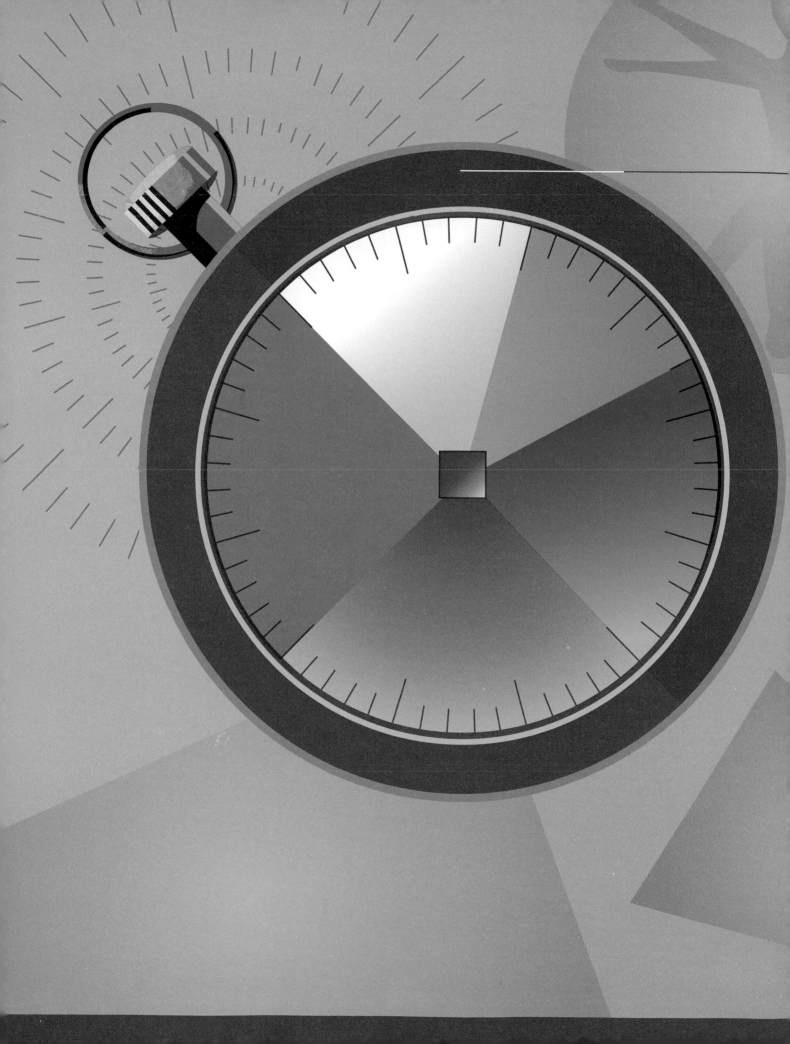

Trauma Systems: The Right Patient in the Right Time to the Right Place

The majority of this text has been devoted to the out-of-hospital recognition and treatment of an individual trauma patient. It is crucial to remember that patient survival actually depends on a system of care, not just the field management. A true trauma system represents the integration of many services, medical specialties, and people, all of whom come together with one idea in mind: optimizing the diagnosis, treatment, and rehabilitation of a victim of traumatic injury to not only save the patient's life but also return him or her to a productive life. Patient access to the EMS trauma system is the 9-1-1 telephone operator followed by the EMS dispatcher.

The EMT is the person and point of first medical contact in the trauma system. The EMT has the major responsibility of recognizing whether the patient in fact needs the services of the trauma system, and if so, enters the patient into the system and activates the system to receive the patient. Once received, emergency physicians, surgeons, nurses, anesthesiologists, radiologists, orthopedic surgeons, neurosurgeons, and a host of other technicians and therapists work side by side to maximize the opportunity for survival and rehabilitation of the patient.

Throughout this text, one particular aspect of the prehospital care has been mentioned—rapid transport to an appropriate facility. Rapid transport is very important because the definitive care of a multisystem or critically injured patient can only be provided in a hospital set up to handle the trauma patient. In most cases, this definitive care involves surgical intervention to control hemorrhage and repair injured organs. As important as prehospital management is, it is only a temporary measure to be provided until definitive care is performed; until that care is provided, the patient will continue to bleed.

THE EMS SYSTEM

Once an incident resulting in personal injury occurs, trauma care will ideally begin the moment the call for medical assistance is placed. Most of the United States has 9-1-1, the "universal" number for help, in place. However, there are still many communities and geographic areas that depend on the use of seven-digit telephone numbers to access public safety services such as police, fire, and ambulance aid.

As EMS systems increased in sophistication over the years, caregivers realized that waiting for the ambulance and EMTs to arrive before instituting medical care only added to the delay in treating a patient. Therefore, many EMS agencies implemented "emergency medical dispatching" and "pre-arrival instructions." These formalized procedures and protocols allow for the emergency medical dispatcher to evaluate the nature of the emergency, tailor the type of response to the incident, and educate and instruct the caller to provide intervention that may help stabilize the medical situation (e.g., applying direct pressure to control hemorrhage).

The sophistication and expertise of the out-of-hospital health care provider has also improved over the years. Although there remain state-to-state variations, relatively standardized training developed over the past 20 years has led to the three levels of emergency medical technicians—basic, intermediate, and paramedic—that are commonly found nationwide.

An essential component of the prehospital care of any patient, including the trauma victim, is medical direction. The care of a trauma patient is ultimately the responsibility of the physician who has medical oversight responsibility for the actions of the EMT. The medical director of the EMS agency or system must have policies, procedures, and protocols in place that define and outline the steps and actions to be performed or provided in caring for a trauma victim. Not only should the medical interventions be specified, but destination protocols, which are integral to the outcome of a trauma patient, should also be defined and known by everyone involved in the prehospital care of the patient. These guidelines should indicate under what circumstances a patient should be taken directly to a trauma center, even if it means bypassing a closer hospital that is not a trauma center. An example of these types of protocols is shown in Figure 16-1.

Every EMS system must also evaluate its performance in responding to and treating the trauma patient. Quality review for improvement of the system will focus on many components of EMS management, such as:

- response time to the scene
- amount of time spent on the scene
- interventions performed on the scene and in the ambulance during transport
- success rate of procedures such as intravenous access and endotracheal intubation
- choice of destination

Only by critically evaluating each call can the agency ensure that quality care in a timely fashion is being provided to critical patients and that patients are being taken to the appropriate facilities.

Finally, it has been recognized that in addition to reviewing the treatment of each individual patient, prehospital care of trauma patients in general must be critically evaluated and all interventions performed in the field must be reviewed to determine the real effect on patient outcome. Thus, in recent years, many researchers have focused their efforts on the provision of care outside of the hospital to determine what works and what does not work.

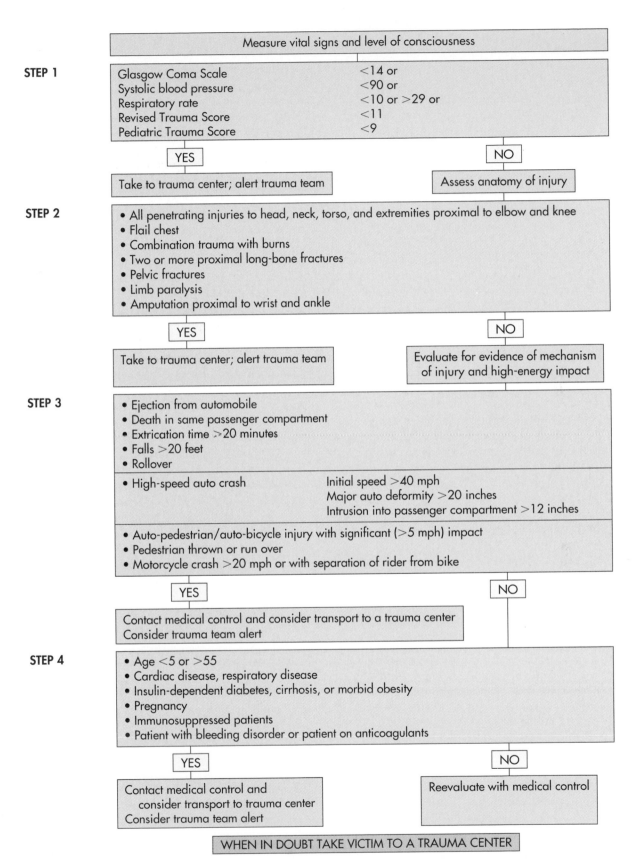

Figure 16-1 Triage decision scheme.

TRAUMA CENTERS

Prehospital evaluation and treatment constitute the introductory phase of the trauma system and are crucial components allowing recognition of the severity of the injury and entry into the trauma system. But, in order to provide definitive care, the trauma patient must be rapidly transported to an appropriate facility. What is an appropriate facility? If the outcome from multisystem trauma is to be optimized, not only must the EMT be trained and prepared to treat the trauma victim, but the receiving facility must also have the appropriate personnel and resources ready and available to accept the patient. The provision of care on the scene is an important first step in the treatment of the patient, but it is only the first step. For the patient to receive the best trauma care possible, a system for trauma care must be in place.

The American College of Surgeons (ACS) is an organization that has taken the lead in describing the resources necessary to provide optimal care for the trauma patient. Every few years, since 1966, the ACS has published and updated a document, now called "Resources for Optimal Care of the Injured Patient." This document delineates the resources, personnel, equipment, and training necessary for an institution to provide quality trauma care. Recognizing that different communities and geographic regions have differing needs and available resources, the document describes several levels of care and preparation, which range from the most comprehensive trauma centers to those facilities that only serve to stabilize a trauma victim while preparing for transfer to a higher level of care.

Trauma centers are categorized based on the resources and programs available at the facility (Figure 16-2). The **Level I** trauma center is a regional resource center that has a full spectrum of services in place, from prevention programs to patient rehabilitation, and serves as the leader in trauma care for a geographic area. Most Level I trauma centers are found in large university-based hospitals because of the requirements for patient care, education and teaching programs, and research. The **Level II** trauma center is expected to provide initial definitive patient care but may not have all of the resources found in a Level I facility. Some complex critical patients may have to be transferred from a Level II trauma center to a Level I facility for comprehensive care. In addition, research is not an essential component of a Level II trauma center's activities. The **Level III** trauma center was designed for communities that do not have the immediate availability of a Level I or II institution. These centers perform evaluation, resuscitation, and operative intervention for stabilization. When necessary, a Level III facility may transfer the patient to a Level I or II trauma center for ongoing or more definitive care. Lastly, **Level IV** facilities, which were created with rural or remote areas in mind, may not be a hospital but rather a clinic-type facility. Level IV facilities provide initial stabilization and will then transfer the patient to a Level I, II, or III trauma center. Ideally, Level III and IV trauma facilities, as well as those acute care hospitals that are not trauma centers, should have preexisting relationships and transfer agreements in place to ensure the rapid and expeditious transfer of patients to Level I or II facilities when indicated.

In 1988, the American College of Emergency Physicians (ACEP) developed a position paper describing the components of a full trauma system (Box 16-1) to complement the ACS document, which originally described only the hospital resources. Together, the two organizations have established the minimum criteria for a comprehensive trauma system. This system begins with access to emergency care via the prehospital phase and continues with the care provided in the emergency department, the operating room, the intensive care unit, the hospital ward, and finally the rehabilitation component. For a patient to return to a full and productive life, all of these components must be present and work together in a coordinated fashion to care for the trauma patient.

Although the ACS has described the resources necessary for trauma centers, it is important to note that recent years have brought changes in the approach to trauma care. In the past, the main focus was on getting the critically injured trauma victim to a trauma center and on the preparation of the facility to be a trauma center. Recently, however, it has been recognized that the majority of

Box 16-1	**Structure of a Trauma Care System**	
Environments	**Components**	**Providers**
Urban	Medical	System man-
Rural	direction	agement
	Prevention	Prehospital
	Communication	providers
	Training	Acute care fa-
	Triage	cilities
	Prehospital care	Rehabilitation/
	Transportation	reconstruc-
	Hospital care	tion services
	Public education	
	Rehabilitation	
	Medical eval-	
	uation	

Adapted with permission from American College of Emergency Physicians. "Guidelines for Trauma Care Systems." *Ann. Emerg. Med.* 16 (1987): 459–463.

The following table shows levels of categorization and their essential (E) or desirable (D) characteristics.

	LEVELS			
	I	II	III	IV
A. HOSPITAL ORGANIZATION				
1. Trauma Service	E	E	E	—
2. Trauma Service Director	E	E	E	—
3. Trauma Multidisciplinary Committee	E	E	D	—
4. Hospital Departments/Divisions/Sections				
a. General Surgery	E	E	E	D
b. Neurologic Surgery	E	E	D	—
c. Orthopedic Surgery	E	E	D	—
d. Emergency Services	E	E	E	D
e. Anesthesia	E	E	E	—
B. CLINICAL CAPABILITIES				
Specialty Availability				
1. In-house 24 hours a day				
a. General Surgery	E	E	—	—
b. Neurologic Surgery	E	E	—	—
c. Emergency Medicine	E	E	E	—
d. Anesthesiology	E	E	—	—
2. On call and promptly available				
a. Anesthesiology	—	—	E	D
b. Cardiac Surgery	E	D	—	—
c. Cardiology	E	E	D	—
d. General Surgery	—	—	E	D
e. Hand Surgery	E	D	—	—
f. Infectious Disease	E	D	—	—
g. Internal Medicine	E	E	E	—
h. Microvascular Surgery (replant/flaps)	E	D	—	—
i. Neurologic Surgery	—	—	D	—
j. Obstetric/Gynecologic Surgery	E	E	D	—
k. Ophthalmic Surgery	E	E	D	—
l. Oral/Maxillofacial Surgery	E	E	—	—
m. Orthopedic Surgery	E	E	D	—

Figure 16-2 Trauma center categorization.

trauma patients do not need the capabilities of a trauma center and that most trauma care can be provided at other acute care hospitals. Therefore, all facilities should be part of the trauma system; efforts in education and trauma care analysis should include all facilities, not just the trauma centers (Figure 16-3).

Integral to a successful trauma system is an ongoing evaluation of the system. Mechanisms must be in place for data collection, quality assessment, review of the care provided, and improvement activities and methodologies to correct identified deficiencies.

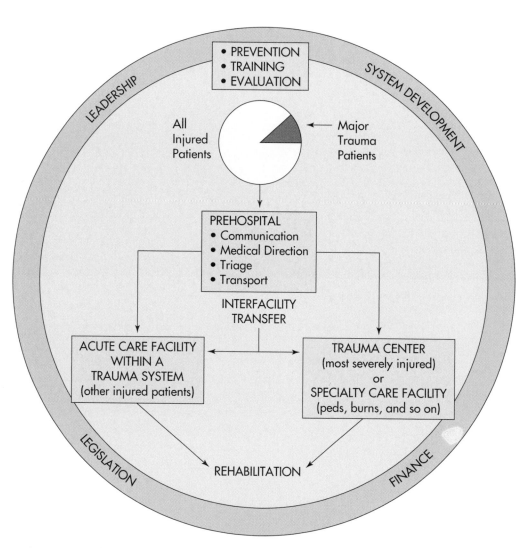

Figure 16-3 The integral nature of the EMS trauma system. (Adapted with permission from the Bureau of Health Services Resources, Division of Trauma and Emergency Medical Services: *Model Trauma Care System Plan*. Rockville, Md.: U.S. Department of Health and Human Services, 1992.)

• Summary •

1. The goal of prehospital trauma care is simple and easily identified—the right patient to the right place at the right time. Every EMS system should identify, in advance, those hospitals that are prepared to receive trauma patients. EMS systems should also have criteria in place to define which patients should be taken directly to these trauma centers. Every EMT is responsible for knowing which facilities are trauma centers and understanding the criteria for determining the appropriate destination.

2. Every member of the trauma care team, including EMTs, emergency physicians, surgeons, and laboratory and radiology personnel, must work together to maximize the opportunity for patient survival and recovery. Political differences, geographic and turf boundaries, and financial considerations should always be subordinate to what is best for the patient.

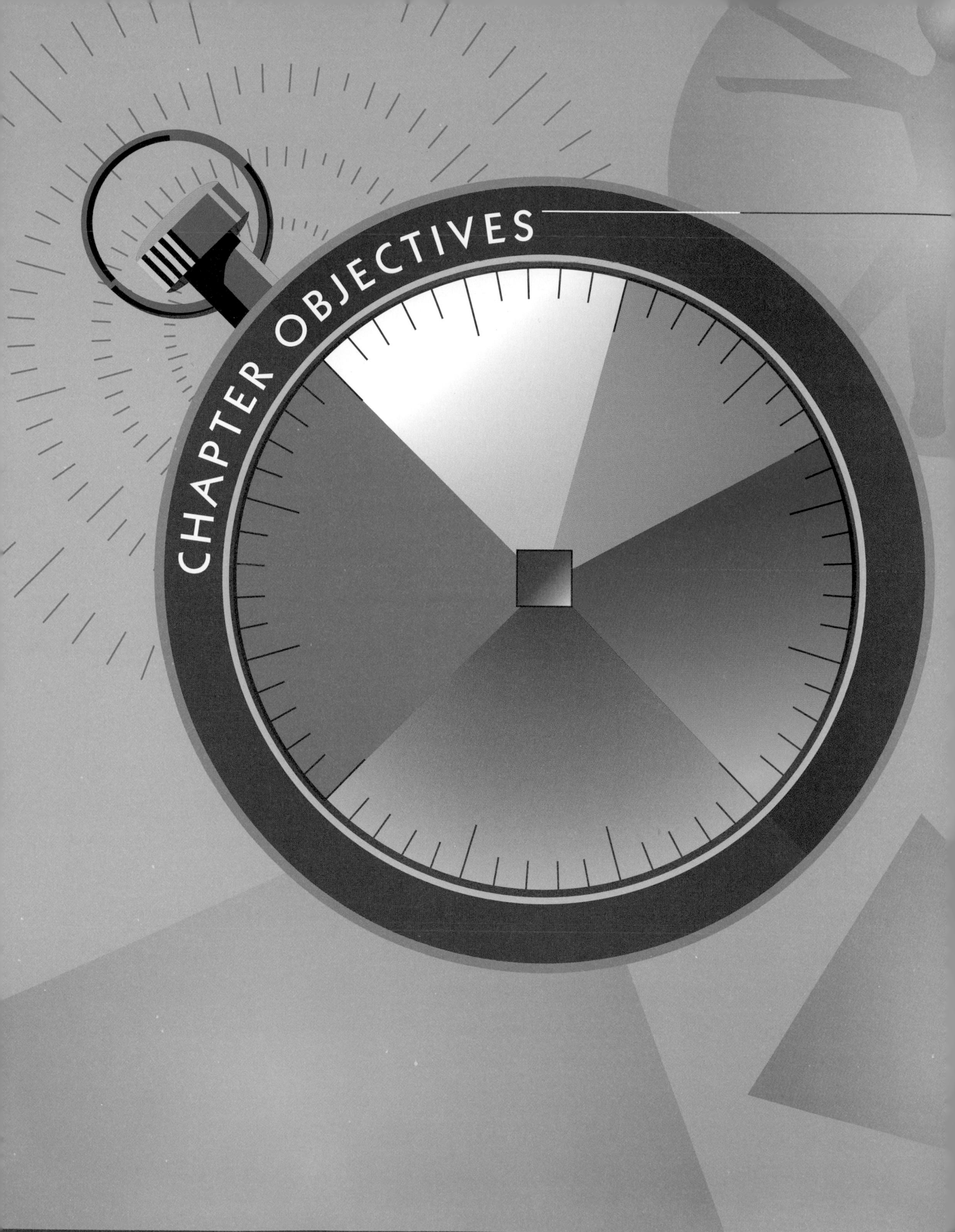
CHAPTER OBJECTIVES

CHAPTER 17

Military Medicine

At the completion of this course the student will be able to:

- Identify significant landmarks in the evolutionary history of the emergency medical service that resulted from the military medical influence.

- Define and describe the differences between military and civilian echelons of care.

- Identify the stages of care associated with battlefield assessment.

- Describe the threat(s) from biologic and chemical weapons of mass destruction.

- Compare and contrast military and civilian mass casualty situations and the conduct of patient triage in these two scenarios.

Scenario

A 24-person Special Operations Forces (SOF) team is ordered to raid a cocaine laboratory in South America. The cocaine lab is located in a dense jungle area protected by an estimated hostile strength of 15 men with automatic weapons. Insertion will be accomplished by a riverine craft approximately 6 kilometers from the target. As the patrol reaches the target area, a booby trap is tripped, injuring the point man (no pulse or respiration) and the patrol leader (massive trauma to the leg with femoral arterial bleeding). There is heavy incoming direct and indirect fire as the lab security force responds to the explosive blast. The planned extraction of the SOF team is by boat, 1 kilometer from the target area.

- As the medic accompanying the SOF team, how would you triage the patients identified in this scenario with regards to treatment and order of evacuation?
- What additional information would be helpful in making medical management decisions at this point?
- Are there any barriers to proper patient management at the scene? How can you work around these barriers?
- Outline the steps you would take to manage these patients.

Modern prehospital trauma life support (PHTLS) had its birth on the battlefields of Europe and the American Civil War. Exigencies of war have driven the evolution of military medical care throughout history with innovations in equipment, principles of care, and training founded on the need to improve combat survivability. Lessons learned in war were applied on the home front as returning medics and corpsmen adapted them to address increasing levels of industrial-based trauma in the civilian sector. The civilian emergency medical system (EMS) would develop from this, maintaining many of the original concepts such as scene safety (avoid becoming a casualty, avoid incurring additional casualties), primary survey (manage life-threatening injuries, avoid additional injuries), and transport (evacuate the casualty as quickly and safely as possible to definitive care).

Despite similarities, significant differences have historically existed between civilian PHTLS and military requirements on the battlefield (Table 17-1). The gap between battlefield trauma management and civilian PHTLS is diminishing, however, as the threat of a terrorist attack grows worldwide. Conventional explosive devices and weapons of mass destruction (chemical, biological, and nuclear) make the civilian population vulnerable to mass casualty situations traditionally faced only by those in combat.

The majority of combat-related deaths occur near the site of injury before the casualty reaches an established medical treatment facility (MTF). Highly trained, nonphysicians provide health care on or near the front lines, and patients are transported to various levels of MTFs for further care. These combat medics have a scope of practice beyond that of their civilian counterparts. Basic first aid is the starting point, but modifications and ingenuity are expected and acceptable when applying basic protocols in a hostile situation. The restrictive environment of the battlefield significantly influences patient care decisions. Mission accomplishment may have a higher priority than immediate evacuation, an apparent conflict with generally accepted patient care standards. Immediate evacuation may not even be an option, and long-term supportive care may be required. Once more, lessons learned in combat can be extended into civilian practice.

Military and civilian health care agencies are increasingly involved in cooperative efforts to provide relief operations in natural or man-made disasters such as hurricanes, floods, earthquakes, chemical spills, or nuclear power plant accidents. Civil-military interoperability has become critical, and the two communities can learn from and complement each other as we continue to fine tune our skills. (For a comparison of civilian and military prehospital care, see Table 17-1.) Familiarity with this chapter will be beneficial to civilian providers as well as their military counterparts.

THE MILITARY MEDIC AND THE EMERGENCE OF PREHOSPITAL CARE

Military and civilian prehospital providers share a common heritage of unparalleled commitment to service at great personal risk and sacrifice. The civilian EMS can be traced to developments and innovations within the military.

MILITARY MEDICINE— THE EARLY YEARS

Armies have not always provided medical care during combat. Wounded soldiers, through most of history, relied on themselves or the compassion of fellow soldiers for any care they might receive. Those on the losing side often faced death at the hands of their victors. Officers sometimes pooled resources and hired a surgeon to accompany them into war, but the common soldier rarely counted on such a luxury.

One notable exception was the Roman Empire, which established a military health care system with hospitals (*valetudinaria*) at their permanent frontier posts, providing institutionalized care for their deployed soldiers. When the Empire fell, however, the idea of an army being responsible for the health of its soldiers was lost for centuries.

Battlefield care reemerged in the first modern nation-states of Europe as the armies of post-revolutionary France organized a system of prehospital care that included a corps of litter bearers *(bracardiers)* to remove the wounded from the field and the flying ambulance or *ambulance volante* of Baron Dominique Jean Larrey to transport surgeons forward and patients to the rear. These concepts of clearing the battlefield and rapidly transporting patients to field hospitals were expanded greatly during the American Civil War.

The early phases of the Civil War clearly illustrated that neither army was adequately prepared for handling battlefield casualties. At the first Battle of the Manassas (or Bull Run), wounded soldiers were left on the battlefield for as long as 5 days. The American people reacted with horror and disgust, leading to the reform of the U.S. Army's medical department. Charles Tripler, medical director of the Army of the Potomac, suggested that some soldiers be trained in the use of litters, and daily litter drills were instituted in 1861. Jonathan Letterman replaced Tripler and established an ambulance corps under the command of a medical officer. Enlisted personnel drilled on evacuation standards, and the senior noncommissioned officer with each ambulance train was examined on his knowledge of bandaging and dressings. This system was extended to all Union armies, by law, for the duration of the war.

Lessons learned during the Civil War had a great impact on civilian care, and many postwar developments were direct outgrowths of wartime experiences. Doctor Edward B. Dalton served as a volunteer medical officer in the Army of the Potomac, worked with the ambulance system, and fully understood the value of prehospital care and dedicated transport. When later appointed sanitary superintendent for New York City, he suggested the establishment, in 1869, of a military-like ambulance system based in city hospitals for handling accident cases. Each ambulance was to carry" . . . a box beneath the driver's seat, containing a quart flask of brandy, two tourniquets, a half dozen bandages, a half dozen small sponges, some splint material, pieces of old blanket for padding, strips of various lengths with buckles, and a 2 ounce vial of persulphate of iron." A young doctor accompanied each ambulance; the idea of a dedicated paraprofessional corps that could provide medical services was not part of the initial U.S. civilian ambulance system. Several European systems, such as those from the British Order of St. John, were staffed with volunteers trained to provide a certain extent of prehospital care.

In the expansion of the American West, military surgeons were faced with a choice of accompanying iso-

Table 17-1 Differences Between Civilian and Military PHTLS

Civilian	Military
1. Patients are usually limited in number, and medical resources are not overwhelmed.	1. Large numbers of injuries can quickly overwhelm available resources.
2. Patients are located in secure areas.	2. Patients are located in nonsecure areas.
3. PHTLS access to supplies and advice is available.	3. There are limited supplies and an isolated provider.
4. The prehospital phase is short.	4. The prehospital phase may be extended.
5. Evacuation times to definitive care are generally short.	5. Evacuations may be delayed.

lated patrols or providing medical care at the base post for soldiers staying behind or those retrieved from combat. Many surgeons resorted to training enlisted personnel to accompany the patrols and to provide initial medical coverage. This extension of medical coverage by paraprofessionals continues today.

THE PARAPROFESSIONAL IN FORWARD CARE

The Battleship Maine was blown up in Havana Harbor in 1898, and the nation mobilized for war with Spain. Hospital corpsmen played a vital role and led volunteer surgeons, like Nicholas Senn, to report: **"The fate of the wounded rest in the hands of the one who applies the first dressing."** The absolute need for prehospital care by trained personnel in the military was universally recognized by World War I. Twentieth-century advances in science and technology enhanced the medics' ability to deliver that care.

Medics and corpsmen leaving the service took their skills into civilian positions. Many went to work for fire and police departments or for mortuaries at a time when undertakers often had the only vehicles in which a patient could be transported. They began to work with ambulance services providing various levels of first aid care. Organized teaching of first aid began to grow under the auspices of the American Red Cross, the Boy Scouts, and other groups reflecting a growing awareness of the value of prehospital care.

THE MODERN DAY EMERGENCY MEDICAL TECHNICIAN (EMT)

The conflict in Vietnam expanded in the 1960s and the evening news graphically revealed the vital role played by the combat medic in saving lives. They were at the site of injury, initiated first aid measures, and participated in rapid patient evacuations back to prestationed trauma hospitals. A transformation occurred in the concept of civilian prehospital care in 1965. There was increasing concern over mass trauma as part of highway safety and civil defense, and the National Academy of Sciences (NAS) published its *Accidental Death and Disability: The Neglected Disease of Modern Society.* This study pointed out that over half the country's ambulance services were provided by morticians, that most of these, as well as most municipal-based ambulances, were geared toward a "collect and run mentality," and no care was provided before or during transport. Supplies were virtually nonexistent, and there were no generally accepted standards for competency or training of ambulance personnel.

The findings of this study led to the Highway Safety Act of 1966 requiring states to develop EMS programs. This was the first comprehensive effort in America to establish a professional, standardized, prehospital EMS. Military manuals were used to compile training programs for EMTs. The first National Registry of EMTs was established in 1970, and certification insured a recognizable civilian profession. A standard EMT textbook, the *Emergency Care and Transportation of the Sick and Injured* was published in 1971.

Many early EMTs were influenced by their military experience where their scope of practice was much wider than civilian agencies allowed. The NAS recommended, in 1970, that ambulance attendants develop advanced EMT medical training programs. Standard EMT-Paramedic training and certification criteria were established in 1977. By 1979, 45 states were participating in paramedic training and all 50 had authorized utilization of advanced EMTs or paramedics in their EMS systems.

MILITARY MEDICAL EVACUATION AND TODAY'S LIFEFLIGHT

The use of helicopters was interjected into civilian EMS programs in 1970 when the NAS recommended an evaluation program using Department of Defense helicopters in conjunction with civilian authorities. Five demonstration areas were established for the Military Assistance to Safety and Traffic (MAST) program. Helicopter evacuation was so successful that despite costs, 22 additional areas were soon added. Air ambulance guidelines were published in 1981 by the Commission of Emergency Medical

Services, the American Medical Association, and the Department of Transportation. Civilian EMS had achieved mature independence.

MILITARY HEALTH SERVICES SUPPORT ORGANIZATION

ECHELONS (LEVELS) OF CARE

Field medical assets of the United States military are organized into five increasingly sophisticated echelons of care. Each echelon builds upon the capabilities of the previous level and adds additional services. Echelons extend from the point of wounding, illness, or injury (usually at the lowest level) and provide a continuum of care. Military medical doctrine is evolving from a fixed facility concept to a more fluid system in order to improve the survivability of wounded soldiers. Advanced capabilities are being moved further forward in the echelons with the idea of balancing maximal care with required mobility.

Echelon of Care I

Echelon I is care at the unit level, accomplished by individual soldiers or a trained medical corpsman. All military personnel are taught basic first aid upon entry into the service. The United States Army augments this capability with its Combat Lifesaver Program, which instructs nonmedical personnel in skills beyond basic first aid. Echelon I also includes mobile aid stations, staffed by medical technicians and a physician or a physician's assistant, that move with the units they support. They function out of small tents or vehicles (such as armored personnel carriers, when in a mechanized unit). Care at this level includes restoration of airway by surgical procedure, administration of intravenous fluids and antibiotics, and stabilization of wounds and fractures. The goal of medical management at the echelon I level is to return the patient to duty or to stabilize the patient for evacuation to the next appropriate level of care.

Echelon of Care II

Echelon II involves a team of physicians, physician's assistants, nurses, and medical technicians capable of basic resuscitation, stabilization, and surgery along with X ray, pharmacy, and temporary holding facilities. Many echelon II facilities have limited laboratories, and this is the first level of care that has transfusion capabilities (group O liquid packed red blood cells). Surgery procedures are limited to emergency procedures to prevent death, loss of limb or body function.

Like echelon I facilities, echelon II units must be small

and mobile. Size is determined by the predicted number and type of casualties during an operation based on previous experience and analysis of the enemy threat. An example of an echelon II unit is the United States Air Force ten-bed facility. It has 51 personnel assigned in support of ten holding beds and one operating room, with enough supplies to perform 50 major surgical cases. Ground or air evacuation is available to transfer the patients to more capable treatment facilities if required.

Echelon of Care III

Echelon III facilities have capabilities normally found in fixed medical treatment facilities and are located in lower enemy threat environments. The goal of the echelon III is restoration of functional health and includes resuscitation, initial or delayed wound surgery, and postoperative treatment. More extensive services such as laboratory, X ray, and pharmacy are available along with a full range of blood products. Care proceeds with greater preparation and deliberation.

Echelon of Care IV

Echelon IV further expands on the capabilities of the echelon III facility by providing definitive therapy within the theater of operations for patients who can be returned to duty within the time set by the theater evacuation policy. Theater evacuation policy (the amount of time a casualty can remain in theater) is dependent upon enemy threat, type of mission, size of the force, air frame availability, bed occupancy, and availability. If the patient cannot be returned to duty within the specified time, evacuation is required, usually to the continental United States (CONUS). Definitive care in an echelon IV facility is normally provided by a fleet hospital ship, a general hospital, or an overseas MTF.

Echelon of Care V

Convalescent, restorative, and rehabilitative care is provided at echelon V. This care is provided by military hospitals, Department of Veterans Affairs (VA) hospitals, or civilian hospitals located in the United States.

Comparison of Military and Civilian Systems of Care

The military system of echeloned medical care may be compared to the civilian trauma system spread out across the theater of operations. If the integrated trauma system used in the civilian community is broken down into parts, it closely matches the military system. Echelon I is comparable to care rendered by paramedics and civilian critical care helicopter units. Echelon II facilities are com-

parable to the resuscitation areas in level 1 trauma centers. Echelons III and IV provide the restorative surgery and medical care provided in acute and intermediate trauma center wards. Finally, echelon V units provide the rehabilitative and support services that are offered in the follow-up phase of care in truly integrated trauma systems.

Echelon Coordination

Military echelon system units are small and geographically separated; superb coordination is required to make the system work. Central control of patient movement within and out of the theater is critical and relies on good communications, visibility of casualty flow through all the medical facilities in theater (to minimize overload of any one facility), and the availability and control of evacuation assets. Proper triage techniques minimize the stress on any one level by ensuring that workloads are appropriate for the degrees of specialization, level of care, and resources. Stable patients, even with serious wounds, may bypass intermediate echelons and be sent directly to definitive care if the transport time is short.

PREHOSPITAL CARE IN THE TACTICAL ENVIRONMENT

TACTICAL COMBAT CASUALTY CARE— GENERAL CONSIDERATIONS

The importance of the prehospital phase in caring for combat casualties is evident from the fact that approximately 90% of those who die from wounds sustained in combat do so on the battlefield before ever reaching a medical treatment facility (MTF).[1] Trauma care training for military corpsmen and medics has in recent years been based primarily on the principles taught in the Advanced Trauma Life Support (ATLS) course.[2] ATLS provides a well thought out, standardized approach to the management of trauma that has proven very successful when used in the setting of a hospital emergency department. ATLS was developed for the in-hospital environment. PHTLS has been developed for the "prehospital" period prior to arrival at a medical facility. The same principles apply but must be used differently. There are differences as well in the combat and noncombat requirements of the prehospital phase.[3-13]

Extrapolation of ATLS principles from the hospital emergency department to the tactical combat setting requires a careful review of the differences that exist between these two settings and how this impacts on the recommended trauma management strategies. The standard

ATLS course currently makes no mention of the exigencies of the battlefield and what modifications to ATLS guidelines might be considered for the combat setting. The need for such modifications is obvious when considering the complicating effect of such factors as darkness, hostile fire, medical equipment limitations, prolonged evacuation times, provider experience levels, mission-related command decisions, hostile environments (aquatic, mountain, desert, and jungle settings), and the unique problems entailed in transporting casualties on the battlefield.

These considerations demonstrate the need for casualty care guidelines that differ somewhat from ATLS guidelines for U.S. Army combat medics. Military as well as civilian organizations have developed recommendations for the care of trauma patients and other medical emergencies that take into account the special conditions encountered by their membership.[13,14]

These observations do not imply any shortcomings in the ATLS course. The ATLS course is well accepted as the standard of care once the patient reaches the Emergency Department of an MTF. Problems arise only as the military attempts to extrapolate the principles of care from civilian ATLS into the battlefield setting. This is an environment for which ATLS was clearly not designed but which PHTLS was set up to do. This section is designed to help address the need of PHTLS in the battlefield setting.

STAGES OF CARE

It is useful to consider the management of casualties that occur during combat missions as being divided into several distinct phases of care as described shortly.[13] This type of approach is essential for combat trauma, because guidelines for combat medics and corpsmen *must* consider not only what the appropriate elements of treatment are but also what is the appropriate time in the continuum of care from battlefield to hospital ship to render each aspect of treatment.

1. *Care Under Fire* is the care rendered by the medic or corpsman at the scene of the injury while both the caregiver and the casualty are still under effective hostile fire. The risk of additional injuries being sustained at any moment are extremely high for both casualty and rescuer. Available medical equipment is limited to that carried by each operator on the mission or by the medical personnel in their medical packs.
2. *Tactical Field Care* is the care rendered by the medic or corpsman once he or she and the casualty are no longer under effective hostile fire. It also applies to situations in which an injury has occurred on a mission, but there has been no hostile fire. Available medical equipment is still limited to that

carried into the field by mission personnel. Time prior to evacuation to an MTF may range from a few minutes to many hours.
3. *Combat Casualty Evacuation Care* is care rendered once the casualty has been picked up by an aircraft, vehicle, or boat for transportation to a higher echelon of care. Additional personnel and medical equipment that have been pre-staged in these assets should be available during this phase of casualty management. The term "CASEVAC" should be used to describe this phase instead of the commonly encountered term "MEDEVAC" because the Air Force reserves the term "MEDEVAC" to describe a noncombat medical transport.

BASIC TACTICAL COMBAT CASUALTY CARE PLAN

Having defined these three phases of casualty management in the tactical combat setting, the next step is to outline in a general way the care that is appropriate to each phase. A basic tactical casualty management plan is presented in Boxes 17-1 through 17-3.[13] This management plan is a generic sequence of steps that will often require modification for specific casualty scenarios, but the basic plan is important as a starting point from which development of individualized scenario-based management plans may begin. A detailed rationale for the steps outlined in the basic management plan for each of these stages of care has been presented.[13] In general, the treatment methods used in the PHTLS course have been followed unless specific combat considerations were felt to justify a departure. A few of the major differences between this recommended combat casualty care plan and PHTLS will be reviewed here and the reasons for these differences discussed.

Box 17-1 Basic Tactical Combat Casualty Management Plan—Phase One: Care Under Fire

1. Return fire as directed or required.
2. Try to keep yourself from getting shot.
3. Try to keep the casualty from sustaining additional wounds.
4. Airway management is generally best deferred until the Tactical Field Care phase.
5. Stop any life-threatening external hemorrhage using necessary means.
6. Take the casualty with you when you leave.

Box 17-2 Basic Tactical Combat Casualty Management Plan—Phase Two: Tactical Field Care

1. Airway management
   - Chin-lift or jaw-thrust
   - Unconscious casualty without airway obstruction: nasopharyngeal airway
   - Unconscious casualty with airway obstruction: cricothyroidotomy
   - Cervical spine immobilization is not efficient for casualties with penetrating head or neck trauma.
2. Breathing
   - Consider tension pneumothorax and decompress if a casualty has unilateral penetrating chest trauma and progressive respiratory distress.
3. Bleeding
   - Control any remaining bleeding using necessary means.
4. IV
   - Start an 18-gauge IV or saline lock.
5. Fluid resuscitation
   - Controlled hemorrhage without shock: no fluids necessary
   - Controlled hemorrhage with shock: Hespan 1,000 cc if available; otherwise lactated Ringer's 2,000 cc
   - Uncontrolled (intra-abdominal or thoracic) hemorrhage: No IV fluid resuscitation
6. Inspect and dress wound
7. Check for additional wounds
8. Analgesia as necessary
   - 5 mg IV of morphine
   - Wait 10 minutes
   - Repeat as necessary
9. Splint fractures and recheck pulse
10. Antibiotics
    - 2 g slow IV push (over 3 to 5 minutes) of cefoxitin for penetrating abdominal trauma, massive soft tissue damage, open fractures, grossly contaminated wounds, or long delays before casualty evacuation
11. Cardiopulmonary resuscitation
    - Resuscitation on the battlefield for victims of blast or penetrating trauma who have no pulse, no respirations, and no other signs of life will not be successful and should not be attempted.

Box 17-3 Basic Tactical Combat Casualty Management Plan—Phase Three: Combat Casualty Evacuation (CASEVAC) Care

1. Airway management
   - Chin-lift or jaw-thrust
   - Unconscious casualty without airway obstruction: nasopharyngeal airway, endotracheal intubation, combitube, or laryngeal mask airway
   - Unconscious casualty with airway obstruction: cricothyroidotomy if endotracheal intubation and/or other airway devices are unsuccessful
2. Breathing
   - Consider tension pneumothorax and decompress with needle thoracostomy if a casualty has unilateral penetrating chest trauma and progressive respiratory distress.
   - Consider chest tube insertion for all penetrating chest trauma.
   - Oxygen
3. Bleeding
   - Consider removing tourniquets and using direct pressure to control bleeding if possible.
4. IV
   - Start an 18-gauge IV or heparin lock if not already done.
5. Fluid resuscitation
   - No hemorrhage or controlled hemorrhage without shock: lactated Ringer's at 250 cc/hr
   - Controlled hemorrhage with shock: Hespan 1,000 cc initially if available; otherwise lactated Ringer's 2,000 cc
   - Uncontrolled (intra-abdominal or thoracic) hemorrhage: no IV fluid resuscitation
   - Head wound patient: Hespan at minimal flow to maintain infusion unless there is concurrent controlled hemorrhagic shock
6. Monitoring
   - Institute electronic monitoring of heart rate, blood pressure, and hemoglobin oxygen saturation
7. Inspect and dress wound if not already done
8. Check for additional wounds
9. Analgesia as necessary
   - 5 mg IV of morphine
   - Wait 10 minutes
   - Repeat as necessary
10. Splint fractures and recheck pulse if not already done
11. Antibiotics (if not already given)
    - 2 g slow IV push (over 3 to 5 minutes) of cefoxitin for penetrating abdominal trauma, massive soft tissue damage, open fractures, grossly contaminated wounds, or long delays before casualty evacuation

CARE UNDER FIRE

A minimum of medical care should be attempted while the casualty and corpsman or medic are actually under effective hostile fire. This is reflected in the recommended care shown in Box 17-1. Suppression of hostile fire and moving the casualty to a position where adequate cover allows more complete evaluation and treatment are major considerations at this point. Significant delays for a detailed examination and meticulous treatment of all aspects of the patient's wounds are ill-advised while under effective hostile fire. It may be critical for the combat medic or corpsman to help suppress the hostile fire before attempting to provide care at all, especially in small-unit operations where friendly firepower is limited and every person is essential to the successful outcome of an engagement. If hostile fire is not effectively suppressed, there is a need to move the casualty to cover. Management of the airway is temporarily deferred inasmuch as this movement will entail the rescuer carrying or dragging the casualty for some distance, during which time airway management will be very difficult or impossible.

The temporary use of a tourniquet to manage life-threatening extremity hemorrhage in this phase may be required. Hemorrhage from extremity wounds is the number one cause of preventable death on the battlefield and was responsible for the deaths of more than 2,500 casualties in Vietnam who had no other major injuries.[15] Use of direct pressure or compression dressings may result in delays in getting the casualty to cover, exposing both casualty and rescuer to increased hazard of additional injury. They may also be less effective than a tourniquet at stopping the bleeding during the initial combat rescue in which the casualty may have to be dragged or carried to cover by the rescuer, making it difficult for the rescuer to simultaneously apply direct pressure to the site of bleeding. Treatment of non–life-threatening bleeding should be deferred until the patient is moved to cover or effective hostile fire is suppressed.

The usual requirement of immobilizing the cervical spine prior to moving a casualty with a penetrating neck or head wound does not apply when moving the casualty out of a fire fight. In less than 2% of patients with penetrating neck injuries in Vietnam would immobilization of the cervical spine have been of possible benefit.[10] The risk of additional hostile fire injuries to both casualty and rescuer while immobilization is being attempted poses a much more significant threat in this setting than that of damage to the spinal cord from failure to immobilize the C-spine.[10]

TACTICAL FIELD CARE

Recommended guidelines for this phase of care are shown in Box 17-2. If a trauma patient is found to be in cardiopulmonary arrest on the battlefield as a result of blast or penetrating trauma, attempts at resuscitation are not appropriate.[13] Prehospital resuscitation of trauma patients in cardiac arrest has been found to be futile even in the urban setting where the victim is in close proximity to trauma centers. Resuscitation of trauma victims in cardiopulmonary arrest should not be attempted on a pulseless nonbreathing trauma patient whose arrest is not secondary to an immediately manageable airway injury. In the tactical combat setting, the cost of attempting to resuscitate patients with inevitably fatal wounds will be measured in additional lives lost as combat medical personnel are exposed to hostile fire during resuscitation efforts and care is withheld from casualties with potentially survivable wounds. Successful completion of the unit's mission may also be unnecessarily jeopardized by these efforts. Only in the case of nontraumatic disorders such as hypothermia, near-drowning, or electrocution should cardiopulmonary resuscitation be performed in the tactical prehospital setting.

Unconscious casualties should have their airways opened with the chin-lift or jaw-thrust maneuvers. If spontaneous respirations are present and there is no respiratory distress, a nasopharyngeal airway is the airway of choice. The two main advantages of this device over an oropharyngeal airway are that it is better tolerated should the patient suddenly regain consciousness and it is probably less likely to be dislodged during transport.

Should an airway obstruction develop or persist despite the use of a nasopharyngeal airway, a more definitive airway is required. The experienced paramedical personnel can quickly insert an endotracheal tube in the field. This technique may be more problematic in the tactical environment, however, for a number of reasons[13]:

1. No studies were found that documented the ability of well-trained but relatively inexperienced paramedical military intubationists to accomplish endotracheal intubation on the battlefield.
2. Many corpsmen and medics have never performed an intubation on a live patient or even a cadaver.
3. Standard endotracheal intubation techniques entail the use of the white light in the laryngoscope, which is tactically compromising on the battlefield, primarily at night.
4. Maxillofacial injuries that cause blood and other obstructions in the airway could make endotracheal intubation more difficult.
5. Esophageal intubations would be much less likely to be recognized on the battlefield and may result in fatalities.

Endotracheal intubation may be difficult to accomplish even in the hands of more experienced paramedical personnel under less austere conditions. First-time intubationists trained with mannequin intubations alone were noted to have an initial success rate of only 42% in the ideal confines of the operating room with paralyzed patients.[16] Most of the previously cited studies documenting the success of paramedical personnel in performing endotracheal intubation noted that they used cadaver training, operating room intubations, supervised initial intubations, or a combination of these methods in training their paramedics. They also stress the importance of continued practice of this skill in maintaining proficiency.

Since significant airway obstruction in the combat setting is likely to be the result of penetrating wounds of the face or neck in which blood or disrupted anatomy precludes visualization of the vocal cords, cricothyroidotomy might be a better next step than intubation if the combat corpsman or medic is trained in this procedure, although this has not been proven under combat conditions either. Cricothyroidotomy has been reported to be safe and effective in trauma victims and may well be the best alternative for any potential intubationist in these very difficult airway management cases.[17] This procedure is not without complications,[18,19] but a prepackaged cricothyroidotomy kit for combat medical use that contains the equipment for an over-the-wire technique has recently been developed at the Walter Reed Army Institute of Research and approved by the FDA. Combat medical personnel should be trained to use this technique in the case of airway obstruction where intubation is not possible. These techniques work well in an urgent environment but not in an emergent setting. The time required to achieve oxygenation can be excessive.

A presumptive diagnosis of tension pneumothorax should be made when progressive, severe respiratory distress develops in the case of unilateral penetrating chest trauma. The diagnosis of tension pneumothorax on the battlefield should not rely on such typical clinical signs as decreased breath sounds, tracheal shift, and hyperresonance on percussion because these signs may not always be present and, even if they are, they may be exceedingly difficult to appreciate on the battlefield. A patient with penetrating chest trauma will generally have some degree of hemo/pneumothorax as a result of his or her primary wound and the additional trauma caused by a needle thoracostomy would not be expected to significantly worsen the patient's condition should he or she not actually have a tension pneumothorax. Combat corpsmen and medics should be trained in this technique and should perform it in this setting. Paramedics are authorized to perform needle thoracostomy in some civilian emergency medical services. Chest tubes are not recommended in this phase of care for the following reasons:

1. They are not needed to provide initial treatment for a tension pneumothorax.
2. They are more difficult and time consuming for relatively inexperienced medical personnel to perform, especially in the austere battlefield environment.
3. Chest tube insertion would be more likely to cause additional tissue damage and subsequent infection than a less traumatic needle thoracostomy.

4. No documentation was found in the literature that demonstrated a benefit from tube thoracostomy performed by paramedical personnel on the battlefield.[13]

Tube thoracostomy is generally not part of the paramedic's scope of care in civilian EMS settings nor were any studies found that address the use of this procedure by corpsmen and medics on the battlefield.

Tourniquets applied during the Care under Fire phase should be replaced with direct pressure or compression dressings when the tactical situation allows, if these measures are equally effective at controlling the hemorrhage in the tactical environment encountered.

Although standard trauma care involves starting two large bore (14 or 16 gauge) intravenous catheters, the use of an 18-gauge catheter is preferred in the field setting because of the increased ease of starting. The larger catheters are necessary to administer large volumes of blood products rapidly, but this is not a factor in the tactical setting since blood products will not be available. Crystalloid solutions can be administered rapidly through the 18-gauge catheters. Although larger bore catheters may subsequently need to be started upon arrival at an MTF, prehospital IVs are often discontinued or changed because of concern about contamination of the IV site.

Despite its frequent use, the benefit of prehospital fluid resuscitation in trauma patients has not been established. The beneficial effect from crystalloid and colloid fluid resuscitation in hemorrhagic shock has been demonstrated largely on animal models where the volume of hemorrhage is controlled experimentally and resuscitation is initiated after the hemorrhage has been stopped. In uncontrolled hemorrhagic shock models, multiple studies have found that aggressive fluid resuscitation in the setting of an unrepaired vascular injury is associated with either no improvement in survival or increased mortality when compared to no fluid resuscitation or hypotensive resuscitation (see Chapter 6: Shock and Fluid Resuscitation). This lack of benefit is presumably due to interference with vasoconstriction and hemostasis as the body attempts to adjust to the loss of blood volume and establish hemostasis at the bleeding site.

A large prospective trial examining this issue in 598 victims of penetrating torso trauma was recently published by Bickell and colleagues.[3,7] They found that aggressive prehospital fluid resuscitation of hypotensive patients with penetrating wounds of the heart was associated with a higher mortality than seen in those for whom aggressive volume replacement was withheld until the time of surgical repair. This difference was most significant in those patients with wounds of the heart; patients with abdominal wounds showed little difference in survival between early and delayed fluid resuscitation. Although confirmation of these findings in other randomized, prospective studies has not yet been obtained, no human studies were found that demonstrated any benefit from fluid replacement in patients with ongoing hemorrhage. Battlefield casualties with penetrating abdominal or thoracic trauma must be presumed to have ongoing hemorrhage prior to surgical repair of their injuries.

If fluid resuscitation is required for controlled hemorrhagic shock in the Tactical Field Care phase, Hespan (6% hetastarch) is recommended as an alternative to lactated Ringer's (LR) solution.[13] Lactated Ringer's solution is a crystalloid, which means that the primary osmotically active particle is sodium. Since the sodium ion distributes throughout the entire extracellular fluid compartment, LR moves rapidly from the intravascular space to the extravascular space. This shift has significant implications for fluid resuscitation. If one infuses 1,000 cc of LR into a trauma patient, one hour later only 200 cc of that volume remains in the intravascular space to replace lost blood volume. This is not a problem in the civilian setting, since the average time for transport of the patient to the hospital in an ambulance is less than 15 minutes.[7,8] Once the patient has arrived at the hospital, infusion of blood products and surgical repair of the patient's injuries can be initiated rapidly. In the military setting, however, where several hours or more typically elapse before a casualty arrives at an MTF, effective volume resuscitation may be difficult to achieve with LR.

In contrast, the large hetastarch molecule in Hespan is retained in the intravascular space and there is no loss of fluid to the interstitium. Hespan actually draws fluid into the vascular space from the interstitium such that an infusion of 500 cc of Hespan results in an intravascular volume expansion of almost 800 cc, and this effect is sustained for 8 hours or longer. In addition to providing more effective expansion of the intravascular volume, a significant reduction in medical equipment weight is achieved by carrying Hespan instead of LR into the field. Four liters of LR weigh almost 9 pounds, while the 500 cc of Hespan needed to achieve a similar sustained intravascular volume expansion weighs just over 1 pound.[13] Hespan in volumes greater than 500 cc produce increased hemorrhage from small vessels. It is used widely in Europe for trauma management but not in the United States.

If the casualty is conscious and requires analgesia, it should be achieved with morphine, preferably administered intravenously. This mode of administration allows for much more rapid onset of analgesia and for more effective titration of dosage than intramuscular administration. An initial dose of 5 mg is given and repeated at 10-minute intervals until adequate analgesia is achieved.

Infection is an important late cause of morbidity and mortality in wounds sustained on the battlefield. Cefoxitin (2 g IV) is an accepted monotherapeutic agent for empiric treatment of abdominal sepsis and should be given without delay to all casualties with penetrating abdominal trauma. Cefoxitin is effective against gram-positive aerobes (except some enterococcus species) and gram-negative aerobes (except for some *Pseudomonas* species). It also has good activity against anaerobes (including *Bacteroides* and *Clostridium* species). Since it is effective against the clostridial species that cause myonecrosis, cefoxitin is also recommended for casualties who sustain wounds with massive soft tissue damage,[20] grossly contaminated wounds, open fractures, or patients for whom a long delay until CASEVAC is anticipated.[21]

CASEVAC CARE

The use of a CASEVAC asset to evacuate the wounded from the battlefield presents the opportunity to bring in additional medical equipment and personnel to treat the casualties. This opportunity led to the recommendation to establish designated Combat Casualty Transportation Teams for Special Operations Forces (SOF).[13] This concept, when implemented, will serve to provide a physician skilled in trauma or critical care management as far forward as possible in the SOF combat environment. This additional medical expertise and equipment will allow for the expanded diagnostic and therapeutic measures outlined in Box 17-3 for the CASEVAC phase of care. The concept of Combat Casualty Transportation Teams and the additional care that they provide needs to be evaluated by the combat units of the conventional forces to determine whether or not this concept might have applicability for their forces as well.

The tactical combat casualty care guidelines described previously have now been implemented in the Naval Special Warfare community[22] and incorporated into the Undersea Medical Officer course conducted by the Navy Bureau of Medicine and Surgery. They are currently scheduled for inclusion in the Textbook of Military Medicine being sponsored by the Office of the Surgeon General of the Army[23] and are being considered for use by units in the Marine Corps and the Air Force. Like all medical management strategies, these guidelines will require periodic review and updating, and the establishment of a standing Department of Defense (DOD) committee on the tactical management of combat trauma has been called for by the commander of the Naval Special Warfare Command.[24] Such guidelines will never be able to anticipate all of the difficulties that may confront the combat medic or corpsman, however, and the need for well-trained combat medical personnel to further modify treatment methods for trauma patients on the battlefield based on the specifics of a given casualty scenario must be recognized. Several scenarios that dramatically illustrate this fact are provided in Boxes 17-4 through 17-7. Scenarios such as these are very useful in the planning phase of combat operations to help medical personnel develop customized management plans. Specialized

Box 17-4 Parachute Insertion Casualty Scenario

- Twelve-person patrol
- Interdiction operation for weapons convoy
- Night static line jump from C-130
- Four mile patrol over rocky terrain to objective
- Planned helo extraction near target
- One jumper has canopy collapse at 40 feet
- Open facial fractures with teeth and blood in oropharynx
- Bilateral ankle fractures
- Open, angulated fracture of the left femur

Box 17-5 Delayed Evacuation Land Warfare Scenario

- Eight-person special operations team
- Dropped into unfriendly Middle Eastern country
- Four-day SCUD hunt
- Planned helo extraction at end of operation
- Lost communications—no CASEVAC or extraction plan changes possible
- Chance encounter on second day
- One soldier shot in abdomen—unconscious
- One soldier shot in leg—external hemorrhage
- One soldier with fragment in eye—light perception vision
- Hostiles all dead

Box 17-6 Combat Swimmer Casualty Scenario

- Limpet mine attack on hostile ship
- Launch from coastal patrol craft 12 miles out
- One hour transit in small boats
- Seven swim pairs using closed-circuit oxygen rigs
- Launch craft approach to approximately 2 miles from the harbor
- Divers wearing wet suits—78° F (26° C) water
- Surface swim for a mile, then begin dives
- One man shot in chest by patrol boat during peek in harbor
- Casualty conscious

Box 17-7 Combined Land Warfare/Diving Scenario

- Two open submersible SEAL Delivery Vehicles (SDVs)
- Eight-person SEAL element
- Insertion from a submarine with 2 hour transit to beach
- Target is heavily defended harbor in a bay
- Divers wearing dry suits in 43° F (6° C) water
- Air temperature 35° F (1° C)
- Boats bottomed for across-the-beach operation
- One man shot in chest at the objective
- Mission plan calls for SEALs to extract by SDV

WEAPONS OF MASS DESTRUCTION

Weapons of mass destruction (WMD) include nuclear devices, biologic agents, and chemical substances. Historically, WMD have been considered as a single class of weapons, but they differ significantly in their use, presentation, and concepts of casualty management. Nuclear weapons may be encountered in the civilian sector as radiation accidents or spills. The technology required to use a nuclear weapon is still substantial in comparison with that required for chemical or biologic agents. A significantly increased threat exists that terrorist groups or hostile nations may use chemical and/or biologic weapons against the United States. These weapons are readily available to determined parties. Each type of weapon will be discussed along with its general management principles.

NUCLEAR WEAPONS

Thermal burns and a variety of traumas complicated by differing degrees of radiological contamination are the most likely injuries to be encountered in survivors of a nuclear blast. Multiple delayed effects may be anticipated, but early treatment will deal with relatively standard trauma management. Decontamination should be conducted as soon as possible but should not delay lifesaving treatment. A radiological spill or incident may occur with or without associated trauma. A simple acronym SWIMS will suffice for most incidents: Stop the spill, Warn others, Isolate the area, Minimize contamination, and Secure ventilation if in an enclosed building. Many civil defense agencies are well versed in the management

workshops that combine the expertise of both physicians and combat medical personnel to review treatment strategies for specific types of casualty scenarios help to provide insights that may be of use to combat medical personnel as they develop these management plans.

of nuclear events, and further information can be obtained through these sources.

BIOLOGIC WARFARE AGENTS

Biologic weapons are among the most insidious and dangerous ever devised by humankind. They have been characterized as the poor person's atomic bomb, a cheaper and less sophisticated alternative to chemical, nuclear, or conventional weapons. Biologic agents may be produced at low cost, in a covert manner, and may be spread easily using readily available equipment. They are capable of producing large numbers of casualties, the first sign of an attack may be days after the actual event when symptoms of a disease begin to appear. Biologic warfare agents (BWAs) fall into four broad categories: true biologic agents, biologic vectors, toxins, and bioregulators.

True biologic agents are living microorganisms (pathogens) that have the ability to cause disease in humans and/or animals and can cause plant destruction. These include viruses, bacteria, fungi, and rickettsiae.

Biologic vectors are insect vectors that have been purposefully infected with a pathogen in an attempt to propagate the spread of a disease. A variety of insect vectors exist within nature, usually endemic to a specific region, and often act as intermediate breeding grounds for local pathogens. Mosquitoes act in this way for the spread of malaria, and infected fleas do the same for plague.

Toxins of biologic origin constitute the third category of BWA. Strictly speaking, these agents are chemicals, but they are generally classified as BWA due to their production within living things. Examples include botulinum and cholera toxins.

The final category of BWA is chemicals that act on the human system as *bioregulators.* These are chemicals that occur naturally, in small amounts within the body, to regulate such functions as heart rate and blood pressure; they may be synthetically derived to achieve the same purposes. In altered concentrations, these agents may lead to a wide variety of adverse actions such as paralysis, loss of consciousness, or death. Given their specificity for use against the human system, they are included as BWA.

The primary means of exposure to most of these agents is via the respiratory tract. The gastrointestinal tract is the second major route of exposure for many infectious agents and toxins, normally through the ingestion of contaminated food or water supplies.

Weight for weight, BWAs are inherently more toxic than either chemical or conventional weapons, have a much higher specificity for their intended targets than chemical weapons and, effectively disseminated, provide the largest area coverage of any type of weapon. Once disseminated, however, BWAs tend to degrade quickly.

There are two primary methods of dissemination of BWAs, both of which depend on weather conditions for maximum effectiveness. The first is from a point source weapon such as a bomb or stationary aerosol generator, which disseminates the agent from a single location. The second is a line source weapon that disseminates the agent from a moving platform such as a spray tank mounted on a vehicle (truck or aircraft). Line source weapons can disperse large amounts of agent over much wider areas than point source weapons and are significantly more effective.

Factors Affecting Dissemination/Spread of BWAs

Atmospheric conditions can dramatically alter the dispersal and subsequent effectiveness of BWA. High winds tend to disperse BWA over a wider area and dilute their concentrations. Unstable winds, especially those with gusty, unpredictable patterns, will provide less uniform spread. Sunlight, particularly the ultraviolet portion, tends to break down toxic agents and kill pathogens through rapid drying. Rain tends to wash an agent out of the air and clear surfaces.

Terrain is equally important in the dispersal patterns and subsequent effectiveness of BWA. Flat, unobstructed territory or an open expanse of water allows for maximum potential distribution. Urban settings or hilly, rugged terrain prevents even distribution, increases vertical dilution, and tends to reduce effective concentrations over distance.

Early detection allows personnel to take protective cover in time to prevent exposure. Limitations in technology, however, make this extremely difficult to achieve. Biologic warfare agent detectors are in development but of questionable reliability at the present time.

Personnel entering a targeted area may lack effective protection, become casualties themselves, and spread the disease further. Delayed effects make it difficult to even discern when and where the attack was conducted. An outbreak of disease may cause significant death or illness yet still mimic a naturally occurring epidemic.

Should biologic agents be of concern, three points should be remembered:

1. Avoid contamination if possible.
2. Decontamination should be conducted, if possible, to eliminate or reduce the hazard from exposed personnel and equipment. Decontamination often involves caustic materials and bleaches to neutralize the agent and thus may damage equipment. The secondary infectious hazard is minimal and treatment may proceed even in the absence of full decontamination.
3. Maintain a high index of suspicion. Look for unusual diseases or patterns of disease if a biologic

incident was possible. Seek treatment early if you develop symptoms after responding to a call. Prompt and effective medical treatment is necessary to counteract the effects of the agents and minimize casualties. Treatment is effective in the majority of commonly used agents but, in some cases, by the time symptoms appear, it may be too late to treat effectively; in others, no effective treatment exists.

Characteristics of BWAs

General characteristics that determine the usefulness of BWAs include:

1. *Infectivity:* This involves the ability of an agent to reliably infect a person or animal exposed to it.
2. *Virulence:* This characteristic relates the agent's ability to incapacitate or kill an intended target once exposure and infection have occurred.
3. *Incubation period:* The incubation period is the lag between the time when infection occurs and the time when symptoms of the disease become apparent. Biologic agents rarely cause instant casualties. With the exception of certain toxins, BWA tend to have effect only after their incubation period.
4. *Stability:* Most biologic agents are unstable when compared to chemical agents. Stability is the ability to maintain virulence and other characteristics over time and under varying ecological conditions.
5. *Environmental persistence:* Persistence is closely related to stability and is the ability of an organism to survive in the environment long enough to have the desired effect.
6. *Resistance:* The ability of an agent to withstand normal medical countermeasures is termed resistance.
7. *Protection:* Protection is the ability of an attacker to protect his or her troops with a vaccine or other protective measure not available to the opponent.
8. *Controllability:* This is the ability to predict, with some measure of assuredness, the extent and nature of the BWA effects given a specific set of employment parameters.
9. *Producibility:* The most likely agents utilized by third world countries will be those that are cheap, easy to produce, and which can be readily obtained on the global market. Only about 30 pathogens have been considered as likely BWA out of the several hundred known to affect humans and animals.

Anthrax

Anthrax is often discussed as the prototypical biologic warfare agent. *Bacillus anthracis,* the causative organism for anthrax, occurs naturally in horses, cattle, and sheep. Anthrax is highly toxic and stable in an aerosolized form.

Once released, exposure can occur through inhalation, ingestion, or wounds in the skin. An inhalation dose of less than a microgram can be fatal in days. The normal incubation period is 3 to 5 days but may be as little as 24 hours with a larger exposure. Cutaneous anthrax has a mortality approaching 20% if left untreated, but less than 1% following treatment. Inhalation anthrax, however, approaches 100% mortality. Treatment of suspected cases must begin prior to the onset of symptoms or it is likely to be ineffective. Even with treatment, survivors may be incapacitated for months and require retreatment due to relapses. Protection against an anthrax attack currently includes the use of personal protective gear and a mask if the attack is detected in time. Current detection methods may be unreliable, however, in warning of an attack early enough to prevent exposure, and detectors are not routinely deployed with at-risk units. An anthrax vaccine is available.

CHEMICAL WARFARE AGENTS

Chemical agents fall into five main categories: nerve agents, vesicants, cyanide, lung agents, and riot control agents. While the potential for terrorist activity exists, these agents may be encountered during cleanup of lands where old chemical munitions were stored or during HAZMAT accidents involving spills of organophosphate insecticides or other industrial chemicals such as phosgene or cyanide. Chemical agents are primarily liquids that produce contact hazards but are even more dangerous as they vaporize. They may be "persistent" (staying on the ground for more than 24 hours) or nonpersistent if they evaporate within 24 hours. In liquid form, these agents are heavier than water and may be covered by puddles. In vapor form, they are heavier than air and tend to collect in low spots. Like biologic agents, the primary considerations are contamination avoidance, decontamination, and movement of decontaminated patients from a contaminated to a clean area. In many circumstances, it is best to treat patients on site and move them after appropriate decontamination is achieved. Failure to do this may result in widespread contamination and increased casualties. Responders to a chemical incident must themselves be protected by appropriate suits and masks, or they risk becoming casualties as well.

Nerve Agents (Box 17-8)

Nerve agents cause involuntary skeletal muscle activity and excessive secretion from lachrymal, nasal, salivary, and sweat glands into the airways and gastrointestinal (GI) tract. Constriction of muscles within the airway produces bronchoconstriction similar to that seen in asthma. In the GI tract it leads to cramps, vomiting, and diarrhea.

Box 17-8 Nerve Agents—Summary

Signs and Symptoms

Small vapor exposure—Miosis, runny nose, shortness of breath

Large vapor exposure—Loss of consciousness, convulsions, apnea, flaccid paralysis

Small to moderate liquid exposure—Localized sweating, fasciculations; nausea, vomiting, diarrhea, feeling of weakness (may start hours later)

Large liquid exposure—Loss of consciousness, convulsions, apnea, flaccid paralysis

Decontamination

Thoroughly flush with hypochlorite and water

Emergency Medical Care

Atropine (2-6 mg); 2 PAMCl; diazepam (depending on severity); ventilation; suction of airways if secretions are copious; supportive care

---

Box 17-9 Vesicants—Summary

Signs and Symptoms

Normally a latent period of hours followed by the onset of erythema and blisters, conjunctivitis, and upper respiratory signs. All may worsen over the following hours. Mustard does not cause pain on contact; lewisite and phosgene oxime cause pain on exposure to liquid or vapor.

Decontamination

Hypochlorite or large amounts of water to flush agent away. Must be within seconds to be maximally effective.

Emergency Medical Care

Immediate decontamination. None otherwise (no early effects). Suspected casualty should be observed for at least 8 hours. Later, symptomatic management of lesions.

The single most effective treatment for exposure to nerve agents is atropine. Atropine will reduce secretions and reduce activity in smooth muscle but has little effect on excess activity of skeletal muscles. Nerve agents penetrate normal clothing and skin to be absorbed into the body. Clinical effects will depend on the route and amount of agent exposure.

Vesicants (Box 17-9)

Vesicants are substances that cause burning of the skin with redness and blistering. These agents are liquids but

Box 17-10 Cyanide—Summary

Signs and Symptoms

Few. After inhalation of a large amount: loss of consciousness, convulsions, apnea, and cardiac arrest.

Decontamination

Not usually necessary in vapor. Wet clothing should be removed, and underlying skin decontaminated (hypochlorite or water).

Emergency Medical Care

Amyl nitrite in bag-valve-mask followed by IV sodium nitrite and sodium thiosulfate; ventilation with oxygen.

---

produce damage in the vapor form as well. Damage begins to occur almost immediately on contact with the skin and the best management is early and thorough decontamination of the affected areas. Clinical effects may be delayed for several hours and increase in severity over several days; death usually occurs due to damage to the respiratory tract. Early responders may not see significant lesions as the effects are often delayed.

Cyanide (Box 17-10)

Cyanide is a common industrial chemical that has been used as a poison for centuries. It is found in cigarette smoke and in some types of foods. Cyanide inhibits the ability of cells to utilize oxygen and causes death by cellular hypoxemia. Although large doses produce rapid death, smaller doses may be effectively treated with rapid administration of the antidotes, support of circulation as necessary, and oxygen.

Lung Agents (Box 17-11)

Lung agents are a class of compounds that cause pulmonary edema. The most important of these is phosgene, a common industrial compound. Teflon, when it burns, may give off perfluoroisobutylene, another agent in this class. Generally, these agents produce damage to the alveolar-capillary membrane with onset of symptoms between 2 and 24 hours depending on the level of exposure. Patients should be observed for a 24-hour period and triaged based on the severity of symptoms that develop.

Riot Control Agents (Box 17-12)

Riot control agents (RCAs) are in common use by law enforcement agencies but are not usually of great concern

Box 17-11 Lung Agents—Summary

Signs and Symptoms

Eye and airway irritation early on in some cases. Later development of pulmonary edema with shortness of breath, cough, and clear sputum.

Decontamination

None usually necessary. Remove wet clothing, decontaminate underlying skin with hypochlorite or water. Fresh air.

Emergency Medical Care

Termination of exposure. Oxygen with positive pressure for respiratory distress. **No physical activity.**

Box 17-12 Riot Control Agents—Summary

Signs and Symptoms

Burning and pain on exposed mucous membranes and skin, causing eye pain and tearing, respiratory discomfort, and stinging on the exposed skin.

Decontamination

Fresh air. Flush eyes with water or saline. Flush skin with alkaline soap and water or weak bicarbonate solution (**not hypochlorite**).

Emergency Medical Care

Usually none needed; effects are self limiting.

to first responders. Medical treatment is not generally indicated following exposure as the effects are self limiting. There are, however, some rare complications worthy of note. Persons with reactive airway disease may develop prolonged bronchospasm following exposure to RCAs. Standard treatment for a severe asthmatic attack may be required. Moderate to severe conjunctivitis has been reported following exposure that occasionally requires treatment by an ophthalmologist. Finally, a delayed onset contact dermatitis may develop that may require follow-up medical care.

Decontamination

Decontamination is vital in any chemical incident and has two main goals. The first is to minimize injury to the casualty. This must be done within minutes after exposure in order to be effective. The best and most effective decontamination is that performed within the first minute after exposure to a liquid chemical agent. If decontamination is delayed 15 to 60 minutes, it may do little to

assist the casualty. If the agent was a nerve agent, the casualty may be dead. The best and often quickest decontamination is physical removal of the agent. Remove any clothing that has been contaminated and clean the skin of any residual. Large amounts of water under pressure or a scraper type object may be effective. Substances that will chemically destroy or detoxify the agent are commonly used for decontamination. Sodium hypochlorite is a primary agent. Undiluted bleach followed by washing may be effective, and specially prepared decontamination kits are available. The second goal is to prevent contamination of rescue personnel, EMS personnel, transport units, and the receiving medical facility. Before a casualty is decontaminated, all personnel in contact with the casualty must wear appropriate protective equipment. There is a significant risk of contaminating vehicles and medical facilities from a chemical casualty. A strict decontamination area must be established with a clean area on one side and the contaminated area on the other. Any person symptomatic or asymptomatic, casualty, or medical care provider who goes from a contaminated area to a clean uncontaminated area, such as a medical treatment area, *must* be decontaminated. Casualties or medical personnel who have not undergone decontamination procedures may contaminate the entire air system of a hospital by spreading a vapor agent.

Specific protective equipment to investigate include the following:

Personal equipment
- Masks, the M40 or older M17A2, and suits
- Self-contained breathing apparatus (SCBA) approved for civilian use
- Standard chemical clothing is available to civilian emergency agencies through the Defense Logistics Agency.
- Civilian responders should have the responder suit.

Detection equipment
- Chemical detection kits

Medical Items
- Mark I nerve agent antidote kit: Decontaminable litter made of monofilament polypropylene fabric, which allows drainage of liquids, does not absorb chemical agents, and is easily decontaminated for re-use
- Fiberglass long spine boards—nonpermeable and easily decontaminated

TRIAGE

The most important concept in successful management of mass casualties is triage. Triage is the sorting of casualties into treatment categories by a designated officer. Categories are determined based on the severity of injury and likelihood of recovery, given limited treatment resources. Resources consist of time, personnel, and equipment. The objective is to provide survival for as many as possible. The triage officer's responsibility is to sort the casualties; he/she does not treat patients and is often alone without equipment. In an ideal situation, a senior experienced trauma or general surgeon should conduct triage as these individuals are most qualified to make the necessary life and death decisions. In practice, many other personnel may be forced to do triage based on circumstances. Patients are triaged and re-triaged at each level of care, and treatment categories may change based on availability of resources. Two of these deserve special mention, field and hospital triage.

FIELD TRIAGE

Field triage occurs near the site of injury. This is the battlefield in wartime or the site of a disaster in peacetime. The triage officer may be a physician but will more likely be a corpsman or nurse. There are three broad categories of patients in the field: those who are about to die, the agonal; those who are more scared than wounded; and all others. Little can be done for the agonal, and the minimally injured should be removed from the scene and returned to duty as soon as possible. Those with more serious injuries need to be treated initially and moved to an MTF as quickly as possible. Two categories are designated based upon injury severity and threat to integrity of airway, breathing, and circulation (the ABCs). These include the traditional "immediate" and "urgent" categories. This determination is based upon the premise that little can be accomplished at the scene in terms of reversing instability and that outcome will be determined at the MTF.

HOSPITAL TRIAGE

Hospital triage is considerably more precise. The triage officer is the surgeon most experienced in trauma care. He or she only sorts patients and rarely treats them. Three categories constitute the simplest, most used method of triage. **"The walking wounded"** are those patients whose injuries would heal with little or no therapy. They constitute approximately 65% of the patients seen. They are moved to a separate area of the MTF where their injuries are treated by a physician and a nurse if staffing permits. **"The expectant"** are those patients who will probably die no matter what treatment is performed and would tie up significant resources in the process. They are moved to a separate area of the MTF and made as comfortable as possible. They number less than 10% of the casualties and are attended by only a single nurse. **"The priority"** are those patients where a meaningful survival can be achieved by immediate or prompt intervention and treatment. They number about 25% of the patient load. Despite obvious differences, military (battlefield) triage and

civilian (disaster) triage adhere to those basic levels of casualty sorting. The next section provides a comparison of casualty management following the terrorist bombing of the U.S. Marine Corps facility in Beirut, Lebanon in 1983 and the terrorist bombing of the A.P. Murrah Federal Building in Oklahoma City in 1995.

COMPARISON OF CIVILIAN VERSUS MILITARY CASUALTY MANAGEMENT

The Beirut bomb resulted in 346 casualties among whom 234 (68%) died immediately. The battalion aid station, located on the fourth floor of the building, was destroyed; the medical officer and numerous corpsmen were killed resulting in a lack of initial medical capability at the scene. Of the 112 survivors, seven subsequently died (6%). Six of these succumbed in association with a delay in treatment secondary to entrapment within the building. Most of the survivors (64%) were flown by helicopter off shore to the USS Iwo Jima where they were triaged. Twenty-four casualties were flown from the scene to Europe and Cypress after the arrival of U.S. and British Air Ambulance Units. Fifteen survivors with minor injuries remained on shore and all survived. Eight casualties were taken to local Lebanese hospitals where one died.

The Oklahoma City bomb caused 759 casualties among whom 167 (22%) died immediately. Of the 83 (11%) survivors who were hospitalized, one died. The remaining 509 casualties were treated as outpatients. The field triage officer in this disaster was an emergency medicine resident from the nearby University Hospital.

EXTENUATING FACTORS RELATED TO BATTLEFIELD TRIAGE

Triage in the combat zone is stressed by obvious extenuating circumstances. The ongoing conflict poses risks to the integrity of the MTF and those components integral to patient transport and evacuation. Casualty care is problematic but may be remarkably efficient despite the difficulties.

Resource limitations are present in both battlefield and domestic occurrences. Contingency planning can minimize shortfalls in both scenarios, and protocols should be established for each. A major treatment facility, whether it be a combat casualty support hospital or a level I trauma center, must have a disaster plan. It should be published, updated routinely, and periodically rehearsed.

ENVIRONMENTAL CONCERNS WITH TRIAGE

Environmental concerns in disaster management include casualty and medical personnel protection against heat, cold, wind, rain, dust, flood, and storm. Sources of water and electricity may be jeopardized, communications disrupted, and transportation rendered impossible. Contingency planning is essential, and these issues should be addressed in standard disaster plans. Exposure to nuclear, biologic, or chemical (NBC) agents has become of increased concern in recent years.

Triage is best done at a distance from the actual scene of a terrorist act. An initial blast may be followed by a second, larger detonation designed to maim and kill those responding to the first.

• Summary •

1. The emergence of prehospital care is deeply rooted in military tradition, dating as far back as the sixteenth century. The modern day EMT is simply an evolution of the *bracardier* of Revolutionary France. The Vietnam conflict was responsible for quantum leaps in what we now regard as prehospital care. With everchanging conditions in the geopolitical picture, future advancements in EMS can already be predicted by what we now see in the Department of Defense.

2. Levels (echelons) of care improve the survivability of wounded soldiers by moving more advanced capabilities further forward in the echelon system. The military-derived system of levels of care is the civilian counterpart spread across a theater of operation.

3. Prehospital care in the tactical environment requires specialized training for physicians, corpsmen, and medics. Due to the complicating effects of battlefield conditions (e.g., darkness, enemy fire, and equipment limitations), scene safety is not always feasible. Care under fire calls for an occasional variance from what we consider normal protocol due to these unique circumstances. Keep in mind that before any combat operation/mission can be undertaken, special attention must be directed at a basic medical care plan.

4. Weapons of mass destruction are the most insidious and dangerous threat devised by humankind. Early detection and decontamination are the most important priorities in countering biological or chemical warfare agents. Treat concurrent injuries as in a conventional setting.

5. The most important concept in successful management of mass casualties, whether in the battlefield or on the home front during peacetime, is triage. Understand that triage in the combat zone is stressed by extenuating circumstances.

Scenario Solution

The point man who sustained the injuries resulting in no pulse or respirations would be placed in the "expectant category." No time or equipment would be used in a resuscitation attempt. The point man will be extracted with the team. The patrol leader with the femoral hemorrhage would be placed in the "immediate category."

Can the patient be stabilized well enough to be extracted with the team as planned? If not, what is the Medical Evacuation Plan (MEDEVAC) plan? How soon can MEDEVAC arrive at the patrol's present location? Does the MEDEVAC aircraft have the necessary equipment to extract the patients from the patrol's present location (i.e. jungle penetrator, Stokes litter)?

Incoming direct and indirect fire make it necessary for the patrol to either suppress hostile fires using fire support (i.e., artillery, naval gunfire, close air support) or break contact and move out of their present position immediately. Transport of the patient is a priority and more definitive care may be delayed until the patrol is in a suitable location.

The patrol leader will receive a pressure dressing or a tourniquet placement until the medic/corpsman can remove him from hostile fire. Later, during movement or at the extraction site, the patient will receive a more definitive dressing and advanced lifesaving procedures including 3:1 volume replacement with lactated Ringer's and a full primary and secondary survey to identify any other conditions that may have previously gone unrecognized.

Review Questions

Answers provided on page 333.

1 The first comprehensive effort in America to upgrade/establish prehospital care was required by states due to which of the following?
   A National Academy of Sciences recommendation in 1970
   B The Commission of Public Charities and Corrections of New York City in 1869
   C The Highway Safety Act of 1966
   D The Commission of EMS or DOT in 1981

2 Which echelon of care is characterized by its mobility and staffing of medical technicians, one physician, and one physician's assistant?
   A echelon I
   B echelon II
   C echelon III
   D echelon IV

3 Which stage of care applies to a situation in which care of an injury is provided while on a mission with no hostile fire?
A Combat Casualty Evacuation Care
B Care Under Fire
C Tactical Field Care
D Battlefield Care

4 Which nerve agent is distinguished with signs of loss of consciousness, convulsions, apnea, and cardiac arrest?
A lung agents
B cyanide
C riot control agents
D anthrax

5 Field triage will most likely be performed by whom?
A surgeon (with the most experience)
B nurse
C physician's assistant
D corpsman

REFERENCES

1. Bellamy, R.F. "The Causes of Death in Conventional Land Warfare: Implications for Combat Casualty Care Research." *Milit. Med.* 149 (1984): 55–62.

2. Alexander, R.H., and Proctor, H.J. *Advanced Trauma Life Support 1993 Student Manual.* Chicago: American College of Surgeons, 1993.

3. Bickell, W.H.; Wall, M.J.; Pepe, P.E.; et al. "Immediate Versus Delayed Fluid Resuscitation for Hypotensive Patients with Penetrating Torso Injuries." *NEJM* 331 (1994): 1105–09.

4. Honigman, B.; Rohwder, K.; Moore, E.E.; et al. "Prehospital Advanced Trauma Life Support for Penetrating Cardiac Wounds." *Ann. Emerg. Med.* 19 (1990): 145–50.

5. Smith, J.P., and Bodai, B.I. "The Urban Paramedic's Scope of Practice." *JAMA* 253 (1985): 544–48.

6. Stern, S.A.; Dronen, S.C.; Birrer, P.; et al. "Effect of Blood Pressure on Hemorrhage Volume and Survival in a Near-Fatal Hemorrhage Model Incorporating a Vascular Injury." *Ann. Emerg. Med* 22 (1993): 155–63.

7. Martin, R. R.; Bickell, W. H.; Pepe, P. E.; et al. "Prospective Evaluation of Preoperative Fluid Resuscitation in Hypotensive Patients with Penetrating Truncal Injury: A Preliminary Report." *J. Trauma* 33 (1992): 354–61.

8. Kaweski, S. M.; Sise, M. J.; and Virgilio, R. W. "The Effect of Prehospital Fluids on Survival in Trauma Patients." *J. Trauma* 30 (1990): 1215–18.

9. Krausz, M. M.; Bar-Ziv, M.; Rabinovici, R.; et al. "'Scoop and Run' or Stabilize Hemorrhagic Shock with Normal Saline or Small-volume Hypertonic Saline?" *J. Trauma* 33 (1992): 6–10.

10. Arishita, G. I.; Vayer, J. S.; and Bellamy, R. F. "Cervical Spine Immobilization of Penetrating Neck Wounds in a Hostile Environment." *J. Trauma* 29 (1989): 332–37.

11. Zajtchuk, R.; Jenkins, D. P.; Bellamy, R. F.; et al., eds. "Combat Casualty Care Guidelines for Operation Desert Storm." Washington, D.C.: Office of the Army Surgeon General Publication, 1991.

12. Ekblad, G. S. "Training Medics for the Combat Environment of Tomorrow." *Milit. Med.* 155 (1990): 232–34.

13. Butler, F. K., Hagmann, J., and Butler, E. G. "Tactical Combat Casualty Care in Special Operations." *Milit. Med.* 161(supp) (1996): 1–16.

14. Wilderness Medical Society. *Practice Guidelines for Wilderness Medical Emergencies.* Indianapolis, 1995.

15. Maughon, J. S. "An Inquiry into the Nature of Wounds Resulting in Killed in Action in Vietnam." *Milit. Med.* 135 (1970): 8–13.

16. Trooskin, S. Z.; Rabinowitz, S.; Eldridge, C.; et al. "Teaching Endotracheal Intubation Using Animals and Cadavers." *Prehosp. and Disaster Med.* 7 (1992): 179–82.

17. Salvino, C. K.; Dries, D.; Gamelli, R.; et al. "Emergency Cricothyroidotomy in Trauma Victims." *J. Trauma* 34 (1993): 503–05.

18. McGill, J.; Clinton, J. E.; and Ruiz, E. "Cricothyrotomy in the Emergency Department." *Ann. Emerg. Med.* 11 (1982): 361–64.

19. Erlandson, M. J.; Clinton, J. E.; Ruiz, E.; et al. "Cricothyrotomy in the Emergency Department Revisited." *J. Emerg. Med.* 7 (1989): 115–18.

20. Bowen, T. E., and Bellamy, R. F., eds. *Emergency War Surgery: Second United States Revision of the Emergency War Surgery NATO Handbook.* Washington, D. C.: United States Government Printing Office, 1988: 175.

21. Ordog, G. J.; Sheppard, G. F.; Wasserberger, J. S.; et al. "Infection in Minor Gunshot Wounds." *J. Trauma* 34 (1993): 358–65.

22. Commander, Naval Special Warfare Command letter of 9 April 1997.

23. Butler, F. K. "Medical Support of Special Operations." In Burr, R. E., Bellamy, R. F., eds. *Medical Operations in Harsh Environments. Textbook of Military Medicine.* Washington, D.C.: Office of the Surgeon General of the Army Publication (In press).

24. Commander, Naval Special Warfare Command letter of 29 May 1997.

Answer Key

1	1. B; 2. C; 3. B; 4. D; 5. B; 6. C; 7. B; 8. D; 9. C; 10. D
2	1. C; 2. Scene Survey, Primary Assessment, Secondary Assessment, Monitoring and Reassessment; 3. C; 4. A; 5. B; 6. B
3	1. A; 2. C; 3. C; 4. B; 5. D
5	1. B; 2. C; 3. C; 4. D; 5. C; 6. A; 7. D; 8. A; 9. C
6	1. A and C; 2. C; 3. A; 4. C; 5. D; 6. A, B, and C; 7. D
7	1. D; 2. B; 3. D; 4. A; 5. C; 6. A
8	1. A; 2. C; 3. B; 4. C; 5. C; 6. D
9	1. D; 2. A; 3. C; 4. B; 5. D
11	1. C; 2. A; 3. C; 4. D; 5. D
12	1. B; 2. D; 3. A; 4. B; 5. C
13	1. D; 2. B; 3. A; 4. C; 5. C; 6. B; 7. D; 8. B
14	1. D; 2. A; 3. B; 4. A; 5. A
17	1. C; 2. A; 3. C; 4. B; 5. D

Glossary

accelerated motion   A sudden surge or increase in motion, e.g., from the transferring of motion in a rear-impact collision; occurs as a slower moving or stationary object is struck from behind.

acetabulum   The cup-shaped hip socket on the lateral surface of the pelvis that holds the head of the femur.

adolescent   A child with the body size and physical development normally found in children from 13 to 16 years of age. An arbitrary grouping of older children based on the similar physical characteristics common to these near-adult ages.

adult   A person (generally 16 years or older) whose body has reached maturity and has finished its progression through the phases of pediatric growth and development.

adult respiratory distress syndrome (ARDS)   Failure of the lungs to function; by loss of O_2 transport ability, usually 24 to 48 hours after injury.

aerobic metabolism   Oxygen-based metabolism that is the body's principal combustion process.

afterload   The pressure against which the left ventricle must pump out (eject) blood at each beat.

air bags   Bags that automatically inflate in front of the driver or passenger upon frontal collisions to cushion the impact. The bags absorb the energy slowly by increasing the body's stopping distance. These bags are only designed to cushion forward motion on the initial impact.

Alzheimer's disease   A form of brain disease commonly associated with premature senile dementia.

amnesia   A loss of memory.

amputation   A severed part or a part that is pathologically or surgically totally separated (removed) from the rest of the body.

anaerobic metabolism   Metabolism not using oxygen.

angina (angina pectoris)   A cramping, crushing midsternal chest pain caused by myocardial anoxia. It often radiates to either arm, most commonly the left, and is associated with a feeling of suffocation and impending death.

anterograde amnesia   Amnesia for events occurring after the precipitating trauma; inability to form new memories.

anticoagulant   A substance or drug that prevents or delays coagulation or the forming of blood clots.

antihypertensive   A drug that reduces high blood pressure (hypertension). Some drugs that increase urine production (diuretics) lower the blood pressure by decreasing blood fluid volume.

aortic tear   Complete or partial tear of one or more layers of tissue of the aorta.

apnea   An absence of spontaneous breathing.

arachnoid mater (arachnoid membrane)   Spiderweb-like transparent membrane between the dura mater and the pia mater. The middle of the three meningeal membranes surrounding the brain.

ataxic respirations   Erratic breathing with no rhythm. Commonly associated with head injury and increased intracranial pressure.

atlas   First cervical vertebra (C1); the skull perches upon it.

avulsion   The ripping or tearing away of a part; a flap or partially separated tissue or part.

axis   Second cervical vertebra (C2); its shape allows for the wide possible range of rotation of the head. *Also,* an imaginary line that passes through the center of the body.

bag-valve device; bag-valve-mask (BVM) device   Mechanical resuscitation device consisting of a self-inflating bag made of plastic or rubber and several one-way valves. Squeezing the bag results in positive pressure ventilation through a mask or endotracheal tube. May be used with or without supplementary oxygen.

baroreceptor   A sensory nerve ending that is stimulated by changes in pressure. Baroreceptors are found in the walls of the atria of the heart, vena cava, aortic arch, and carotid sinus.

Battle's sign   Discoloration posterior and slightly inferior to the outer ears due to bleeding into the subcutaneous tissue caused by an occipital basilar skull fracture.

blunt trauma   Nonpenetrating trauma caused when there is a temporary cavity in the body caused by a rapidly moving object with a small frontal projection concentrating its energy in one area.

body surface area (BSA)   Outer surface of the body covered by the skin. Percentage of the body's total surface area represented by any body part. Used as one factor in determining size of a burn.

brain stem   The stemlike part of the brain that connects the cerebral hemispheres with the spinal cord.

Broselow Resuscitation Tape   A commercially available system for estimating pediatric medication dosing and equipment sizing based on patient length.

capillaries   The smallest blood vessels. Minute blood vessels that are only one cell wide, allowing for diffusion and osmosis through the capillary walls.

cardiac output   The volume of blood pumped by the heart at each contraction (reported in liters per minute).

cardioaccelerator center   The brain center that activates the sympathetic response that increases the rate of the heart.

cardioinhibitory center   A part of the medulla that slows or inhibits the heart's activity.

cardiovascular   Referring to the combination of the heart and blood vessels.

catecholamines   Group of chemicals produced by the body that work as important nerve transmitters. The main catecholamines made by the body are dopamine, epinephrine (also called adrenaline), and norepinephrine. They are part of the body's sympathetic defense mechanism used in preparing the body to act.

caudad   Toward the tail (coccyx).

cavitation   Forcing tissues of the body out of their normal position; to cause a temporary or permanent cavity, e.g., when the body is struck by a bullet, the acceleration of particles of tissue away from the missile, producing an area of injury where the large temporary cavity occurs.

cell wall   The outer wall of each cell.

central neurogenic hyperventilation (CNHV)   Pathologic rapid and shallow respiratory pattern associated with head injury and increased intracranial pressure.

cephalad   Toward the head (away from the tail).

cerebellum   A portion of the brain that lies dorsal to the medulla oblongata and is concerned with coordination of movement.

cerebrospinal fluid (CSF)   A fluid found in the subarachnoid space and dural sheath; acts as a shock absorber protecting the brain and spinal cord from jarring impact.

cerebrum   The largest part of the brain; responsible for the control of specific intellectual, sensory, and motor functions.

cervical flexion   Rotating the head forward or downward causing bending of the neck.

cervical spine   The neck area of the spinal column containing seven vertebrae (C1–C7).

chemoreceptors   A sensory nerve ending that is stimulated by and reacts to certain chemical stimuli; located outside of the central nervous system. Chemoreceptors are found in the large arteries of the thorax and neck, the taste buds, and the olfactory cells of the nose.

chemoreceptor cells   Cells that stimulate nerve impulses by reacting to chemical stimuli. Certain chemoreceptor cells control the respiratory rate.

Cheyne-Stokes respiration   Pathologic respiratory pattern with periods of shallow, slow breathing increasing to rapid, deep breathing and then returning to shallow, slow breathing followed by a short apneic period. Commonly associated with head injury and increased intracranial pressure.

chin lift   A way to open the airway of a patient with suspected cervical spine compromise. Adaptation of chin lift airway maneuver that includes manual immobilization of the head in a neutral in-line position.

coccygeal spine   The most caudad part of the spinal column; contains the three to five vertebrae that form the coccyx.

Colles' fracture   Fracture of the wrist. If the victim falls forward onto his outstretched hands to break his fall, this may result in a silver fork deformity.

compartment syndrome   The ischemia and compromised circulation that can occur from vascular injury. The cellular edema produces increased pressure in a closed facial or bony compartment.

compensated shock   Inadequate peripheral perfusion as evidenced by signs of decreased organ perfusion, but with normal blood pressure.

complication   An added difficulty that occurs secondary to an injury, disease, or treatment. Also, disease or accident superimposed upon another without being specifically related, yet affecting or modifying the prognosis of the original disease.

compression   Type of force involved in impacts resulting in a tissue, organ, or other body part being squeezed between two or more objects or body parts.

compression injuries   Injuries caused by severe crushing and squeezing forces; may occur to the external structure of the body or to the internal organs.

consensual reflex   The reflexive constriction of one pupil when a strong light is introduced into the other eye. A lack of consensual reflex is considered a positive sign of brain injury or eye injury.

contraindication   Any sign, symptom, clinical impression, condition, or circumstance indicating that a given treatment or course of treatment is inappropriate and therefore outside of accepted medical practice. *Relative contraindication:* something usually considered as a contraindication but that under special circumstances may be overruled by a physician as an accepted medical practice on a case-by-case basis.

contusion   A bruise or bruising.

cyanosis   Blue coloring of skin, mucous membranes, or nail beds indicating unoxygenated hemoglobin and a lack of adequate oxygen levels in the blood; usually secondary to inadequate ventilation or decreased perfusion.

decerebrate posturing   Characteristic posture present in an individual with decerebrate rigidity. When a painful stimulus is introduced, the extremities are stiff and extended, and the head is retracted. One of the forms of pathologic posturing (response) commonly associated with increased intracranial pressure.

decorticate posturing   A characteristic pathologic posture of a patient with increased intracranial pressure; when a painful stimulus is introduced the patient is rigidly still with the back and lower extremities extended while the arms are flexed and fists clenched.

definitive care   In-hospital care that resolves the patient's illness or injury after a definitive diagnosis has been established. Clear and final care that is without question what the particular patient needs for his individual problem.

density   The number of particles in each given area of tissue.

diaphragmatic rupture (diaphragmatic herniation)   A tearing or cutting of the diaphragm so that the abdominal and thoracic cavity are no longer separated, allowing abdominal contents to enter the thoracic cavity. Usually a result of increased intra-abdominal pressure producing a tear in the diaphragm.

diastolic blood pressure   The resting pressure between ventricular contractions measured in millimeters of mercury (mm Hg).

Don Juan syndrome   The pattern that often occurs when victims fall or jump from a height and land on their feet. Bilateral calcaneus (heel bone) fractures are often associated with this syndrome. After the feet land and stop moving, the body is forced into flexion as the weight of the still-moving head, torso, and pelvis come to bear. This can cause compression fractures of the spinal column in the thoracic and lumbar areas.

down-and-under pathway   When a vehicle ceases its forward motion the occupant usually continues to travel downward into the seat and forward into the dashboard or steering column.

dura mater   The outer membrane covering the spinal cord and brain; the outer of the three meningeal layers. Literally means "tough mother."

dysrhythmia (cardiac)   Abnormal, disordered, or disturbed rhythm of the heart.

ecchymosis   A bluish or purple irregularly formed spot or area resulting from a hemorrhagic area below the skin.

edema   A local or generalized condition in which some of the body tissues contain an excessive amount of fluid; generally includes swelling of the tissue.

endotracheal intubation   Insertion of a large cuffed tube into the trachea for direct ventilation from outside of the body. The most desirable way of achieving definitive control of respirations and a protected airway in trauma patients.

epidural space   Potential space between the dura mater surrounding the brain and the cranium. Contains the meningeal arteries.

esophageal obturator airway (EOA) An airway device that includes a tube (containing a cuff) that is blindly inserted into the esophagus; the cuff obstructs the esophagus and holds the tongue out of the airway; connects to a mask through which ventilation of the oropharynx occurs.

exsanguination Total loss of blood volume producing death.

FiO$_2$ Fraction of oxygen in inspired air stated as a decimal. An FiO$_2$ of 0.85 means that 85/100ths or 85% of the inspired air is oxygen.

fight-or-flight response A defense response that the sympathetic nervous system produces that simultaneously causes the heart to beat faster and stronger, constricts the arteries to raise blood pressure, and increases the ventilatory rate.

flail chest A chest with an unstable segment produced by multiple ribs fractured in two or more places or including a fractured sternum.

flexion A bending movement around a joint that decreases the angle between the bones at the joint. In the cervical region it is a forward bending motion of the head bringing the chin nearer to the sternum.

foot-pounds of force A measure of mechanical force brought to bear. Force equals mass times deceleration or acceleration.

foramen magnum The opening at the base of the skull.

fracture A broken bone. A simple fracture is closed without a tear or opening in the skin. An open fracture is one where the initial injury or bone end has produced an open wound at or near the fracture site. A comminuted fracture has one or more free-floating segments of disconnected bone.

gastric ventilation Air undesirably forced down the esophagus and into the stomach rather than into the lungs.

geriatric Dealing with aging and the diagnosis and treatment of injuries and diseases affecting the elderly.

G force (gravitational force) Actual force of acceleration or deceleration or of centrifugal force.

Glasgow Coma Scale A scale for evaluating and quantifying the level of consciousness or unconsciousness by determining the best responses to standardized stimuli that the patient is capable of.

global overview The simultaneous 15- to 30-second overview of the patient's condition. The global overview focuses on the patient's immediate respiratory, circulatory, and neurologic status.

hemianesthesia Loss of sensation on one side of the body.

hemiparesis Weakness limited to one side of the body.

hemiplegia Paralysis on one side of the body.

hemorrhage Bleeding. *Also,* a loss of a large amount of blood in a short period of time, either outside or inside the body.

hemothorax Blood in the pleural space.

homeostasis A constant, stable internal environment. Balance necessary for healthy life processes.

hyperextension Extreme or abnormal extension. A position of maximum extension. Hyperextension of the neck is produced when the head is extended posterior to a neutral position and can result in a fracture or dislocation of the vertebrae or spinal cord damage in patients with an unstable spine.

hyperflexion Extreme or abnormal flexion. A position of maximum flexion. Increased flexion of the neck can result in a fracture or dislocation of the vertebrae or spinal cord damage in patients with an unstable spine.

hypertension Having a blood pressure greater than the upper limits of the normal range. Generally considered to exist if the patient's systolic pressure is greater than 150 mm Hg.

hypertensive crisis A sudden severe increase in blood pressure exceeding 200/120 mm Hg.

hyperthermia Body temperature much higher than normal range.

hypertonic Osmotic pressure greater than serum or plasma.

hypoperfusion Inadequate perfusion (bathing) of cells with properly oxygenated blood.

hypotension Blood pressure below normal acceptable range.

hypothenar eminence Fleshy part of the palm along the ulnar margin.

hypothermia Subnormal core body temperature below normal range, usually between 78° and 90°F (26° and 32.5°C).

hypotonic A solution of lower osmotic pressure than another. *Also,* having a lower osmotic pressure than normal serum or plasma.

hypovolemia Inadequate (below normal range) fluid blood volume.

hypoxia (hypoxemia) Deficiency of oxygen. Inadequate available oxygen. Lack of adequate oxygenation of the lungs due to inadequate minute volume (air exchange in the lungs) or a decreased concentration of oxygen in the inspired air. *Cellular hypoxia:* inadequate oxygen available to the cells.

immune system A related group of responses of various body organs that protects the body from disease organisms, other foreign bodies, and cancers. The main organs of the immune response system are the bone marrow, the thymus, and the lymphoid tissues, spleen, and liver.

incisura (tentorial incisura) Opening in the tentorium cerebelli at the junction of the midbrain and the cerebrum. The brain stem is inferior to the incisura.

infant A child between 7 weeks to 1 year of age.

interstitial fluid The extracellular fluid located between the cell wall and the capillary wall.

intubation Passing a tube into a body aperture. Endotracheal intubation is the insertion of a breathing tube through the mouth or nose into the trachea to provide an airway for oxygen or an anesthetic gas.

ischemia Local and temporary deficiency of blood supply due to obstruction of circulation to a body part or tissue.

ischemic sensitivity The sensitivity of the cells of a tissue to the lack of oxygen and usefulness of anaerobic metabolism before cell death occurs.

jaw thrust A maneuver that enables the EMT to open the airway of a trauma patient while the head and cervical spine are manually maintained in a neutral in-line position.

jugular vein distention (JVD) Backup of pressure on the right side of the heart resulting in venous pooling and neck vein distention (engorgement) due to decreased filling of the left heart and reduced left heart output.

kinematics The process of looking at an accident and from the mechanism of injury determining what injuries are likely to have resulted from the forces and motion and changes in motion involved. The science of motion.

kinetic energy (KE) Energy available from movement. Function of the weight of an item and its speed. KE = one-half of the mass times the velocity squared.

kyphosis A forward, humplike curvature of the spine commonly associated with the aging process. Kyphosis may be caused by aging, rickets, or tuberculosis of the spine.

laws of motion Scientific laws relating to motion. Newton's first law of motion: A body at rest will remain at rest and a body in motion will remain in motion unless acted upon by some outside force.

ligamentum arteriosum A remnant of fetal circulation and point of fixation at the arch of the aorta.

logroll A way to turn a person with a possible spine injury from one side to the other or completely over while manually protecting the spine from excessive, dangerous movement. Used to place patients with a suspected unstable spine onto a longboard.

lucid interval Period of normal mental functioning between periods of disorientation, unconsciousness, or mental illness.

lumbar spine Part of the spinal column found at the lower back inferior to the thoracic spine, containing the five lumbar vertebrae (L1–L5).

mass The victim's weight.

mass casualty incident (MCI) An incident (such as a plane crash, building collapse, or fire) that produces a large number of victims from one mechanism, at one place and at the same time.

mechanical energy Form of energy dealing with movement.

mediastinum The middle of the thoracic cavity containing the heart, the great vessels, the trachea, the mainstem bronchi, and the esophagus.

medulla (medulla oblongata) Part of the brain stem. The medulla is the primary regulatory center of autonomic control of the cardiovascular system.

meninges Three membranes that cover the brain tissue and the spinal cord.

metabolism The sum of all physical and chemical changes that take place within an organism; all energy and material transformations that occur within living cells.

minute volume The amount of air exchanged each minute; calculated by multiplying the volume of each breath (tidal volume) by the number of breaths per minute (rate).

myocardial contusion A bruising of the heart or the heart muscle.

myocardium The middle and thickest layer of the heart wall; composed of cardiac muscle.

nares (singular: naris) The openings in the nose that allow passage of the air from the outside to the throat. The anterior nares are the nostrils. The posterior nares are a pair of openings in the back of the nasal cavity where it connects with the upper throat.

nasopharyngeal airway An airway that is placed in the nostril and follows the floor of the nasal cavity directly posterior to the nasopharynx. This airway is commonly tolerated by patients with a gag reflex.

newborn A child from birth to 6 weeks of age.

nonpatent airway An obstructed airway.

non-rebreather reservoir mask (NRB) An oxygen mask with a reservoir bag and non-rebreather valves that allow the exiting of exhaled air. It delivers high oxygen concentrations of between 80%–100% to the patient when attached to a high-liter flow oxygen source.

occipital condyles The two rounded knuckle-like bumps at the end of the occipital bone at the back of the head.

oculomotor nerve The third cranial nerve; controls pupillary/constriction.

odontoid process The toothlike protrusion on the upper surface of the second vertebra (axis) around which the first cervical vertebra (atlas) turns, allowing the head to rotate through approximately 180°.

oncotic pressure Pressure that determines the amount of fluid within the vascular space.

open pneumothorax (sucking chest wound) A penetrating wound to the chest causes the chest wall to be opened, producing a preferential pathway for air moving from the outside environment into the thorax.

oropharyngeal airway An airway that when placed in the oropharynx superior to the tongue holds the tongue forward to assist in maintaining an open airway. *It is only used in patients with no gag reflex.*

osmosis The movement of water (or other solvent) across a membrane from an area that is hypotonic to an area that is hypertonic.

osteoporosis A loss of normal bone density with thinning of bone tissue and the growth of small holes in the bone. The disorder may cause pain (especially in the lower back), frequent broken bones, loss of body height, and various badly formed parts of the body. Commonly a part of the normal aging process.

palpation Process of examining by application of the hands or fingers to the external surface of the body to detect evidence of disease, abnormalities, or underlying injury.

para-anesthesia Loss of sensation in lower extremities.

paradoxical pulse Condition in which the patient's systolic blood pressure drops more than 10–15 mm Hg during each inspiration usually due to the effect of increased intrathoracic pressure.

paraplegia Paralysis of the lower extremities.

paresis Undue localized weakness or partial (less than total) paralysis related in some cases to nerve inflammation or injury.

PASG Pneumatic antishock garment; (MAST—military or medical antishock trousers).

patent airway An open unobstructed airway of sufficient size to allow for normal volumes of air exchange.

pathophysiology The study of how normal physiological processes are altered by disease, or injury.

PEARRL Pupils equal and round, reactive to light. The term used when checking the patient's eyes to determine if they are round and normal appearing and that they appropriately react to light by constricting, or whether they are abnormal and unresponsive. Generally the presence of consensual reflex is included in this examination term.

pediatric Dealing with children; dealing with injuries and diseases affecting children (birth to 16 years of age).

pediatric trauma score (PTS) A clinical scoring system based on clinical information available at the time of initial assessment that has been known to be predictive of severity of injury and can be used for triage decision making.

penetrating trauma Trauma when an object penetrates the skin. Generally produces both a permanent and a temporary cavity.

percutaneous transtracheal ventilation (PTV) A procedure where a 16-gauge or larger needle is inserted directly into the lumen of the trachea through the cricothyroid membrane or directly through the tracheal wall through which the patient is ventilated.

perfusion Fluid passing through an organ or a part of the body. *Also,* the surrounding and bathing of a tissue or cell with blood or fluid parts of the blood.

pericardial space A potential space existing between the heart muscle (myocardium) and the pericardium.

pericardial tamponade Compression of the heart by blood collecting in the pericardial sac, which surrounds the heart muscle (myocardium); also sometimes called cardiac tamponade.

pericardium A tough fibrous, flexible but inelastic membrane that surrounds the heart.

peritoneal space Space in the anterior abdominal cavity that contains the bowel, spleen, liver, stomach, and gallbladder. The peritoneal space is lined with the peritoneum.

pharynx The throat; a tubelike structure that is a passage for both the breathing and digestive tracts. *Oropharynx:* area of the pharynx posterior to the mouth; *nasopharynx:* area of the pharynx beyond the posterior nares of the nose.

pia mater A thin vascular membrane closely investing the brain and spinal cord and proximal portions of the nerves. The innermost of the three meningeal membranes that cover the brain.

pleura Thin membrane that lines the inner side of the thoracic cavity and the lungs. The part that lines the thoracic cavity is called the *parietal pleura;* the fold covering the lung is called the *visceral pleura.*

pneumothorax Injury that produces air in the pleural space; commonly associated with a collapsed lung. A pneumothorax can be open with an opening through the chest wall to the outside or closed resulting from blunt trauma or a spontaneous collapse.

preload The volume and pressure of the blood coming into the heart from the systemic circulatory system (venous return). The process outside of the heart in the vena cava.

premature ventricular contraction A premature irregular extra contraction of the ventricles due to an ectopic stimulus causing a contraction rather than the normal stimuli from the normal pacing node. Second most common abnormal rhythm of the heart.

preschooler A child with the body size and physical development normally found in children from 2 to 6 years of age. An arbitrary grouping of children based on the similar physical characteristics common to these ages.

priapism The penis remains erect usually for a long period. It may be caused by a urinary stone, or an injury to the lower spinal column.

pulmonary contusion A bruising of the lungs. This can be secondary to blunt or penetration trauma.

pulmonary diffusion Movement of oxygen from the alveoli across the alveolar capillary (A-C) membrane and into the red blood cells (RBCs) or the plasma.

pulmonary function Controlled patent airway, ventilation, diffusion, and perfusion resulting in arterial blood that contains adequate oxygen for aerobic metabolism and a proper level of carbon dioxide to maintain tissue acid-base balance.

pulse pressure The increase in pressure (surge) that is created as each new bolus of blood leaves the left ventricle. *Also,* the difference between the systolic and diastolic blood pressure (systolic pressure − diastolic pressure = pulse pressure).

quadriplegia Paralysis of all four extremities.

raccoon eyes (periorbital ecchymosis) Very distinct ecchymotic area around each eye, limited by the orbital margins.

rapid deceleration mechanism A series of three collisions that occur when a vehicle suddenly ceases forward motion. Collision of (1) the vehicle, (2) the occupant inside the vehicle, and (3) the occupant's internal organs.

rapid sequence intubation A method of patient preparation for intubation including pharmacologic adjuncts for sedation and muscle relaxation.

respiration The total ventilatory and circulatory steps involved in the exchange of oxygen and carbon dioxide between the outside atmosphere and the cells of the body. Sometimes in medicine limited to meaning breathing and the steps in ventilation.

respiratory tract The pathway for air movement between the outside air and the alveoli; includes the nasal cavity, oral cavity, pharynx, larynx, trachea, bronchi, and lungs.

retrograde amnesia Loss of memory for events and situations just preceding the time (immediate preinsult period) of the patient's injury or illness. *Also,* loss of memory for past events.

retroperitoneal space Space in the posterior abdominal cavity that contains the kidneys, ureters, bladder, reproductive organs, inferior vena cava, abdominal aorta, pancreas, a portion of the duodenum, colon, and rectum.

rotational impact When one car strikes the front or rear side of another, causing it to rotate away from the point of impact. *Also,* when one corner of the car strikes an immovable object or one moving slower or in the opposite direction of the auto, resulting in it rotating.

rule of nines A topographic breakdown (mostly of 9% and 18% portions) of the body in order to estimate the amount of body surface covered by burns.

sacral spine Part of the spinal column below the lumbar spine containing the five sacral vertebrae (S1–S5), which are connected by immovable joints to form the sacrum. The sacrum is the weight-bearing base of the spinal column and is also a part of the pelvic girdle.

safety Evaluation of all possible dangers and ensuring that no unreasonable threats or risks still exist.

SAR Search and rescue.

scene Environment to be evaluated in which injury occurred. In a motor vehicle accident this includes evaluation of the number of vehicles, what forces acted upon each, and the degree and type of damage to each.

school age A child with the body size and physical development normally found in children from about 6 to 12 years of age. An arbitrary grouping of children based upon the similar physical characteristics common to these ages.

secondary assessment Head-to-toe evaluation of the trauma patient. This assessment is only done when the EMT is sure there are no immediate life-threatening problems; in urgent patients usually done en route.

semipermeable membrane Membrane that will allow fluids (solvents) but not the dissolved substance to pass through it.

sensory exam A gross examination of sensory capability and response to determine the presence or absence of loss of sensation in each of the four extremities.

sepsis Infection.

shear Change-of-speed force resulting in a cutting or tearing of body parts.

sinoatrial node Node at junction of superior vena cava with right cardiac atrium; regarded as the pacing or starting point of the heartbeat. In healthy patients, pacing from this node causes atrial contraction, is slowed, and then results in producing ensuing contraction of the ventricles.

situation Events, relationships, and roles of those parties who, with the patient, were involved in a call. The situation (e.g., domestic dispute, single-car accident without an apparent reason, elderly person living alone, a shooting) is important in evaluating the EMT's safety and as a part of properly assessing the event (incident) and the patient.

spinal shock Injury to the spinal cord causing interruptions to the nervous system's communication between the brain and the blood vessels served by nerves that branch from the cord below the point of injury; this results in a loss of ability of the vessels to constrict inferior to the point of disruption of the cord, producing hypotension without blood loss.

stroke volume The volume of blood pumped out by each contraction (stroke) of the left ventricle.

subarachnoid space Space between the pia mater proper and arachnoid membrane; contains cerebrospinal fluid and meningeal veins. The subarachnoid space is a common site of subdural hematomas.

systolic blood pressure Peak blood pressure produced by the force of the contraction (systole) of the ventricles of the heart.

tachycardia Abnormally fast rate of heartbeats; defined as a rate over 100 beats per minute in an adult.

tension pneumothorax Condition when the air pressure in pleural space exceeds the outside atmospheric pressure and cannot escape. The affected side becomes hyperinflated, compressing the lung on the involved side and shifting the mediastinum to partially collapse the other lung. A tension pneumothorax is usually progressive and is an imminent life-threatening condition.

tertiary injuries The third group of injuries sustained in a sequence (or pattern) of injury-producing events, such as explosions. Injuries that occur when the victim becomes a missile and is thrown against some object. These injuries are similar to those sustained in ejections from automobiles, falls from significant heights, or when the victim is thrown against an object by the force wave resulting from an explosion. Tertiary injuries are usually obvious injuries.

tentorium cerebelli (tentorium) An infolding of the dura that forms a covering over the cerebellum. The tentorium is a part of the floor of the upper skull just below the brain (cerebrum).

tentorial herniation Normally the cerebrum (brain) is supra-tentorial. When, due to increased intracranial pressure, part of the brain is pushed down through the incisura, tentorial herniation occurs.

thoracic spine The part of the spinal column between the cervical spine (superiorly) and the lumbar spine (inferiorly) containing the twelve thoracic vertebrae (T1–T12). The twelve pairs of ribs connect to the thoracic vertebrae.

thorax (thoracic cavity) Hollow cylinder supported by twelve pairs of ribs that articulate posteriorly with the thoracic spine and ten pairs that articulate anteriorly with the sternum. The two lowest pairs are only fastened posteriorly (to the vertebrae) and are called floating ribs. The thoracic cavity is defined and separated inferiorly by the diaphragm.

tidal volume Normal volume of air exchanged with each ventilation. About 500 cc of air is exchanged between the lungs and the atmosphere with each breath in a healthy adult at rest.

toddler A child with the body size and physical development normally found in children from about 1 to 2 years of age.

tonsil-tip catheter Rigid suction catheter designed for rapid removal of large amounts of fluids, vomitus, blood, and debris from the mouth and pharynx to avoid aspiration.

toxemia Distribution throughout the body of poisonous products of bacteria (toxins) growing in a focal or local site.

traumatic aneurysm An abnormal dilation, bursting, or tearing of a major blood vessel (usually an artery) caused by or related to an injury.

traumatic asphyxiation Blunt and crushing injuries to the chest and abdomen with marked increase of intravascular pressure, producing rupture of the capillaries.

Trendelenburg position Simultaneous lowering of the patient's head while elevating the patient's legs. Usually done by raising the foot end of a flat bed or longboard higher than the head end. This position uses gravity to counter shock by improving circulation to the head and other vital organs. In this position (with the abdomen higher than the thorax) the weight of the abdominal contents presses on the diaphragm, producing some respiratory difficulty. Often EMTs use a *modified Trendelenburg position* with the head and torso horizontal and only the legs elevated, which will not produce respiratory problems.

triage French word meaning "to sort"; a process in which a group of patients is sorted according to their priority of need for care. When only several patients are involved, triage involves alternating from patient to patient meeting all patients' highest priority needs first, then moving to lower priority items. In a mass casualty incident with a large number of patients involved, triage is done by determining both urgency and potential for survival.

tumble End-over-end motion. Bullets commonly tumble when resistance is met by the leading edge of the missile.

up-and-over pathway The body's forward motion carries it up and over the steering wheel; the chest or abdomen commonly impacts the steering wheel, while the head strikes the windshield. In the semisitting position common in passenger cars, once the down-and-under motion has ended as the knees are stopped by the dashboard, the body then continues in an up-and-over movement. In some trucks, where the driver is sitting fully upright with his feet stopped by the pedals, the up-and-over movement may occur initially.

vagal Dealing with stimulation of the vagus (tenth cranial) nerve. The parasympathetic system's response that slows the heart rate and reduces the force of contractions, keeping the body within workable limits. This response can normally override the sympathetic system's chemical release, keeping the heart rate in an acceptable range. Accidental vagal stimulation, however, can result in producing an undesirable bradycardia, further reducing the patient's cardiac output and circulation.

vagus nerve   The tenth cranial nerve; when stimulated, slows the heart rate regardless of levels of catecholamines. It contains motor and sensory functions and a wider distribution than any of the other cranial nerves.

velocity   Quickness of motion. Speed, as in the speed of a moving mass.

ventilation   Movement of air into and out of the lungs through the normal breathing process. The mechanical process by which air moves from the atmosphere outside the body through the mouth, nose, pharynx, trachea, bronchi, and bronchioles, and into and out of the alveoli. To ventilate a patient is to provide positive pressure inspirations with a ventilating device such as a bag-valve-mask device, and then alternately allowing time for passive exhalation to occur; used in patients who are apneic or who cannot provide adequate ventilation for themselves.

whistle-stop catheter (whistle-tip catheter)   A soft catheter used for suctioning the nasal passage, deep oropharynx, or endotracheal tube; allows for controlled intermittent suction. Its name is derived from the opening (whistle-stop) found in the side of the proximal end of the catheter. Suction is not produced at the distal tip until this hole or port is covered with one of the operator's fingers, producing a closed system to the opening at the distal tip.

zygomatic arches   The bones that form the superior area of the cheeks of the face. Laterally, superior to the molars, these extend more anteriorly than the maxilla, giving the individual some of his unique facial structure; commonly called the cheekbones.

Note: Due to limits of space, a glossary cannot include every term used in a text or replace a complete medical dictionary. The editors have limited inclusion to key terms or terms that may be unique to or uniquely used in this text.

Anatomic terms are carefully identified and defined in the section on anatomy and physiology of the chapter in which they are introduced; only a few are also included in the glossary.

The definitions found for each entry in this glossary may not represent the most common primary definition or all of the possible medical uses and definitions for that term. The definition felt to be the most useful and most relevant to trauma and the term's use in this text have been selected. The glossary only provides a brief reference. For a more complete understanding, the reader should refer back to the primary chapter in which the term is used.

For terms not included or for alternate definitions, the EMT may wish to consult a medical dictionary, guide to medical terminology, or a textbook of anatomy and physiology for more information.

Bibliography

American Academy of Orthopaedic Surgeons. *Emergency Care and Transportation of the Sick and Injured.* 6th ed. Park Ridge, IL, 1994.

American College of Emergency Physicians. "Guidelines for Trauma Care Systems." *Ann. Emerg. Med.* 16 (1987): 459–63.

American College of Surgeons Committee on Trauma. *Advanced Trauma Life Support Program.* Chicago, 1993.

American Heart Association and American Academy of Pediatrics. *Textbook of Pediatric Advanced Life Support.* Dallas: The American Heart Association, 1988.

American Trauma Society. *Trauma Facts.* 1987.

Arshita, Bellamy, and Vayer. "Cervical Spine Immobilization of Penetrating Neck Wounds in a Hostile Environment." *J. Trauma* 29(3).

Aughey, K.; Hess, D.; Eitel, D.; et al. "An Evaluation of Pulse Oximetry in Prehospital Care." *Ann. Emerg. Med.* 20(8) (1991): 887–91.

Bachulis, B.L., et al. "Clinical Indications for Cervical Spine Radiographs in Traumatized Patient." *Am. J. Surg.* 153(5) (May 1987): 473.

Bickell, W.H. "Are Victims of Injury Sometimes Victimized by Attempts at Fluid Resuscitation?" *Ann. Emerg. Med.* 22 (1993): 225–26.

Bove and Davis. *Diving Medicine.* 3d ed. WB Saunders Co., 1997.

Bureau of Health Services Resources, Division of Trauma and Emergency Medical Services. *Model Trauma Care System Plan.* Rockville, MD: U.S. Department of Health and Human Services, 1992.

Butler, F.K.; Hagman, J.; and Butler, E.G. "Tactical Combat Casualty Care in Special Operations." *Milit. Med.* 161(suppl) (1996): 1–16.

Butman, A.M., and McSwain, N.E., Jr. "Emergency Patient Removal." *J. of Pre-Hosp. Care* 1(3) (July/Aug 1984): 22–26, 45.

Cales, R.H., and Trunkey, D.D. "Preventable Trauma Deaths." *JAMA* 245 (1985): 1059–63.

Caroline, Nancy. *Emergency Care in the Streets.* 5th ed. Boston: Lippincott-Raven Publishers, 1995.

Cayten, C.G.; Murphy, J.G.; and Stahl, W.M. "Basic Life Support Versus Advanced Life Support for Injured Patients with an Injury Severity Score of 10 or More." *J. Trauma* 35(3) (1993): 460–67.

Champion, H.R., and Sacco, W.J. "Measurement of Injury Severity and Its Practical Application." *Trauma Quarterly* 1 (1984): 25–36.

Champion, H.R.; Sacco, W.J.; Copes, W.S.; et al. "A Revision of the Trauma Score." *J. Trauma* 29 (1989): 623–29.

Corry, J. "Emergency Oxygen Administration." *NAUI* (1989).

Curry, G.J. *Immediate Care and Transport of the Injured.* Charles C. Thomas, 1965.

Cwinn, A.A.; Pons, P.T.; Moore, E.E.; et al. "Prehospital Advanced Trauma Life Support for Critical Blunt Trauma Victims." *Ann. Emerg. Med.* 16(4) (1987): 399–403.

Daugherty, G. *Field Guide for the Diver Medic.* 2d ed. Coastal Aquatics Publications, 1992.

Davidson, J.S., and Birdsell, D.C. "Cervical Spine Injury in Patients with Facial Skeletal Trauma." *J. Trauma* 29(9) (Sept 1989): 1276–78.

Douglas, G.J., and Simpson, J.S. "The Conservative Management of Splenic Trauma." *J. Pediatr. Surg.* 6 (1971): 545.

Eastman, A.B. "Blood in Our Streets: The Status and Evolution of Trauma Care Systems." *Arch. Surg.* 154 (1992): 677–81.

Eichelberger, M.R.; Pratsch, G.L.; et al. *Pediatric Trauma Care.* Rockville, MD: University Park Press, 1988.

Feliciano, D.V.; Mattox, K.L.; Jordan, G.L.; et al. "Management of 1000 Consecutive Cases of Hepatic Trauma (1979–1984)." *Ann. Surg.* 204 (1986): 438–45.

Fleisher, G.; Templeton, J.; and Delgado-Paredes, C. "Fluid Resuscitation Following Liver Laceration: A Comparison of Fluid Delivery About and Below the Diaphragm in a Pediatric Animal Model." *Ann. Emerg. Med.* 16, 147–52.

Garcia, V.; Gotschall, C.S.; Eichelberger, M.R.; et al. "Rib Fractures in Children: A Marker of Severe Trauma." *J. Trauma* (Dec. 1989): 1726.

Gilliam, B. *Deep Diving: An Advanced Guide to Physiology, Procedures and Systems.* Watersport Publishing, 1992.

Gilliam, B. *Diving Accident Management Field Guide.* Ocean Tech, 1989.

Gilliam, B. "Evaluation of Decompression Sickness Incidence in Multi-day Repetitive Diving for 77,680 Sport Dives." Proceedings of the 1991 Repetitive Diving Conference, American Academy of Underwater Sciences.

Hadley, M.N.; Zabramski, J.M.; Browner, C.M.; et al. "Pediatric Spinal Trauma." *J. Neurosurg.* 68 (Jan 1988): 18–24.

Halvorsen, L.; Bay, B.K.; Perron, P.R.; et al. "Evaluation of an Intraosseous Infusion Device for the Resuscitation of Hypovolemic Shock." *J. Trauma* 29 (1989): 1029.

Harris, G.J., and Soper, R.T. "Pediatric First Rib Fractures." *J. Trauma* 30 (1990): 343–45.

Heiskell, L.E., and Carmona, R.H. "Tactical Emergency Medical Services: An Emerging Subspecialty of Emergency Medicine." *Ann. Emerg. Med.* 23 (1994): 778–85.

Herzenberg, J.E.; Hensinger, R.N.; Dedrick, D.K.; et al. "Emergency Transport and Positioning of Young Children Who Have an Injury of the Cervical Spine." *J. Bone Joint Surg.* 71A(1) (1989): 15–22.

Honigman, B.; Rohwder, K.; Moore, E.E.; et al. "Prehospital Advanced Trauma Life Support for Penetrating Cardiac Wounds." *Ann. Emerg. Med.* 19 (1990): 145–50.

Hoyt, D.B.; Shackford, S.R.; McGill, T.; et al. "The Impact of In-house Surgeons and Operating Room Resuscitation on Outcome of Traumatic Injuries." *Arch. Surg.* 124 (1989): 906–10.

Jones, S.A.; Weigel, A.; White, R.D.; McSwain, N.E.; and Breiter, M. *Advanced Emergency Care for Paramedic Practice.* Philadelphia: J.B. Lippincott Company, 1992.

Karp, M.P.; Cooney, D.R.; Pros, G.A.; et al. "The Nonoperative Management of Pediatric Hepatic Trauma." *J. Pediatr. Surg.* 18 (1983): 512–18.

King, H., and Shumacker, H.B. "Susceptibility to Infection after Splenectomy Performed in Injury." *Ann. Surg.* 136 (1952): 239–42.

Kraus, J.F.; Fife, D.; Cox, P.; et al. "Incidence, Severity and External Causes of Pediatric Brain Injury." *AJDS* 140 (1986): 687–93.

Krebs, Henry Gabriele. *When Violence Erupts.* St. Louis: Mosby, 1990.

Lippman, J. *DAN Emergency Handbook.* Divers Alert Network, 1991.

Luten, R. "Pediatric Resuscitation Chart and Equipment Shelf: Aids to Mastery of Age-related Problems." *J. Emerg. Med.* 4 (1986): 9–14.

McCabe, J.B., and Nolan, D.J. "Comparison of the Effectiveness of Different Cervical Immobilization Collars." *Ann. Emerg. Med.* vol. 15, no. 1 (Jan 1986): 50–53.

McSwain, N.E., and Kerstein, M.D. *Evaluation and Management of Trauma.* East Norwalk, CT: Appleton & Lange, 1987.

Mallonee, S.; Shariat, S.; Stennies, G.; et al. "Physical Injuries and Fatalities Resulting from the Oklahoma City Bombing." *JAMA* 276 (1996): 382–87.

Mateer, J.R.; Olson, D.W.; Stueven, H.A.; and Aufderheide, T.P. "Continuous Pulse Oximetry during Emergency Endotracheal Intubation." *Ann. Emerg. Med.* 22(4) (1993): 675–79.

Mount, T., and Gilliam, B. *Mixed Gas Diving.* Watersport Publishing, 1993.

Mullins, R.J.; Veum-Stone, J.; Hedges, J.R.; et al. "Influence of a Statewide Trauma System on Location of Hospitalization and Outcome of Injured Patients." *J. Trauma* 40 (1996): 536–46.

National Highway Traffic Safety Administration. *1988 Traffic Fatality Facts.* U.S. Department of Transportation, July 1989.

National Highway Traffic Safety Administration. *Occupant Protection Facts.* National Center for Statistics and Analysis, U.S. Department of Transportation, June 1989.

National Safety Council. *Accident Facts—1984 Edition.* National Safety Council, 1984.

NAVSEA. *U.S. Navy Air Decompression Table Handbook and Recompression Chamber Operator's Handbook.* Best Publishing, 1980.

Neifeld, G.L.; Keene, J.G.; Hevesy, G.; et al. "Cervical Injury in Head Trauma." *J. Emerg. Med.* 6 (1988): 203–07.

O'Malley, K.F., and Ross, S.E. "The Incidence of Injury to the Cervical Spine in Patients with Craniocerebral Injury." *J. Trauma* 28(10) (Oct 1988): 1476–78.

Overgaard, J., and Tweed, W.A. "Cerebral Circulation after Head Injury." *J. Neurosurgery* 41 (1974): 531.

Pal, J.M.; Mulder, D.S.; Brown, R.A.; et al. "Assessing Multiple Trauma: Is the Cervical Spine Enough?" *J. Trauma* 28(8) (Aug 1988): 1282–84.

Pang, D., and Pollack, I.F. "Spinal Cord Injury Without Radiographic Abnormality in Children—The SCIWORA Syndrome." *J. Trauma* 29(5) (May 1989): 654–64.

Pfenninger, E.G.; Reith, A.; Breitig, D.; et al. "Early Changes of Intracranial Pressure, Perfusion Pressure, and Blood Flow after Acute Head Injury." *J. Neurosurg.* 70 (1989): 774–79.

Plant, M., and Gifford, R. "Trivial Head Trauma and Its Consequences in a Perspective of Regional Health Care." *Milit. Med.* 141 (1976): 244–47.

Polley, T.Z., and Coran, A.C. "Special Problems in Management of Pediatric Trauma." *Critical Care Clinics* 2 (1986): 775–89.

Pons, P.T.; Honigman, B.; Moore, E.E.; et al. "Prehospital Advanced Trauma Life Support for Critical Penetrating Wounds to the Thorax and Abdomen." *J. Trauma* 25(9) (1985): 828–32.

Powell, J.N.; Waddell, J.P.; Tucker, W.S.; et al. "Multiple-level Noncontiguous Spinal Fractures." *J. Trauma* 29(8) (Aug 1989): 1146–51.

Ramenofsky, M.L.; Luterman, A.; Quindlen, E.; et al. "Maximum Survival in Pediatric Trauma: The Ideal System." *J. Trauma* 24 (1984): 818–23.

Reid, D.C.; Henderson, R.; Saboe, L.; et al. "Etiology and Clinical Course of Missed Spine Fractures." *J. Trauma* 27(9) (Sept 1987): 980–86.

Resources for Optimal Care of the Injured Patient. Committee on Trauma, American College of Surgeons, Chicago, 1993.

Rice, D.P.; MacKenzie, E.J.; and associates. "Cost of Injury in the United States: A report to Congress 1989." San Francisco: Institute for Health & Aging, University of California, and Injury Prevention Center, The Johns Hopkins University, 1989.

Rimel, R.; Geordani, B.; Barth, J.; et al. "Disability Caused by Minor Head Injury." *J. Neurosurg.* 9 (1981): 221–28.

Ringenberg, B.J.; Fisher, A.K.; Urdanata, L.F.; et al. "Rational Ordering of Cervical Spine Radiographs Following Trauma." *Ann. Emerg. Med.* 17(8) (Aug 1988): 792–96.

Rivara, F.P.; Parish, R.A.; and Mueller, B.A. "Extremity Injuries in Children: Predictive Value of Clinical Findings." *Pediatrics* 78 (1986): 803–11.

Rosemurgy, A.S.; Norris, P.A.; Olson, S.M.; et al. "Prehospital Traumatic Cardiac Arrest: The Cost of Futility." *J. Trauma* 35(3) (1993): 468–74.

Roye, W.P., Jr.; Dunn, E.L.; and Moody, J.A. "Cervical Spinal Cord Injury—A Public Catastrophe." *J. Trauma* 28(8) (Aug 1988): 1260–64.

Ruge, J.R.; Sinson, G.P.; McLone, D.G.; et al. "Pediatric Spinal Injury: The Very Young." *J. Neurosurg.* 68 (Jan 1988): 25–30.

Rutkowski, D. *Recompression Chamber Life Support Manual.* Hyperbarics International, 1991.

Shilling, Carlston, and Mathias. *The Physician's Guide to Diving Medicine.* Plenum Press, 1984.

Sidell, F.R. "Management of Chemical Warfare Agents. A Handbook for Emergency Medical Services."

Stablein, D.M.; Miller, J.D.; Choi, S.C.; et al. "Statistical Methods for Determining Prognosis in Severe Head Injury." *Neurosurgery* 6 (1989): 243–48.

Stamler, K.D. "Effect of Crystalloid Infusion on Hematocrit in Non-bleeding Patients with Applications to Clinical Traumatology." *Ann. Emerg. Med.* 18: 747–49.

Swan, K.G., and Swan, K.G., Jr. "Triage: The Past Revisited." *Milit. Med.* 161 (1996): 448–52.

Tepas, J.J.; DiScala, C.; Ramenofsky, M.L.; et al. "Mortality and Head Injury: The Pediatric Perspective." *J. Pediatr. Surg.* In press.

Tepas, J.J.; Mollitt, D.L.; Talbert, J.L.; et al. "The Pediatric Trauma Score as a Predictor of Injury Severity in the Injured Child." *J. Pediatr. Sur.* 22 (1987): 14–18.

Tepas, J.J.; Ramenofsky, M.L.; Mollitt, D.L.; et al. "The Pediatric Trauma Score as a Predictor of Injury Severity: An Objective Assessment." *J. Trauma* 28 (1988): 425–29.

Trunkey, D.D., and Lewis, F.R. *Current Therapy of Trauma.* St. Louis: Mosby, Inc., 1991.

U.S. Army Medical Research Institute of Infectious Diseases. *Medical Management of Biological Casualities Handbook.* Frederick, MD: Fort Detrick.

Waite, C. *Case Histories of Diving and Hyperbaric Accidents.* UHMS, 1988.

Walker, M.L.; Starrs, B.; and Mayer, T.A. *Head Injuries in Emergency Management of Pediatric Trauma.* Edited by T. Mayer. Philadelphia: WB Saunders, 1985: 272–77.

Wienke, B. *Basic Decompression Theory and Application.* Best Publishing, 1991.

Woodring, J.H.; Lee, C.; and Jenkins, K. "Spinal Fractures in Blunt Chest Trauma." *J. Trauma* 28(6) (June 1988): 789–93.

Index